ecade of vigor and two of se-
tion of ills at the cost of some
effects do, or do not, include
le, specific serotonin reuptake
rectile and orgasmic dysfunc-
e. The SSRIs are useful in treat-

Phosphodiesterase inhibitors,
ffects that are generally mild
ack, provoking all those jokes
's database shows no general
ocardial infarction (excepting

be read with profit by anyone
s concise, up-to-date descrip-

f drugs – is not a page turner,
ons. In exhaustively catalogu-
ts on male sexual health, *and*
gives the best demonstration
some deserving trust, others
s, but I suspect it will surprise
ould spend some time in the
indings reported in the press

nd fraud in medical research.
archers, one can only wonder
ble overview of the research
port, as Professor Krause has
by a better source on drugs

Allan Mazur
Professor of Public Affairs
The Maxwell School
Syracuse University
Syracuse, NY

Walter Krause

Drugs Compromising Male Sexual Health

Walter Krause, Em. Prof. Dr. med.
Universitätsklinikum Gießen und Marburg
Klinik für Dermatologie und Allergologie
35033 Marburg
Germany

Additional material to this book can be downloaded
ISBN 978-3-642-44090-8 Springer Berlin Heidell

Springer is a part of Springer Science+Business Media
springer.com

Softcover re-print of the Hardcover 1st edition 2008

Editor: Marion Philipp, Heidelberg, Germany
Desk Editor: Ellen Blasig, Heidelberg, Germany
Reproduction, typesetting and production: LE-TEX J
GbR, Leipzig, Germany
Cover design: Frido Steinen-Broo, EStudio, Calamar, S

SPIN 11932864

Printed on acid-free paper 24/3180/YL 5 4 3 2 1 0

There is really no Achillean choice between one c
nescence. Medicine offers lesser trade-offs: some allevi
side effects. Professor Krause shows us when the side
compromising "that most male of activities". For examp
inhibitors (SSRIs), while relieving depression, promote
tion. Sometimes side effects can be turned to advantag
ing premature ejaculation.

Occasionally the trade-off is too good to pass up.
most famously Viagra, restore potency with adverse e
and self-limiting. Initial fears of increased risk of heart at
about dying happy, are not sustained. Professor Krause
cardiac side effects in most studies, and no increase in m
men taking nitrate medications).

In overview, the first part of this book is short and wil
inclined to open the volume in the first place. It contair
tions of testicular function, erection and ejaculation.

The second, bulky part of this book – the database o
but readers will be rewarded by digesting selected porti
ing and summarizing the literature on adverse drug effe
evaluating the quality of each study, Professor Krause
I have seen of inconsistency among research reports –
not. This may not be big news to experienced researcher
many clinicians. (I wish science and health journalists w
database, because it might help them realize that novel
and on television are often irreproducible.)

Readers must turn elsewhere for discussions of bias a
Here, even stipulating the honesty and objectivity of rese
how some of their work made it into print. In any sensi
literature, it is essential to consider the quality of each re
done. It will be a long time before this volume is replaced
that affect male sexual function.

Preface

Adverse effects of drugs on sexual functions are often neglected in practical medicine, because they are usually mild or moderate and rarely prompt hospital admissions, denominated as severe ADEs. In addition, standard textbooks of pharmacology and those which discuss drug side effects consider these topics only marginally, and well-known sexual side effects are not mentioned. There are, of course, a number of review articles on the possible adverse effects of drugs on sexual dysfunction, in particular on erectile dysfunction. But delineations of the exact figures of the incidence of sexual adverse effects in a concrete drug are often lacking in these papers. Reviews also frequently do not describe the database of the reported adverse effects, thus leaving the quality of evidence uncertain.

This book summarizes quotations from the literature which describe particular effects of drugs on male sexual functions. A special concern of the composition is the information on the quality rating of the reports quoted, and to reflect the overall quality of evidence that supports a specific adverse effect of a pharmacological or therapeutic subgroup of drugs. The quality rating is expressed in analogy to the grading system for clinical studies of the Scottish Intercollegiate Guidelines Network (SIGN). The systematic of drugs follows the ATC/DDD system published by the WHO.

The book is intended to encourage physicians who use any of the drugs mentioned for treatment in their patients to ask their patients about adverse effects, and to give attention to possible observations in their patients. A collection of these observations will enhance our knowledge of the compromising of male sexual health by drugs.

Marburg, October 2007
Walter Krause

Contents

Acronyms and Abbreviations Used in the Text

Acronym/abbreviation	Definition
19NT-HPP	19-nortestosterone hexyloxyphenylpropionate
5-ASA	5-amino salicylic acid
5-PDE	5-phosphodiesterase
ABVD	Bleomycin, dacarbazine, doxorubicin, vinblastine
ADEs	Adverse drug effects, adverse drug events
BSFI	Brief Male Sexual Function Inventory
CASA	Computer-assisted semen analysis
CI	Confidence interval
CIVPP	Lomustine, prednisone, procarbazine, vinblastine
COPP	Cyclophosphamide, prednisone, procarbacine, Vincristine
CPA	Cyproterone acetate
CVB	Cisplatin, vindesine, bleomycin
DHEA	Dehydroepiandrosterone
DSG	Desogestrel
e.d.	Erectile dysfunction
FISH	Fluorescence in-situ hybridization
FSH	Follicle-stimulation hormone
GnRH	Gonadotropin-releasing hormone
Gy	Gray
hCG	Human chorionic gonadotropin
HDL	High-density lipoprotein
hMG	Human menopausal gonadotropin
ICSI	Intracytoplasmatic sperm injection
ICSI-TESE	Intracytoplasmatic sperm injection after testicular Sperm extraction

IELT	Intravaginal ejaculation latency time
IHH	Idiopathic hypogonadotropic hypogonadism
IIEF	International index of erectile function
IPSS	International prostate symptom score
IU	International unit
IVF	In-vitro fertilization
LH	Luteinizing hormone
LNG	Levonorgestrel
LUTS	Lower urinary tract symptoms
MOPP	Mechlorethamine, vincristine, procarbazine, Prednisone
MPA	Medroxprogesterone acetate
MVPP	Mustine, vinblastine, procarbazine, prednisolone
n.g.	Not given
NETE	Norethisterone enanthate
NIH	National Institutes of Health (Bethesda, Maryland)
NOVP	Mitoxantrone, prednisone, vinblastine, vincristine
NPT	Nocturnal penile tumescence
OR	Odds ratio
PADIC	Cisplatin, dacarbazine, doxorubicin
POMB-ACE	Bleomycin, cisplatin, cyclophosphamide, Dactinomycin, etoposide, methotrexate, vincristine
PTSD	Post-traumatic stress disorder
RCT	Randomized control trial
RR	Relative risk
SHBG	Sexual hormone binding globulin
T	Testosterone
TESE	Testicular sperm extraction
VBP±A	Vinblastine, bleomycin, cisplatin, adrimycin, Zona pellucida

1 Male Sexual Health

Male sexual health was defined by the 1994 International Conference on Population and Development in Cairo and the 1995 Fourth World Conference on Women held in Beijing. The conferences expanded the right to family planning to include the right to better sexual and reproductive health. On the basis of the World Health Organization's definition of health, the Cairo Programme defines reproductive health as:

a state of complete physical, mental and social well-being and … not merely the absence of disease or infirmity, in all matters relating to the reproductive system and to its functions and processes. Reproductive health therefore implies that people are able to have a satisfying and safe sex life and that they have the capability to reproduce and the freedom to decide if, when and how often to do so. Implicit in this last condition are the right of men and women to be informed and to have access to safe, effective, affordable and acceptable methods of family planning of their choice, as well as other methods of their choice for regulation of fertility which are not against the law, and the right of access to appropriate health-care services that will enable women to go safely through pregnancy and childbirth and provide couples with the best chance of having a healthy infant (paragraph 72).

(Published by the United Nations Department of Public Information – DPI/1877 – February 1997)

Reproductive rights are further elucidated by the UNFPA (source: UNFPA website):

Attaining the goals of sustainable, equitable development requires that individuals are able to exercise control over their sexual and reproductive lives. This includes the rights to:

- *Reproductive health as a component of overall health, throughout the life cycle, for both men and women*
- *Reproductive decision-making, including voluntary choice in marriage, family formation and determination of the number, timing and spacing of one's children and the right to have access to the information and means needed to exercise voluntary choice*
- *Equality and equity for men and women, to enable individuals to make free and informed choices in all spheres of life, free from discrimination based on gender*
- *Sexual and reproductive security, including freedom from sexual violence and coercion, and the right to privacy.*

In this sense, the term "male sexual health" comprises satisfying sexual function including the social aspects of partnership and gender identification, the psychological conditions of libido and arousal, as well as the physiological reactions of erection and ejaculation, but also the undisturbed function of androgen production and sperm maturation by the testes leading to the ability to induce a pregnancy in the female partner.

1.1 Structure and Physiology of the Testis

1.1.1 Introduction

The testis is a paired organ located in the scrotum. It consists of two different functional compartments: (a) the seminiferous tubules; and (b) the interstitial tissue. The tubules contain the spermatogenetic tissue, the volume of which amounts to up to 90% of the testicular volume. The interstitial tissue contains the blood and lymph vessels, the nerves, the connective tissue and the immune cells, and the Leydig cells, in which the testosterone biosynthesis takes place.

The tubuli seminiferi are surrounded by a wall containing myofibroblasts. There contractions, which support the transport of the spermatozoa, are probably moderated by oxytocin. In the lumen of the tubules, there are two cell types, the Sertoli cells and the germ cells. The process of germ cell development in the male from the primordial germ cells, through spermatogonia, spermatocytes and spermatids to the mature haploid spermatozoa is called spermatogenesis

The Sertoli cells have different functions: (a) forming of the blood–testis barrier, which guarantees the intratubular milieu; (b) "feeding" of the germ cells and facilitating their differentiation in the spermatogenesis; (c) phagocytosis of the residues of the sperm cytoplasm as well as of apoptotic germ cells; and (d) secretion of steroid hormones and inhibin. Sertoli cells yield an exclusive structure: the ectoplasmic specialization (Toyama et al. 2003), which comprises the plasma membrane, a subsurface cistern formed by the endoplasmic reticulum and a layer of microfilaments that consists of actin between the two structures. One type of the ectoplasmic specialization is localized in the adjoining parts of the Sertoli cells (Sertoli–Sertoli junction); another type is present in that region of the Sertoli cells which faces the acrosomal region of the differentiating spermatids. It is similar to the hemidesmosomes of the basal cells of the epidermis (Sertoli–spermatid junction; Fig. 1.1.1).

Within the ectoplasmic specialization there are several proteins, in part specific to the two types of junctions: ZO-1; ZO-2; ZO-e; occludin, which binds to ZO-1; the claudin family; and symplektin. Some of these proteins are found also in other junctional regions of epithelial cells. Fimbrin, vinculin and espin are found as actin-binding or actin-bundling proteins. Disturbance of one of the types of ectoplasmic specialization by different toxins leads to defects in the sper-

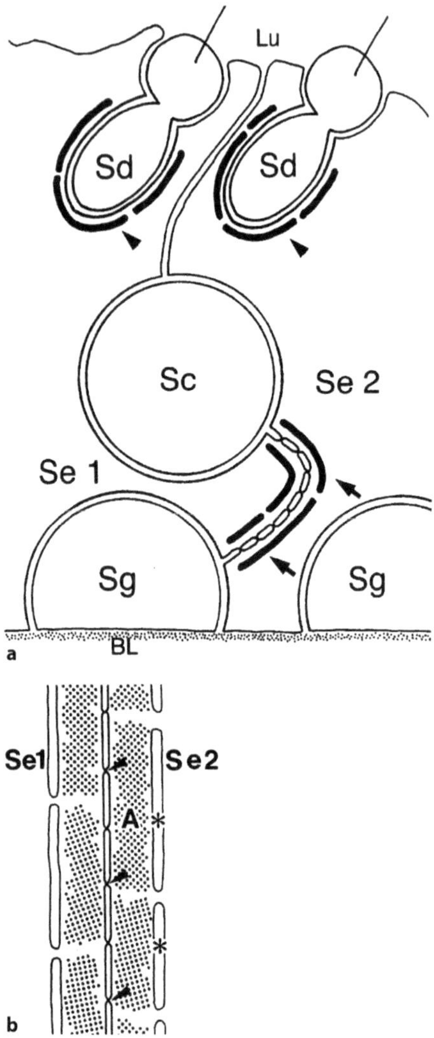

Fig. 1.1.1 There are two types of ectoplasmic specialization in the Sertoli cells (*Sc*): (a) one between Sertoli cells and spermatids (*Sd; arrowheads*), placed near the tubular lumen (*Lu*), and those between two Sertoli cells (*Se 1, Se 2; arrows*) and the spermatogonia (*Sg*), localized at the basal lamina (*BL*); and (b) the ectoplasmic specialization between adjoining Sertoli cells, which is composed of tight junctions (bottom, *arrowheads*). *Asterisks* represent the subsurface cistern of the endoplasmic reticulum. (From Toyama et al. 2003)

matogenesis. Compounds acting in this way are oestrogens. Also genetic alterations may influence the proteins of ectoplasmic specialization. In this sense, Sertoli cells are the most relevant cells of the testis in terms of protection of spermatogenesis, but also in terms of vulnerability.

Another type of cell-to-cell interaction among Sertoli cells, and between Sertoli cells and germ cells, is mediated by gap junctions, which link the neighbouring cells to each other. As channels, they allow direct transportation of molecules with a molecular mass of up to approximately 1 kDa, a process by which the cells exchange signals of metabolism and cell differentiation. The constituents of the gap junctions are connexins, a protein family of at least 20 members in mammals. In the rat testis, transcripts for 11 connexins have been identified. Connexin 43 and connexin 31 are of particular importance. In the seminiferous tubules, gap junctions containing connexin 43 form an intercellular network, which possibly coordinates the metabolic influences of Sertoli cells on germ cell differentiation. The state of gap junctions between the testicular cells is controlled by endocrine and paracrine messengers, such as gonadotropins, steroid hormones and thyroid hormones. Environmental toxins and endocrine disruptors may impair the gap junctions (Pointis and Segretain 2005).

The other cell types of the tubules are classified as germ cells. The germinal stem cells lie in the niche on the basal lamina of seminiferous tubules. Culturing these cells in vitro is now possible, but the goal of a spermatogenesis in vitro is still far away (Ogawa et al. 2005). The cells differentiate through four mitoses and the meiosis to the haploid spermatozoa. During these processes, the germ cells are embedded in the Sertoli cells and migrate from the basement of the tubules to the adluminal compartment. Spermatogonia type A pale are the stem cells, which remain in the tubules for further generations. Spermatogonia type A dark are the first type of differentiating cells. They divide mitotically to spermatogonia type B; they divide again to form the primary spermatocytes. These spermatocytes undergo the first meiotic division in a long-standing process of chromosome arrangement as zygotene, leptotene and pachytene spermatocytes, leading to secondary spermatocytes which contain half of the chromosomes but a diploid amount of DNA. The secondary spermatocytes divide mitotically into the haploid spermatides, which differentiate during spermiogenesis to the mature spermatozoa. The spermatids are interconnected by intercellular bridges, which dissolve with maturation. During spermiogenesis (a) the nucleus is condensed to about 10% of the original volume, mainly by replacing the different histones by four types of protamines, (b) the acrosome evolves from the Golgi apparatus, forming the acrosomal cap of the mature spermatozoa and (c) the flagellum is fortified (Kim et al. 2002). An important factor in the regulation of spermatid maturation is cAMP-responsive element modulator (CREM). When the mature spermatids leave the testis, they are designated as spermatozoa.

Gene expression of spermatids ceases after replacement of histones by protamines. The transcription takes place in the round spermatides, and a translation of transcripts is possible in later spermatids, e.g. for production of new proteins used in maturating spermatids such as protamines. Genes expressed during spermiogenesis avoid methylation in male germ cells, even if they are methylated in somatic cells. The methylation in germ cells is somewhat similar to the gene methylation in cancer cells (Tanaka and Baba 2005).

Cells of spermatogenesis may undergo apoptosis at all cell stages; more than half of cells of the different stages of differentiation are eliminated by apoptosis. By morphological criteria, the peak has been observed in type-A spermatogonia, in primary spermatocytes and in maturing spermatids. Apoptosis is important also for the cessation of the prepuberal germ cell wave, which occurs in many mammalian testes. Apoptotic cells are either shed into the lumen of the tubules or they are phagocytosed by Sertoli cells. Sertoli cells express the Fas ligand, which helps to eliminate Fas-positive germ cells, and the phagocytosis of spermatogenic cells, when they externalize the phosphatidyl serine as a marker of apoptosis, is performed also by Sertoli cells via a class-B scavenger receptor. They also attack Fas-positive immune cells, thus possibly supporting the maintenance of the testis as an immune-privileged region. CREM, which is highly expressed in postmeiotic cells, is also involved in apoptosis (Nakanishi and Shiratsuchi 2003).

The process of spermatogenesis, including mitoses, meiosis, differentiation and apoptosis, is regulated not only by the gonadotropins FSH, LH and testosterone, but also by local control signals that regulate cell function (Lamb and Niederberger 1994), among which are epidermal growth factor, fibroblast-like growth factors, transforming growth factors, interleukin and insulin-like growth factors I and II. There are also growth factors unique to the testis secreted by Sertoli cells; among these are inhibins, activins and the Muellerian-inhibiting substance. The FSH receptors are found in the Sertoli cells and spermatogonia.

1.1.2 The Spermatozoa

The spermatozoa transport the male genome through the female genital tract in order to procreate the embryo after fusion with the oocyte. The spermatozoa are motile cells that consist of the head, which contains the DNA, the midpiece, which contains mitochondria, which produce the kinetic energy, and the tail, which gives the spermatozoa their motility. The spermatozoa undergo multiple changes of their surface and their general characteristics on their (mainly passive) passage through the male genital tract as well as on their (mainly active) migration through the female genital tract.

The cytoplasm of mature spermatozoa contains practically none of the cellular machineries necessary for protein synthesis. The constituent proteins of spermatozoa are generally synthesized in spermatocytes and/or spermatids (Toshimori 2003), but they are pivotally altered during epididymal passage. During the passage, the spermatozoa gain motility, the ability to bind to the zona pellucida and fuse with the oocyte membrane by changes in their plasma membrane. They undergo intense changes in protein composition: some proteins of testicular origin are removed or altered, whereas others are added from epididymal sources. Some major proteins secreted in the epididymis have been identified in different species, among them lactoferrin, clusterin and different enzymes acting in the carbohydrate metabolism, e.g glycosidases and glycosyltransferases. Clusterin is most common among the species as a whole; the other proteins are secreted in species-specific amounts. Some of the proteins are bound to, or integrated into, the sperm membrane, e.g. the cysteine-rich secretory protein (CRISP), which is found in the postacrosomal region of ejaculated sperm. Also in human spermatozoa, proteins of epididymal origin were identified in the membrane (HE1-5). There is a high concentration of enzymes in the epididymal fluid, which may contribute to the remodelling of the sperm membrane. Epididymal proteins are also involved in protection of sperm against oxidative injury (e.g. the gamma-glutamyl transpeptidase, GGT), in immune protection (e.g. clusterin protection against complement-induced cell lysis) and in antimicrobial activity of semen (e.g. hCAP-18). On the other hand, also proteins dissolved from the spermatozoa activate the epididymal secretions. A better understanding of the role of epididymal proteins in sperm maturation will allow the development of male contraceptives and will also facilitate the understanding of untoward effects of drugs (Dacheux et al. 2003).

Some of the proteins are secreted in an apocrine manner by the epididymal epithelium and appear in exosomes, called epididymosomes (Sullivan et al. 2005). These epididymosomes interact with spermatozoa. Among the proteins are two enzymes involved in the polyol pathway: an aldose reductase and a sorbitol dehydrogenase, as is the macrophage migration inhibitory factor (MIF). Also, one of

1

the surface proteins, P25b, which is necessary for the binding to the surface of the egg, is added to spermatozoa by epididymosomes. In-vitro studies showed that the transfer of epididymosomal proteins to specific membrane domains of spermatozoa is saturable, as well as temperature- and pH-dependent, and is optimal at pH 6.5. The presence of zinc in the incubation medium, but not of calcium or magnesium, significantly increases the efficiency of protein transfer.

Mature sperm cells in the adult male show a great morphological variety, in particular of the head. There is, however, no association with aberrations of the genetic information. In fertile men, no significant association between the number of morphologically abnormal spermatozoa and those bearing chromosomal abnormalities as evaluated by the hamster-oocyte penetration test was found. This association was also lacking in men with known chromosomal translocations. By fluorescence in-situ hybridization analysis (FISH), no association of abnormal morphology and abnormal chromosomes in spermatozoa could be shown. Also in defined morphological abnormalities, such as globozoospermia or multiflagellate sperm, no increased rate of chromosomal abnormalities could be found (Sun et al. 2006).

1.1.3 Sperm Motility

Sperm motility throughout the female genital tract is guaranteed by sperm-innate sources. The migration is directed by physical and chemical entities; among them are substances which bind to an olfactory receptor (Serrano and Garcia-Suarez 2001). Spermatozoa move in a symmetrical, lower-amplitude waveform that drives them in a more or less straight line. In certain conditions, spermatozoa gain "hyperactivated motility", which enables them to move progressively also in a more viscous environment, such as the fallopian tube. This special form of movement is associated with the ability of sperm to fertilize the oocyte (Turner 2006).

A prerequisite for successful sperm motility is the flagellar ultrastructure. In the midpiece of the flagellum there are nine outer dense fibres right inside the plasma membrane and the mitochondrial sheath. The axoneme is situated within this ring, which contains other microtubule doublets with associated dynein arms, radial spokes and a central pair of microtubule doublets (Fig. 1.1.2). The axoneme is highly conserved structure consisting mainly of α and β tubulins. The motor proteins are the dyneins, which cause a sliding of the microtubules along one another, and which lead to a bending of the flagellum. The outer dense fibres store the kinetic energy and adds it via elastic return to the movement.

The energy transfer requires glycolysis; spermatozoa are able to store glycogen and may even be capable of gluconeogenesis. In the mitochondrial sheath, sperm-specific isoforms of the lactate dehydrogenase and the hexokinase are present. In some species, the presence of the key gluconeogenic enzyme fructose-1,6-bisphosphatase was demonstrated. Biophysically, a diffusion of ATP from mitochondria along the sperm tail as far as to the tip over a length

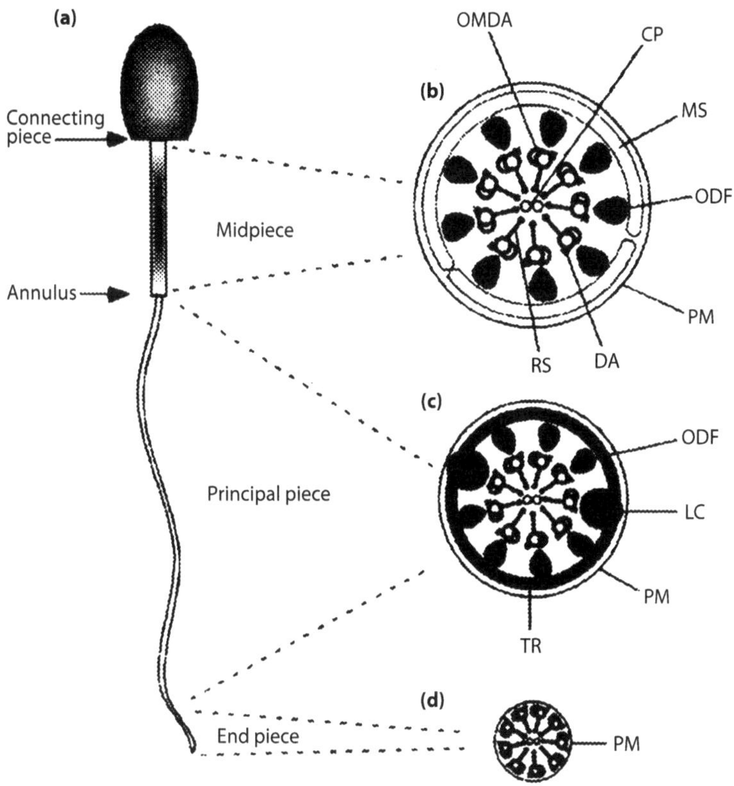

Fig. 1.1.2 **a** Representation of the spermatozoon and the ultrastructure of the flagellum. **b** A section of the midpiece shows outer dense fibres (*ODF*) below the mitochondrial sheath (*MS*) and the plasma membrane (*PM*). Two ODFs have been replaced by two longitudinal columns (*LC*), connected by transversal ribs (*TR*), In the centre, there are the nine outer microtubule doublets of the axoneme (*OMDA*) with dynein arms (*DA*) and radial spokes (*RS*) and the central pair of microtubule doublets (*CP*). **c** At the end of the principal piece the structure is similar, but there is no longer a mitochondrial sheath. **d** In the end piece, no more ODF are left. (From Turner 2006)

of 48 μm in human spermatozoa is possible. Creatine kinase, adenylate kinase and phosphoglycerate kinase are able to transfer ATP away from the mitochondria and return ADP. For the transport of hydrogen ions and phosphate, carbonic anhydrase and GAPDH are present. The enzymes are innate components of the spermatozoa from the spermatogenesis (Ford 2006).

Sperm motility is also regulated by changes in the intracellular Ca(2+) concentrations. Several types of Ca(2+)-permeable channels in the sperm plasma membrane have been demonstrated. There are voltage-operated channels of different types and specific distribution over the sperm cell, store-operated channels, cyclic nucleotide-gated channels and CatSpers, a novel family of ion channels expressed exclusively in spermatozoa. There are also Ca(2+)-clearing mechanisms: ATP-utilizing Ca2+ pumps of different types and the Na+–Ca2+ exchanger, which may be blocked by verapamil. At least two different stores enables the intracellular modulation of Ca(2+) (Jimenez-Gonzalez et al. 2006).

1.1.4 Capacitation and Acrosome Reaction

In the female reproductive tract, spermatozoa undergo a series of biochemical transformations, collectively called capacitation. The first event in capacitation is cholesterol efflux leading to the elevation of intracellular calcium and bicarbonate, which activates adenylyl cyclase (AC) to produce cyclic-AMP. The next step is the activation of a protein kinase A (PKA) to indirectly phosphorylate certain proteins on tyrosine. During capacitation, there is also an increase in protein tyrosine phosphorylation-dependent actin polymerization and the membrane-bound phospholipase C (PLC). Sperm binding to zona-pellucida causes further activation of cAMP/PKA and protein kinase C (PKC), respectively. The PKA together with inositol-trisphosphate activates calcium channels in the outer acrosomal membrane, which allows an influx of calcium ions to the cytosol. This results in F-actin dispersion, which enables the outer acrosomal and the plasma membrane to come into contact and fuse, thus leading to exocytosis of acrosomal contents (Breitbart 2003). This process, called acrosome reaction, is physiologically induced by progesterone from the follicle fluid. Spermatozoa contain a non-G-protein coupled membrane progesterone receptor, which is distinct from the cytosolic receptor which induces hormone responses of target cells. The rise of Ca2+ ions during acrosome reaction is the most important step in the process; experimentally, it can be mimicked by the incubation with calcium ionophore (Serrano and Garcia-Suarez 2001).

A number of voltage-gated Ca2+ channels have been described, but the contribution of each of them to sperm physiology is not clear. The knowledge would be a prerequisite for a pharmacological alteration of sperm function via specific ion channels. Ca2+ channel blockers, which are used, for example, in hypertension, indeed influence sperm function, but they do not induce infertility. For other ion channels, some insights into their role in sperm function are present (e.g. K+ channels are relevant for volume regulation), but only compounds applicable in vitro are known to be effective up to now, and side effects of systemically applied drugs have never been observed (Fig. 1.1.3; Zhang and Gopalakrishnan 2005).

1.1.5 Fertilization of the Oocyte

Capacitation takes place usually in the vicinity of the cumulus oophorus. After this, they bind to the zona pellucida (ZP) mediated by special adhesion proteins. Following binding, the spermatozoa undergo acrosome reaction, by which

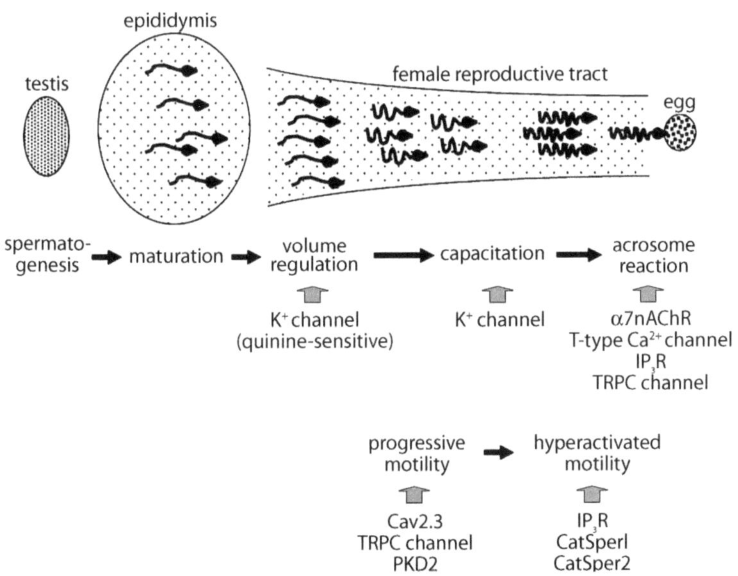

Fig. 1.1.3 Different ion channels are implicated in sperm function. (From Zhang and Gopalakrishnan 2005)

the acrosomal contents are liberated in order to enable the spermatozoa to penetrate the ZP. The most relevant oocyte proteins involved are the zona pellucida glycoproteins 1–3 (ZP 1–3). In mice, the protein ZP3 functions as a sperm receptor, but it is inactivated in fertilized eggs by using special oligosaccharides attached to the peptide. ZP3 also appears to induce acrosome reaction after binding of sperm to the ZP. Members of the ADAM (a disintegrin and metalloprotease) family, ADAM1, ADAM2, ADAM3, and also the epididymal protein DE/cysteine-rich secretory protein 1 (CRISP) from the spermatozoa, are involved in sperm-oocyte binding and membrane fusion. The corresponding proteins ("sperm receptors") of the oocyte seem to be integrins. The process is similar to a fusion of virus particles to infected cells (Brewis et al. 2005; Wassarman et al. 2005). Also CD9, an integral plasma membrane protein from the oocyte, takes part in sperm–egg fusion. CD9 is a member of the tetraspanin family of proteins, which are ubiquitous parts of living cells. The proteins are characterized by four transmembrane regions and two extracellular loops. They interact with integrins, immunoglobulins, proteoglycans, complementary regulatory proteins, and growth factor receptors (Kaji and Kudo 2004). Recent data in mice suggest that the three-dimensional structure of the zona pellucida is responsible for sperm binding, rather than a single protein or carbohydrate (Hoodbhoy and Dean 2004).

After binding, the spermatozoa actively pass through the ZP. The passage is mediated mainly by the proteolytic enzyme acrosine. A second adhesion process takes place at the oolemma: the sperm–oocyte attachment starts at the equatorial region of the spermatozoa. Several integrins have been identified which modulate the attachment. The adhesion is immediately followed by sperm–egg fusion. After sperm entry into the oocyte, a sperm factor induces calcium oscillations of the oocyte, which lead to egg activation to form the female pronucleus. From the sperm chromatin, the male pronucleus is formed. The two pronuclei ultimately fuse at syngamy, by which process fertilization is complete.

1.1.6 Testing Substances that Compromise Spermatogenesis and Fertility (adapted from Creasy 1997)

There are a large number of structurally diverse chemicals that cause testicular damage in laboratory animals, but the effects of only relatively few have been proven in humans. The most meaningful studies have been performed with dibromochloropropane (DBCP), which compromises male fertility, but it has long been known to induce testicular atrophy in rats.

A number of regulatory guidelines for studies on reproduction and fertility exist. For drug registration, the results of the International Conference on Harmonization (ICH) have been accepted by the governments of the United States, the European Union and Japan. For male reproductive toxicity, the guidelines require a premating dosage for at least 4 weeks, and an evaluation of testicular histology after fixation with Bouin's solution and staining with PAS (periodic acid Schiff). The guidelines do not include two-generation studies, which would probably be useful for the detection of oestrogenic effects; these are recommended by guidelines of the Environmental Protection Agency (EPA) and the Organization for Economic Co-operation and Development (OECD).

A testicular toxicant will usually result in germ cell loss. This is easy to verify because of histological observation. Also, germ cell degeneration, which produces different features in different generations of spermatogenic cells, may be observed. The particular event of delayed spermiation is more difficult to detect. It can be observed only when the stages of the spermatogenetic cycle are specifically evaluated. Sertoli cells and Leydig cells may also be affected.

As a practical approach for the assessment of testicular damage, the following qualitative measures are recommended:

1. Check which are the most differentiated form of germ cells, i.e. spermatogonia or spermatocytes.
2. Check for inhibited sperm release.
3. Check for disorganization of the normal spermatogenic stages.
4. Look for an increased number of abnormal cells.
5. Check the epididymis for cell changes of spermatozoa.

As quantitative parameters, the following measurements can be acquired:

1. Tubular diameter
2. Cell counts of spermatocytes or other cells, expressed as a ration to Sertoli cell number
3. Counting homogenization-resistant spermatids (which is the most rapid and sensitive method)

A particular question concerns the genetic transfer of sperm abnormalities to the offspring. More than 100 chemicals which induce detrimental effects to sperm-parameter quality were known by 1983 (Wyborek et al. 1983). It is likely that these substances are also able to induce numerical and structural chromosomal defects or even single-gene defects.

Table 1.1.1 DNA and chromosomal alterations that can be transmitted by sperm (from Wyborek et al. 2005)

Aneuploidy
Of sex chromosomes
Of autosomes
Structural aberrations
Duplications/deletions
Rearrangements
Chromosome breaks
Epigenetic modifications
Imprinting
Premutational lesions
DNA adducts
Protamine adducts
Single- and double-strand breaks
Nucleotide
Gene mutations

The possible genomic alterations are listed in Table 1.1.1 Alterations of the genome of the postmeiotic, haploid cells may be transported to the zygotes. In human sperm, transient increased chromosomal abnormalities were observed by FISH within the first months after chemotherapy with antineoplastic drugs. The knowledge of the mechanisms underlying the alterations is limited, since only few compounds have been tested sufficiently. It is also unknown which drugs produce transient, and which produce possibly permanent, alterations of maturing germ cells.

1.1.7 Testosterone Production and Testosterone Effects

Testosterone is the most relevant of the androgens, compounds that interact with androgen receptors in target tissues to bring about the androgenic effects. Target tissues are male reproductive organs, spermatogenesis, secondary male sex characteristics, libido, development of muscle mass, strength and power (Medline's definition).

The largest part (about 95%) of the testosterone amount of 6–7 mg, which is produced in the body daily, originates from the approximately 500 million Leydig cells of the testis. The biosynthesis of testosterone starts from cholesterol, which is transported in the LDL fraction of the serum lipoproteins. The transport of cholesterol to the mitochondria is mediated by the StAR protein (steroidogenesis activator). The first steroid prohormone produced is pregnenolone. Several defined enzymes catalyze the further steps of biosynthesis in the endoplasmic reticulum. All enzymatic reactions, which require energy, depend on cytochrome P450. All the testosterone precursors also are delivered to the blood, because the metabolism to testosterone is limited (Rommerts 1998). Leydig cells store only little testosterone; nearly all of the produced amount is delivered to the blood. In this way, hormone levels of 3–10 ng/ml (10.4–34.8 nmol/l) are maintained in the blood serum.

The most relevant control instrument of Leydig cell function is the luteinizing hormone (LH) from the hypophysis. The embryonic and fetal development of the number and structure of Leydig cells is probably independent of LH, but even in an early postnatal period its stimulatory role is important. The Leydig cells possess membranous receptors for LH. They stimulate an adenyl cyclase and thus the production of cAMP. The binding to the receptor also stimulates protein kinases, which among others regulate the expression of certain genes in order to mediate the tropic effects of LH. An increase of mRNA production leads to a rise in steroid production via a regulation of the StAR production and the enzyme activities. The end point of the LH effect is an increase in the production of testosterone. The effect is demonstrable in the human by an increase of testosterone serum levels, which is also achieved with human chorionic gonadotrophin (hCG).

Hormonal control of Leydig cell function forms an "endocrine cascade". The hypothalamus produces the gonadotropin-releasing hormone (GnRH) and secretes it via the hypophyseal portal system. The secretion is not continuous, but instead occurs in pulses with 60- to 120-min intervals. After binding of GnRH to the specific receptors, the gonadotropic cells of the anterior pituitary gland produce and secrete the gonadotropins FSH and LH. In particular LH is secreted in pulses following the GnRH pulses, thus forming a characteristic pulse pattern in the peripheral blood. The amount and pulsatility of LH is mediated by gonadal steroids at the pituitary level (Amory and Bremner 2001).

Within the endocrine cascade leading to testosterone production in the Leydig cells, there are several mechanisms that lower the production in ageing. Firstly, the GnRH release from the hypothalamus declines. As a consequence, the LH episodic peaks have a lower amplitude, but the same frequency, as in younger men; thus, the stimulation of testosterone production decreases. The same defect attenuates the feedback response of the hypothalamus to testosterone. In addition, also the GH secretion decreases, which is an important factor in steroid production by the Leydig cells, acting synergistically with LH. The pituitary function, however, appears to be uninfluenced.

The steroid production by the Leydig cells is influenced by the local cytokine milieu. The concentration of all the cytokines increases with age, and most of them have an inhibiting effect on steroidogenesis. The concentration of insulin-like growth factor I, on the other hand, which increases steroidogenesis, declines with age. Several mechanisms within the Leydig cell itself act in the same direction. The induction of cAMP formation and phosphokinase-A activity, which is important for the intracellular signalling in the Leydig cell, decreases in ageing cells due to defects – which are unknown up to now – in the signalling pathway. The production of the StAR protein decreases with age. A tonic inhibition of StAR gene expression is mediated by the cyclooxygenase-2 activity, and again this enzyme activity increases with age (Fig. 1.1.4; Wang and Stocco 2005).

Proinflammatory cytokines derived from testicular macrophages also mediate Leydig cell functions. Testicular macrophages are found in close vicinity to the Leydig cells in the interstitial tissue. Cytoplasmic processes of Leydig cells have been observed to lead to membrane invagination of adjacent macrophages. Macrophage-secreted cytokines, such as interleukin-1 and tumor growth factor-α, have been shown to stimulate the proliferation immature Leydig cells. On the other hand, the steroidogenic acute regulatory protein (StAR) is inhibited by transforming growth factor-ß, tumor necrosis factor, interferon-γ, reactive oxygen species and others. Similarly, the key enzyme of testosterone biosynthesis, the 3ß-hydroxysteroid dehydrogenases, has been shown to become inhibited by tumor necrosis factor, reactive oxygen species and others, and the same factors have also inhibited cytochrome P450 in the Leydig cell (Hales 2002).

Testosterone is transported to the target organs via the blood stream. The quick efflux into the extracellulary space is avoided by testosterone binding serum proteins. There is the sexual hormone binding globulin (SHBG), binding testosterone with high affinity but low capacity, and albumin, which binds testosterone with low affinity but high capacity. Ninety-eight percent of the blood testosterone is bound to such proteins; only 2% are available to the peripheral metabolizing enzymes and the testosterone receptors in the target cells, but a decrease of free testosterone is quickly replaced by diffusion from the protein-bound steroid.

Testosterone action in the target organs is mediated by the androgen receptors (AR). They are present in nearly all tissues; they mediate the testosterone effect in the testes, the male accessory glands, the skin, the muscles, the liver and possibly also in the bone. The AR gene is located on the X chromosome; thus, only a single copy exists in males. Each mutation of the AR gene is followed by alterations of the androgen target structures, because no co-dominant allele exists. Mutations are more frequent than in other genes,

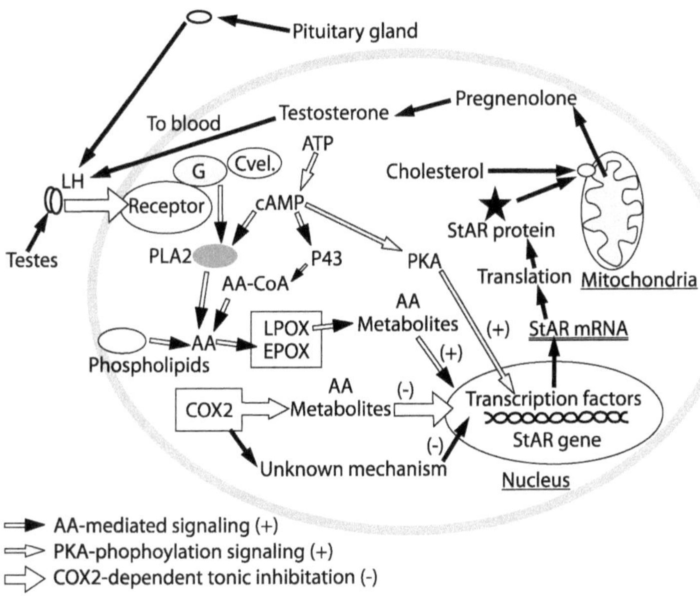

Fig. 1.1.4 Luteinizing hormone (LH) stimulates testosterone biosynthesis in Leydig cells. It binds to the LH receptor in the cell membrane and activates a G protein. From there, signal transduction to the nucleus is performed by two separate pathways, the PKA phosphorylation pathway and the AA-medicated pathway. The StAR protein transports cholesterol to the mitochondria, where it is converted to different steroids. The PKA phosphorylates transcription factors regulating SzAR gene transcription. G proteins activate phospholipase A, which catalyzes AA release from phospholipids. After its release, AA is metabolized by three families of enzymes, the lipoxygenases (*LPOX*), the epoxygenases (*EPOX*) and the cyclooxygenases (*COX*). Metabolites produced by LPOX and EPOX enhance StAR gene expression, while those induced by COX2 inhibit StAR gene expression. (From Wang and Stocco 2005)

because AR is not essential for a viable human organism. Mutations in the AR gene are usually followed by decreased androgen sensitivity of the target organs, the complete lack of function of which is known as the complete androgen insensitivity syndrome (Gelmann 2002).

The AR protein contains four functional domains: the NH2-terminal transactivation domain; the DNA-binding domain (DBD); the hinge region; and the ligand-binding domain (LBD). The NH2-terminal domain is the most variable region. The region contains a polymorphic polyglutamine repeat that ranges from 8 to 31 repeats in normal individuals. Longer polyglutamine tract length results in decreased AR transcriptional activity in vitro. Clinically, men with a long polyglutamine tract have an increased incidence of impaired spermatogenesis. A length of the polyglutamine tract to more than 40 repeats causes the rare Kennedy syndrome, which consists of neuromuscular disorder, spinal and bulbar muscular atrophy and decreased virilization. The hinge region of AR links the DBD and LBD, which contain the nuclear localization signal (NLS). Single amino acid exchange in this region has been shown to produce partial or complete androgen insensitivity (Heinlein and Chang 2002).

The binding of testosterone induces new conformation of the receptor protein, which afterwards is able to bind to the hormone-responsible element of a gene, thus enhancing the transcription rate of this gene. The transcriptional activity of AR is modulated by co-regulatory proteins, of which a large number have been identified. Co-regulators may enhance transactivation (co-activators) or reduce transactivation (co-repressors) of target genes. Co-regulators can be divided into two major types: type-I co-regulators influence the binding of the AR to the target genes; and type-II co-regulators function primarily in the appropriate structural conformation of the AR after ligand binding (Heinlein and Chang 2002).

In some organs, testosterone is reduced to 5-α-dihydrotestosterone by the 5-α-reductase prior to the binding to the receptor. The enzyme 5-α-reductase is of relevance mainly in the skin and the prostate. There are two isoenzymes: they show poor homology, and they have different chromosomal localization and different expression patterns in the prostate and skin. Substances which inhibit both types of the enzyme are known and clinically used in diseases of the prostate and skin (Occhiato et al. 2004). Men with 5-α-reductase-2 deficiency have ambiguous genitalia, but normal male libido with normal spermatogenesis, and may be able to father children by assisted reproduction (Imperato-McGinley 2002).

The role of oestrogens in the male is less clear and less well examined than that of testosterone (Abney 1999). Oestrogens are involved in the physiology of testicular functions as "paracrine" factors. They act via a specific receptor [oestrogen receptor α (Erα) and oestrogen receptor β (Erβ)]. Oestrogens are synthesized by means of the cytochrome-P450-dependent aromatase, a product of a single gene: Cyp19. The enzyme is localized mainly in Leydig cells. The known effects of oestradiol on the Leydig cells depend on their developmental stage. In the fetal cell, oestradiol blocks the development from precursor cells, whereas in the adult Leydig cell, the androgen production is diminished by the inhibition of several enzymes involved in testosterone synthesis. Sertoli cells take part in oestrogen production, and also the spermatogenic cells contain aromatase, and transcripts are demonstrable to the point of sperm cytoplasmic droplets. Consequently, it has been shown that human-ejaculated spermatozoa contain Erα (Carreau et al. 2006).

Oestrogens are considered to be survival factors for germ cells. In the Rhesus model, an inhibition of spermatid maturation is observed after treatment with aromatase inhibitor. Also in men, in very rare cases mutations of the aromatase gene lead to sterility. Oestrogens, however, have a mainly inhibitory effects on male fertility, thus explaining the influences of endocrine disruptors (Carreau et al. 2003).

References

1. Abney TO. The potential roles of estrogens in regulating Leydig cell development and function: a review. Steroids. 1999 Sep;64(9):610–7.
2. Amory JK, Bremner W. Endocrine regulation of testicular function in men: implications for contraceptive development. Mol Cell Endocrinol. 2001 Sep;182(2):175–9.
3. Breitbart H. Signaling pathways in sperm capacitation and acrosome reaction. Cell Mol Biol (Noisy-le-grand). 2003 May;49(3):321–7.
4. Brewis IA, Van Gestel RA, Gadella BM, Jones R, Publicover SJ, Roldan ER, Frayne J, Barratt CL. The spermatozoon at fertilisation: current understanding and future research directions. Hum Fertil (Camb). 2005 Dec;8(4):241–51.
5. Carreau S, Lambard S, Delalande C, Denis-Galeraud I, Bilinska B, Bourguiba S. Aromatase expression and role of estrogens in male gonad: a review. Reprod Biol Endocrinol. 2003 Apr 11;1:35.
6. Carreau S, Delalande C, Silandre D, Bourguiba S, Lambard S. Aromatase and estrogen receptors in male reproduction. Mol Cell Endocrinol. 2006 Feb 26;246(1–2):65–8.
7. Creasy DM. Evaluation of testicular toxicity in safety evaluation studies: the appropriate use of spermatogenic staging. Toxicol Pathol. 1997 Mar–Apr;25(2):119–31.
8. Dacheux JL, Gatti JL, Dacheux F. Contribution of epididymal secretory proteins for spermatozoa maturation. Microsc Res Tech. 2003 May 1;61(1):7–17.

9. Ford WC. Glycolysis and sperm motility: Does a spoonful of sugar help the flagellum go round? Hum Reprod Update. 2006 May–Jun;12(3):269–74.
10. Gelmann EP. Molecular biology of the androgen receptor. J Clin Oncol. 2002 Jul 1;20(13):3001–15.
11. Hales DB. Testicular macrophage modulation of Leydig cell steroidogenesis. J Reprod Immunol. 2002 Oct–Nov;57(1–2):3–18.
12. Heinlein CA, Chang C. Androgen receptor (AR) coregulators: an overview. Endocr Rev. 2002 Apr;23(2):175–200.
13. Hoodbhoy T, Dean J. Insights into the molecular basis of sperm–egg recognition in mammals. Reproduction. 2004 Apr;127(4):417–22.
14. Imperato-McGinley: 5α-reductase-2 deficiency and complete androgen insensitivity: lessons from nature. Adv Exp Med Biol. 2002;511:121–31.
15. Jimenez-Gonzalez C, Michelangeli F, Harper CV, Barratt CL, Publicover SJ. Calcium signalling in human spermatozoa: a specialized "toolkit" of channels, transporters and stores. Hum Reprod Update. 2006;12(3):253–67.
16. Kaji K, Kudo A. The mechanism of sperm-oocyte fusion in mammals. Reproduction. 2004 Apr;127(4):423–9.
17. Kim ED, Barqawi AZ, Seo JT, Meacham RB. Apoptosis: its importance in spermatogenic dysfunction. Urol Clin North Am. 2002 Nov;29(4):755–65, vii.
18. Lamb DJ. Growth factors and testicular development. J Urol. 1993 Aug;150(2 Pt 2):583–92.
19. Nakanishi Y, Shiratsuchi A. Phagocytic removal of apoptotic spermatogenic cells by Sertoli cells: mechanisms and consequences. Biol Pharm Bull. 2004 Jan;27(1):13–6.
20. Occhiato EG, Guarna A, Danza G, Serio M. Selective nonsteroidal inhibitors of 5 alpha-reductase type 1. J Steroid Biochem Mol Biol. 2004 Jan;88(1):1–16.
21. Ogawa T, Ohmura M, Ohbo K. The niche for spermatogonial stem cells in the mammalian testis. Int J Hematol. 2005 Dec;82(5):381–8.
22. Pointis G, Segretain D. Role of connexin-based gap junction channels in testis. Trends Endocrinol Metab. 2005 Sep;16(7):300–6.
23. Rommerts FFG. Testosterone: an overview of biosynthesis, transport, metabolism and nongenomic actions. In: Testosterone, Action, Deficiency, Substitution. Eds E Nieschlag, HM Behre, Springer, Berlin Heidelberg New York, 1998
24. Serrano H, Garcia-Suarez D. Molecular aspects of mammalian fertilization. Asian J Androl 2001;3: 243–9.
25. Sullivan R, Saez F, Girouard J, Frenette G. Role of exosomes in sperm maturation during the transit along the male reproductive tract. Blood Cells Mol Dis. 2005 Jul–Aug;35(1):1–10.

26. Sun F, Ko E, Martin RH. Is there a relationship between sperm chromosome abnormalities and sperm morphology? Reprod Biol Endocrinol. 2006 Jan 25;4:1.
27. Tanaka H, Baba T. Gene expression in spermiogenesis. Cell Mol Life Sci. 2005 Feb;62(3):344–54.
28. Toshimori K. Biology of spermatozoa maturation: an overview with an introduction to this issue. Microsc Res Tech. 2003 May 1;61(1):1–6.
29. Toyama Y, Maekawa M, Yuasa S. Ectoplasmic specializations in the Sertoli cell: new vistas based on genetic defects and testicular toxicology. Anat Sci Int. 2003 Mar;78(1):1–16.
30. Turner RM. Moving to the beat: a review of mammalian sperm motility regulation. Reprod Fertil Dev. 2006;18(1–2):25–38.
31. Wang X, Stocco DM. The decline in testosterone biosynthesis during male aging: a consequence of multiple alterations. Mol Cell Endocrinol. 2005 Jun 30;238(1–2):1–7.
32. Wassarman PM, Jovine L, Qi H, Williams Z, Darie C, Litscher ES. Recent aspects of mammalian fertilization research. Mol Cell Endocrinol. 2005 Apr 29;234(1–2):95–103.
33. Wyborek AJ, Gordon LH, Burkhart JG et al. An evaluation of human sperm as indicators of chemically induced alteration of spermatogenic function. A report of the U.S. Environmental Progection Agency Gene-Tex Program. Mutat Res 1983;115: 73–148.
34. Wyrobek AJ, Schmid TE, Marchetti F. Relative susceptibilities of male germ cells to genetic defects induced by cancer chemotherapies. J Natl Cancer Inst Monogr. 2005;(34):31–5. Review.
35. Zhang D, Gopalakrishnan M. Sperm ion channels: molecular targets for the next generation of contraceptive medicines? J Androl. 2005 Nov–Dec;26(6):643–53.

1.2 Physiology of Erection

1.2.1 Introduction

Erection is defined as "the state of the penis when the erectile tissue becomes filled or swollen (tumid) with blood and causes the penis to become rigid and elevated. It is a complex process involving central nervous system; peripheral nervous systems; hormones; smooth muscles; and vascular functions" (Medline's definition).

Efficient erection is a marker of good health. In a teleological sense, it may be taken as a physical trait which prompts females to mate with individuals that demonstrate efficient erection, assuming they are of superior fitness, which is inherited. Erectile dysfunction, on the other hand, indicates individuals with lower phenotypic qualities (Cellerino and Jannini 2005).

The two paired corpora cavernosa contain the erectile tissue. They are sponge-like, expandable organs that form the greater part of the penis. There crura are fixed to the osseous pelvis near the tuberosity of the os ischium. Towards the tip of the penis the corpora cavernosa are connected to each other, and the septum between them becomes porous. The corpora cavernosa are surrounded by a strong fibrous envelope, the tunica albuginea, which consists of superficial, longitudinal collagen fibres and deep fibres, which are arranged circularly. At the ventral (urethral) and dorsal part of the longitudinal layer there are two thickenings that originate from the insertion of the bulbospongiosus and the ischiocavernosus muscles (Hsu 2006). Blood filling of the corpora cavernosa, the tumescence, leads to an elongation and hardening of the penis. Tumescence and rigidity are clinically classified into five stages, E1–E5, whereby E5 designates full erection sufficient for vaginal penetration.

A similar organ surrounds the urethra, including the glans penis, called corpus spongiosum, which remains softer with blood filling in order to allow the extension of the urethra during ejaculation. The sponge-like tissue contains irregular blood-filled spaces lined by a specified endothelium and separated by connective tissue.

The blood supply of the spaces is ensured by the A. penis profunda. Its branches divide further into small arteries which have two purposes: firstly, arteries breaking up into capillaries supply the connective tissue, and secondly, the helicinal arteries draining directly into the cavernous sinuses. Balancing between these two systems helps to achieve and sustain

1

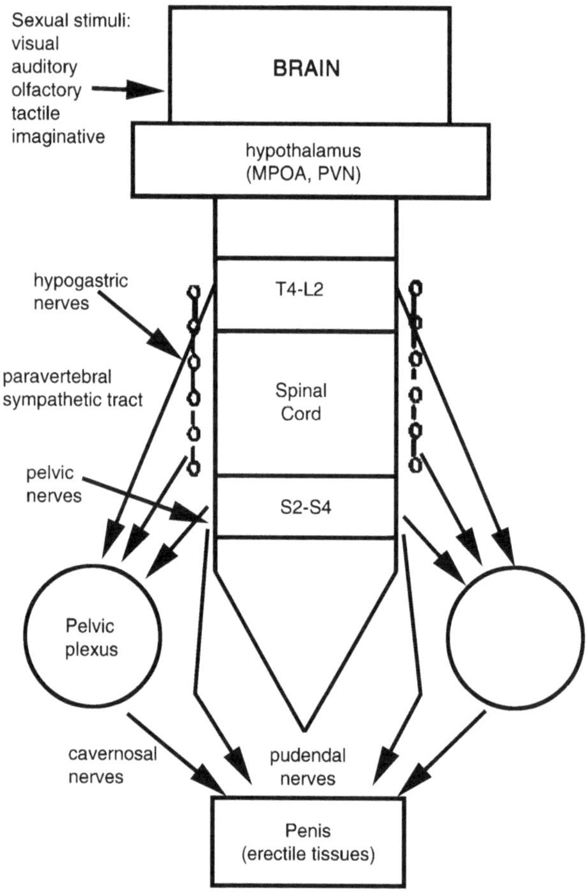

Fig. 1.2.1 The neuroanatomy of the male genital apparatus. Sexual stimuli activate the brain. From there, neuronal impulses travel through the medulla oblongata and the spinal cord to the genital apparatus. This is innervated mainly by pudendal nerves, which originate from the sacral tract and contain afferent sensory and motor pathways, and by the cavernosal nerves, which contain sympathetic and parasympathetic pathways that originate from the pelvic plexuses. The supplying hypogastric nerves originate in the thoraco-lumbar tract and from pelvic nerves which originate in the sacral tract of the spinal cord. *MPOA* medial preoptic area, *PVN* paraventricular nucleus of the hypothalamus. (From Argiolas and Melis 2005)

tumescence. The capillaries are collected into the subalbugineal venular plexus, while the outflow from the cavernous sinuses is collected into venules at the periphery of the corpus cavernosum. The blood can leave the erectile tissue only through a drainage system of veins around the outside wall of the corpus cavernosum. In the flaccid penis, these veins are open, but during erection they are constricted by the expanding spongy tissue.

Also a variety of nerve elements of the sympathic and parasympathetic systems are relevant for erection. An important integration centre is the paraventricular nucleus of the hypothalamus (Fig. 1.2.1). Among others, it contains vasopressin- and oxytocin-producing neurons, which seem to play a key role in sexual behaviour in general. Oxytocinergic neurons project to the spinal cord, being relevant for erection by means of synapses to peripheral nerves. The sum of spinal neurons which control erection, and which also receive sensory information from the genital skin, is called "spinal erection centre" (Guiliano and Rampin 2004).

A number of neurotransmitters and neuropeptides have been shown to stimulate the oxytocinergic neurons in the paraventricular nucleus, among them dopamine, nitric oxide (such as in peripheral erectile tissue), hexarelin peptides, VGF peptides and a cannabinoid antagonist (Fig. 1.2.2). The neurons contain, for example, G-protein-coupled dopamine D2 receptors, which explains the effects of apomorphine in erectile dysfunction. The effect of the cannabinoid antagonist stimulating erection is associated with its effects in pain reception, motor disturbance and temperature regulation. Another group of neurotransmitters and neuropeptides which inhibit the paraventricular oxytocinergic neurons and impair erection are γ-amino-butyric acid (GABA), and opioid peptides, among others. In opioid addicts, the impairment of erectile function is well known. The central role of oxytocinergic neurons is supported by the observation that oxytocin knockout mice mated and copulated normally. There is probably a redundancy of the integrated systems (Giuliano and Rampin 2004).

There are also melanocortin peptides derived from the pro-opiomelanocortin (POMC) active in erection. A melanocortin-receptor agonist, MT-II (which activated four of the five known melanocortin receptors), has been able to induce erectile activity in men with psychogenic or vascular erectile dysfunction. It has been effective in the peripheral erectile tissue, in stimulating the nerve action of the cavernosal smooth muscle, in the spinal level as well as centrally via the neurons of the paraventricular nucleus. It is unknown, however, whether the melanocortin receptors play a physiological role in penile erection (Martin and MacIntyre 2004).

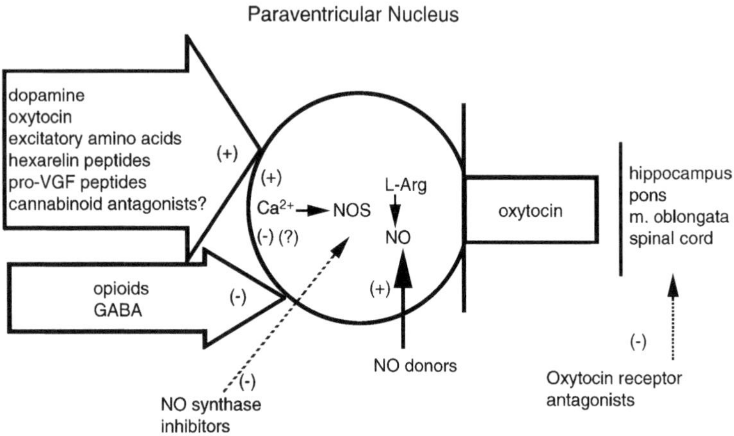

Fig. 1.2.2 Central control of erection: the oxytocinergic neurons of the paraventricular nucleus of the hypothalamus project to the spinal cord. These neurons are activated by dopamine, amino acids, oxytocin itself, hexarelin analogue peptides and pro-VGF-derived peptides, or by the blockade of cannabinoid CB1 receptors, and are inhibited by the opioid and GABAergic receptors. A nitric oxide synthetase takes part in the activation. Activation of the neurons induces erection, and inhibition leads to loss of erection. (From Argiolas and Melis 2005)

The nerve impulses spreading along the systems are usually induced by sexual arousal as a consequence of visual or tactile sexual stimuli. Erection occurs also in other conditions, e.g. there are also sleep-related erections or those induced by drugs. Different neural mechanisms trigger erections on different occasions (Argiolas and Melis 2005). Neurotransmitters and similar agents which are active in the erectile tissue are summarized in Table 1.2.1.

Filling of the cavernous spaces and increase of blood flow depends on cavernous smooth muscle cell relaxation, which is principally regulated by cyclic nucleotide signalling. Firstly, soluble guanyl cyclase is activated by nitric oxide (NO), which is released from the endothelium or nerve endings and enters the muscle cell by diffusion. Other guanyl cyclases located in the membrane are activated by natriuretic peptides. Adenyl cyclases in the cytoplasmic membrane are indirectly activated via a G-protein-coupled receptor, causing augmentation of guanosin triphosphate (GTP) binding to the G protein. As a consequence, the production of cAMP and cGMP increases (Lin et al. 2005). The binding of the cyclic phosphates activates protein kinases, which phosphorylate

Table 1.2.1 Neurotransmitters, neuropeptides and other agents that act on erectile tissues at local level. (Adapted from Argiolas and Melis 2005)

Compound	Effect on cavernosal smooth muscle	Effect on penile vasculature
Noradrenaline	Contraction	Contraction
Acetylcholine	Relaxation	
Nitric oxide	Relaxation	Relaxation
Vasoactive intestinal polypeptide	Relaxation	Relaxation
Neuropeptide Y	Unknown	Contraction
Endothelins	Contraction	Contraction
PGE2, PGF2a, PGD, PGI2, TXA2	Contraction	Unknown
PGE1	Relaxation	Unknown
Phosphodiesterase-V inhibitors	Relaxation	None
Soluble guanylate cyclase activators	Relaxation	Relaxation
RhoA–Rho kinase inhibitors	Relaxation	Relaxation

specific targets, e.g. ion channels. The cGMP-dependent protein kinase activates – besides other ion channels – a high-conductance Ca2+ sensitive K+ channel (Archer 2002). The reduced Ca2+ concentration in the corporal smooth muscle cell produces a decline in myosin light-chain kinase activity, thus decreasing the actin–myosin cross-bridges.

The cAMP signalling pathway includes (and uses or is influenced by) adenosine, calcitonin gene-related peptides, prostaglandins, vasoactive intestinal polypeptide (VIP) and their specific receptors. The cGMP signalling pathway includes natriuretic peptides, NO and the specific receptors. In each episode of nucleotide signalling, the intracellular concentration typically increases two- or threefold over the basal level and then declines rapidly. The decline is due to the hydrolysis of cyclic nucleotides by phosphodiesterases (PDE), of which PDE5 is the principal enzyme in the corpus cavernosum and is specific for cGMP hydrolysis. When the PDE5 is phosphorylated by cGMP, its catalytic activity is increased, and also the non-catalytic sites, which bind cGMP and gain binding activity; thus, the PDE5 control of cGMP is regulated in the sense of a short-loop feedback (Corbin 2004). An inhibition of the PDE5, which is clinically achieved by, for example, sildenafil, decreases the nucleotide hydrolysis and sustains the relaxation of the smooth muscle, resulting in prolonged erection (Lin et al. 2005).

Nitric oxide is synthesized in specialized neurons from L-arginine by means of the NO-synthetase (NOS) and acts as a neurotransmitter in nitroxidergic nerves innervating smooth muscles of the corpus cavernosum. The NO is also produced by sinusoidal endothelial cells, and both the endothelial and the nerval NO induce additionally vasodilation of the penile vessels (Toda et al. 2005). Predominantly the neuronal form of the NOS initiates the erection, whereas the endothelial form helps to maintain it (Burnett and Musicki 2005). Substances which inhibit NO synthesis or enhance its degradation thus impair penile erection.

The NOS isoforms influence the biology of the penis continuously in addition to the intermittent erections. A lack of this continuous tonic activity may also be a cause for priapism, if brief episodes of neurostimulation induce erection in this case. The NO effects in the penis are additionally regulated by a number of factors such as neurotransmitters, hormones, growth factors and cytokines, mediating influences from other parts of the body and of general diseases (Burnett and Musicki 2005).

1.2.2 Role of Androgens in Erection

Androgens are essential for development and function of the corpus cavernosum penis. Testosterone is more active following conversion to 5α-dihydrotestosterone in the erectile tissue. Locally applied 5α-DHT is able to promote penile growths in children with 5α-reductase deficiency (Traish and Kim 2005).

The role of androgens in erectile function of adult men is less clear. Undoubtedly, there are androgen receptors in the corpus cavernosum. A threshold level of testosterone is necessary to enable erections, but higher levels do not improve erectile function. At least in levels below this threshold, erectile function is directly correlated with circulating testosterone levels (Mikhail 2006). Long-lasting severe testosterone deficiency compromises erectile function, but the mechanisms in humans are not fully elucidated.

A direct correlation of normal testosterone levels to the efficacy of treatments for erectile dysfunction, particularly in elderly men, has been proven, however, by some well-conducted studies. In general, the threshold for testosterone levels in order to maintain normal sexual functions appears to be higher in elderly men. In therapeutic failure of PDE5 inhibitors, a restoration of testosterone levels to the normal range is advisable (Gooren and Saad 2006).

Androgens may play a role in maintaining the innervation of erectile tissue. In laboratory animals, the NO synthetase activity in the corpus cavernosum declines after castration. Also in the animal model, androgens were able to upregulate the PDE5 activity, indicating that erection induction, as well as termination, is facilitated when supply of androgens is normal. Also the maintenance of the trabecular architecture of the smooth muscles is androgen dependent, possibly by blocking apoptosis of fibrocytes, which is increased in androgen deficiency. There is also evidence for a role of androgens in the fibroelastic properties of the corpus cavernosum by influencing connective tissue protein synthesis and degradation. A direct comparison of these observations of a severe androgen deficiency, induced by castration in experimental animals, to the gradual decline of androgen levels in different phases of human diseases, however, is not possible (Traish and Kim 2005).

1.2.3 Priapism

Priapism is the persistence of erection in the absence of sexual stimulation. The complete pathophysiology is unclear. Primarily, priapism was associated with venous occlusion (low-flow priapism), such as occurs, for example, in sickle cell disease, as a consequence of the injection of vasoactive drugs, which are associated with neoplastic diseases and haemotological malignancies, but also with traumata. Another form is high-flow priapism, in which arterial overflow is considered to be the pathogen. Priapism may also originate from neurological diseases by disturbance of the neuroregulatory mechanisms responsible for erection. On a molecular level, an altered balance of the interaction between NO-induced relaxation and adrenergic stimulation contraction of smooth muscle is of relevance. This concerns also other local factors which influence the erectile tissue, such as endogenous vasoactive substances (e.g. oxygen supply, endothelial factors), neurotransmitters (e.g. NO, vasoactive intestinal peptide VIP), and metabolic events (e.g. androgenic milieu, abnormal expression of ion channels of the smooth muscle cell, abnormal enzyme activities; Burnett 2003).

References

1. Archer SL. Potassium channels and erectile dysfunction. Vascul Pharmacol. 2002 Jan;38(1):61–71.
2. Argiolas A, Melis MR. Central control of penile erection: role of the paraventricular nucleus of the hypothalamus. Prog Neurobiol. 2005;76(1):1–21.
3. Burnett AL. Priapism pathophysiology: clues to prevention. Int J Impot Res. 2003 Oct;15 Suppl 5:S80–5.
4. Burnett AL, Musicki B. The nitric oxide signaling pathway in the penis. Curr Pharm Des. 2005;11(31):3987–94.
5. Cellerino A, Jannini EA. Why humans need type 5 phosphodiesterase inhibitors. Int J Androl. 2005;28 Suppl 2:14–7.
6. Corbin JD. Mechanisms of action of PDE5 inhibition in erectile dysfunction. Int J Impot Res. 2004 Jun;16 Suppl 1:S4–7.
7. Giuliano F, Rampin O. Neural control of erection. Physiol Behav. 2004 Nov 15;83(2):189–201.
8. Gooren LJ, Saad F. Recent insights into androgen action on the anatomical and physiological substrate of penile erection. Asian J Androl. 2006 Jan;8(1):3–9.
9. Hsu GL. Hypothesis of human penile anatomy, erection hemodynamics and their clinical applications. Asian J Androl. 2006 Mar;8(2):225–34.
10. Lin CS, Lin G, Lue TF. Cyclic nucleotide signaling in cavernous smooth muscle. J Sex Med. 2005;2(4):478–91.
11. Martin WJ, MacIntyre DE. Melanocortin receptors and erectile function. Eur Urol. 2004 Jun;45(6):706–13.
12. Mikhail N. Does testosterone have a role in erectile function? Am J Med. 2006 May;119(5):373–82.
13. Toda N, Ayajiki K, Okamura T. Nitric oxide and penile erectile function. Pharmacol Ther. 2005 May;106(2):233–66.
14. Traish A, Kim N. The physiological role of androgens in penile erection: regulation of corpus cavernosum structure and function. J Sex Med. 2005 Nov;2(6):759–70.

1.3 Physiology of Ejaculation

Ejaculation is "the emission of semen to the exterior, resulting from the contraction of muscles surrounding the male internal urogenital ducts" (Medline's definition). It is closely connected to the male orgasm. Sexual behaviour has components of rewarding behaviour, and ejaculation appears to be the most reinforcing component. Little is known about the neurochemical basis of this rewarding experience. Some relations to opioids and their receptors have been shown (Coolen et al. 2004).

Ejaculation consists of two phases. In the initial phase, emission, smooth muscles of the vas deferens, the seminal vesicles and the prostate, as well as their secretions, are involved. At the end, the mixture of spermatozoa from the epididymis and the vas deferens with the secretions of the seminal vesicles, forming about 50% of the ejaculate, and the prostate, which secretes nearly the other half of the semen, is made available in the prostatic (posterior) urethra. The sperm progression in the seminal tract during ejaculation, and the contractions of the epididymis, is supported by oxytocin, a potent stimulator of epididymis contractility. It also induces the release of another potent stimulator of epididymal contractility, endothelin-1 (Filippi et al. 2003).

The neural regulation of this process is guided by sympathic and parasympathetic nerves. The neurons of the sympathic nerves involved are located in the intermediolateral cell columns and the central grey of the spinal cord from T12 to L2, the fibres are part of the hypogastric nerves. In paraplegic men, stimulation of superior hypogastric plexus causes seminal emission. As transmitters, norepinephrine, acetylcholine, vasoactive intestinal peptide (VIP) and NO have been identified (Giuliano and Clement 2005). The parasympathis neurons are located in the sacral portion of the intermediolateral cell columns (sacral parasympathetic nucleus). The emission process is influenced by central mechanisms via sensory stimuli from the genital skin and from visual stimuli of the central mechanisms (Giuliano and Clement 2005).

The emission is inevitably followed by the second phase of the ejaculation, in which the ejaculate is expulsed through the external urethra, performed by a rhythmic contraction of striated perineal muscles. Although the bulbocavernosus and ischiocavernosus are striated muscles, their neurons share some similarities with autonomic muscles. They exhibit susceptibility to autonomic motor neuron disorders, they depend trophically on the presence of testosterone, and their dendritic arbors may cross the midline. Many spinal interneurons have been identified, which participate in the reflex activation of these motoneurons (Johnson 2006).

The second phase is considered to be a spinal cord reflex. The spinal ejaculation centre, which is located in the lumbar part of the spinal cord, is the commander of the peripheral organs involved in ejaculation and probably also integrates the sexual inputs during sexual activity. During this process, smooth muscle of the bladder neck contract in order to inhibit seminal reflux into the bladder, and the bulbospongiosus and ischiocavernosus muscles display the rhythmic contractions. The origin of the rhythmic contraction of the pelvic floor muscles is still unclear (Giuliano and Clement 2005).

The spinal circuits regulating ejaculation involve both the parasympathetic and sympathetic autonomic motor nerve system, the somatic motor system and afferent fibres of the visceral, somatic and mucocutaneous nerve fibres. Penile mechanoreceptors respond to vibratory and tangential surface tactile stimulation, to increased blood flow in the erectile tissue and stretching of the internal corpora cavernosa, and they increase their sensitivity during ongoing erection. The penile sensory nerves are essential for ejaculation (Giuliano and Clement 2005).

The neuroanatomical organization of the circuitry of ejaculation is described by afferent and efferent neural structures. The nerves triggering this process contain sympathetic and parasympathetic fibres. The coordinating neural centres are located in the dorsomedial and dorsolateral motor nuclei of the ventral horn of sacral segments. Sensory stimuli are guided via n. pudendus into the upper sacral and lower lumbar segments of the spinal cord. Spinal neurons, which receive sensory input from the penis, are located throughout T12 to S1. A second afferent pathway is represented by sensory fibres along the hypogastric nerves entering the spinal cord via thoracolumbar roots. The cell bodies of the efferent preganglionic nerves are located in thoracolumbar segments of the spinal cord, and the postganglionic cells are located in the pelvic plexus (Fig. 1.3.1)

Impulses from the spinal cord centre are additionally coordinated by supraspinal sites. Several supraspinal regions are involved in the control of spinal centres for ejaculation by direct axonal projections. The neurons are mainly oxytoninergic and project to the spinal cord. Oxytocin is also liberated from the neural tissue, because after ejaculation the oxytocin levels are elevated.

The anatomical sites of the supraspinal regions are the medial preoptic area of the hypothalamus, which is of pivotal importance, the paraventricular nucleus and the nucleus paragigantocellularis in the medullary reticular formation. By use of positron emission tomography (PET) the strongest activation has been shown to occur in the mesodiencephalic

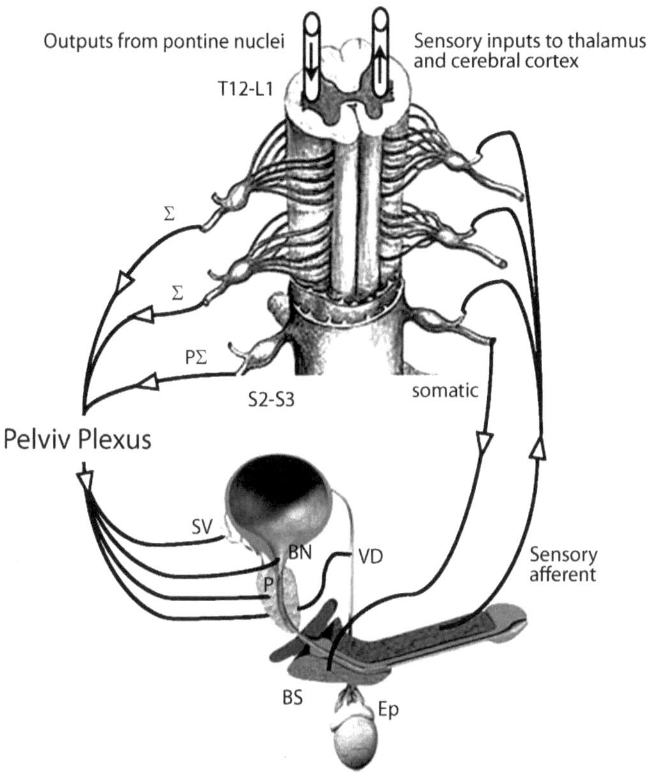

Fig. 1.3.1 Neural pathways controlling ejaculation. Sympathetic (Σ), parasympathetic (*P*Σ) and somatic nerves from lumbosacral spinal nuclei command anatomical structures responsible for ejaculation. Sensory afferent fibres from the genital areas are integrated at the spinal and brain level. *BN* bladder neck, *BS* bulbospongious muscle, *Ep* epididymis, *P* prostate, *SV* seminal vesicle, *VD* vas deferens. (From Giuliano and Clement 2005)

transition zone. The PET has also shown that mainly the ventral tegmental area and the cerebellum seem to be activated during ejaculation, whereas the amygdala region is deactivated (Holstege 2005).

Recently, a group of neurons in the lumbar spinal cord originating in the thalamus (LSt cells) were demonstrated to be an integral part of the spinal ejaculation generator. Lesions of LSt cells completely inhibited ejaculation. The LSt cells were found to be activated following ejaculation, but not following other components of sexual behaviour (Allard et al. 2005).

Signals to the central structures induce the psychological feelings of orgasm. The anatomical structures are found in cortico-limbic centres. In the opposite direction, these centres also control the tone of the spinal ejaculation generator (Allard et al. 2005).

Anatomically, the sites commanding erection and ejaculation are close in proximity. In the experimental animals, using the Fos expression, it was demonstrated that specific sub-divisions of the neural regions were activated with respect to different elements of sexual behaviour.

Interneuronal connection of these systems is realized mainly via serotoninergic pathways. Serotonin generally is inhibitory to ejaculation, explaining the clinical effect of selective serotonin reuptake inhibitors (SSRI) in patients with premature ejaculation. Other neurons use GABA as a neurotransmitter; thus, the inhibition of ejaculation by baclofen may be explainable (Giuliano and Clement 2005).

References

1. Allard J, Truitt WA, McKenna KE, Coolen LM. Spinal cord control of ejaculation. World J Urol. 2005 Jun;23(2):119–26.
2. Coolen LM, Allard J, Truitt WA, McKenna KE. Central regulation of ejaculation. Physiol Behav. 2004 Nov 15;83(2):203–15.
3. Filippi S, Vignozzi L, Vannelli GB, Ledda F, Forti G, Maggi M. Role of oxytocin in the ejaculatory process. J Endocrinol Invest. 2003;26(3 Suppl):82–6.
4. Giuliano F, Clement P. Physiology of ejaculation: emphasis on serotonergic control. Eur Urol. 2005 Sep;48(3):408–17.
5. Holstege G. Central nervous system control of ejaculation. World J Urol. 2005 Jun;23(2):109–14.
6. Johnson RD. Descending pathways modulating the spinal circuitry for ejaculation: effects of chronic spinal cord injury. Prog Brain Res. 2006;152:415–26.

2 Drugs Which Compromise Male Sexual Health

A great many drugs affect male sexual functions. The standard textbook of clinical pharmacology, Goodman and Gilman's *The Pharmacological Basis of Therapeutics*, in its first edition, defines a drug as follows: "A drug may be broadly defined as any chemical agent which affects living protoplasm, and few substances would escape inclusion by this definition". In this sense, the definition includes not only drugs used in the treatment of diseases, but also lifestyle drugs and environmental toxins.

Herein, primarily those drugs intended for other diseases, which happen to exert adverse effects on sexual functions, are reviewed. In general, there are sufficient data of pharmacodynamics for most drugs used in medicine, including the concentration at the site and the organ of the adverse effects, and of pharmacokinetics, including the metabolism and possibly effective metabolites, to explain their effects on a cellular and molecular level; however, there are a number of drugs intended for the treatment of sexual dysfunction. For example, drugs which improve erection have been designed to improve sexual health, which is not a severe or life-threatening condition, and treated patients are often otherwise healthy persons. In these drugs, the absence of severe adverse effects, which would compromise their effectiveness, is essential. An exclusion of risks originating also from dose-regimen errors is mandatory for security reasons; thus, also these adverse effects are to be included in the list of drugs which compromise male sexual health.

2.1 Adverse Drug Effects

Adverse drug effects are often detected in phase-II and phase-III studies, and they are frequently explainable from the mode of action of the drug tested. In addition, there are "idiosyncratic" adverse reactions, which may not be deduced from the pharmacological effects of the drug. The incidence may be below 1 in 1000, and these effects will not be detected in phase-II and phase-III studies. The population at risk may not be distributed evenly across the general population, e.g. because of genetic heterogeneity (Goodman Gilman 2005). The spontaneous reporting of adverse reactions is thus an effective way to shed light on potential adverse reactions. Most national and supranational authorities in the Western world have introduced a reporting system for adverse drug events.

In general, there are sufficient data of pharmacodynamics for most drugs used in medicine, including the concentration at the site and the organ, of the adverse effects, and of pharmacokinetics, including the metabolism and possibly effective metabolites, to explain their effects on a cellular and molecular level. In these drugs, an explanation of the adverse effects at these levels is often possible. A number of these adverse effects will also be detected in phase-II and phase-III studies.

In addition, however, there are "idiosyncratic" adverse reactions, which may not be deduced from the pharmacological effects of the drug. The incidence may be less than 1 in 1000, and these effects will not be detected in phase-II and phase-III studies. The population at risk may not be distributed evenly across the general population, e.g. because of genetic heterogeneity (Goodman and Gilman 2005). The spontaneous reporting of adverse reactions is thus an effective way to shed light on potential adverse reactions. Most national and supranational authorities in the Western world have introduced a reporting system for adverse drug events (ADEs).

Adverse drug events are the most frequent type of iatrogenic disease. Patient's age, gender, number of drugs, as well as co-morbidity influence the incidence of ADEs. The absolute number of adverse events and their relation to the amount of drugs applied, however, differs with respect to quantify. For example, it has been estimated that 3–5% of all hospitalizations (or perhaps more) are a consequence of adverse drug reactions, and a patient hospitalized for internal diseases has a chance of 30% to experience and adverse drug reaction. Although some ADEs are the result of medication errors, most ADEs result from drugs which were correctly prescribed and applied (Scott-Evans et al. 2005; Goodman and Gilman 2005).

According to a survey published in the "Journal of American Pharmacists' Association" in 2001, the cost of detected drug-related morbidity and mortality in the United States exceeded US$177 billion in 2000, with hospital admissions accounting for about 70% of total costs. Since 1995, the costs associated with drug-related problems have more than doubled (WHO 2002). A 2004 study in the United Kingdom carried out a prospective analysis of 18,820 patients admitted into hospital over 6 months to assess the cause of admission. There were 1225 admissions related to an ADE, giving a prevalence of 6.5%, with the ADE directly leading to admission in 80% of cases. The projected annual cost of such admissions to the National Health Service was £466 million (US$847 million, €666 million; Pirmohamed et al. 2004).

For all medicines there is a trade-off between the benefits and the potential for harm. The harm can be minimized by ensuring that medicines of good quality, safety and efficacy be prescribed and used rationally. Pharmacovigilance is the science and activities relating to the detection, assessment, understanding and prevention of adverse effects or any other drug-related problems (WHO 2002).

As a measure of ADE severity, it has become increasingly relevant to consider alterations of the subjective quality of life of patients in the treatment of diseases, in addition to the healing or improvement of the medical aspects. From a disease perspective, quality of life has been said to refer to social, emotional and physical well-being of patients following treatment. Also pharmaceutical companies follow this trend and collect information on possible changes of quality of life in order to assess the properties and compatibility of their products. The measurement of quality of life needs elaborated instruments. A standardized questionnaire for the rating of quality of life in different diseases was elaborated by the WHO (Angermeyer et al. 2000; Bowling 2001).

The ADEs are considered in nearly all publications on new drugs and in all textbooks of pharmacology. There is also a standard textbook, *Meyler's Side Effects of Drugs*, which is updated every year (Dukes et al. 1996), available online since 2006. It summarizes the untoward effects observed in any applied drugs. There are a number of websites for information on adverse drug reactions, drug interactions, drug toxicity, special risk situations and pharmacological or patient-dependent factors associated with the occurrence of side effects. The most extensive database is SEDBASE. It is a full-text database that critically analyzes the published drug-side-effect literature on drugs currently in use. Permanent renewal of the database is performed by recognized authorities. Each year approximately 9000 articles on adverse drug reactions are published in the scientific literature. The database is organized by drug-class chapters and does not contain any speculative or unsubstantiated statements.

http://library.dialog.com/bluesheets/html/bl0070.html-The access carries a fee (cost per dial unit: $8.40, cost per minute: $1.40).

http://www.rxlist.com/: Profiles of particular drugs are available. Each entry contains a chapter "Side Effects", which summarizes very briefly (about one page of text) the most important ADEs.

www.drugdigest.org; www.drugs.com: On these sites, non-professional users may look for adverse effects of particular drugs.

http://www.akdae.de/ (Arzneimittelkommission der Deutschen Ärzteschaft). Access to particular drug adverse effects also exists in German.

References

1. Angermeyer MC, Kilian R, Matschinger H. WHO-QOL – 100 und WHOQOL – BREF: Handbuch für die deutschsprachige Version der WHO-Instrumente zur Erfassung von Lebensqualität . Göttingen, Hogrefe, 2000
2. Bowling A. Measuring disease, 2nd Ed., Open University Press, Buckingham, Philadelphia, 2001
3. Dukes MNG et al. (Eds) Meyler's side effects of drugs, 13th Ed. Elsevier, Amsterdam, 1996
4. Goodman LS, Gilman A. The pharmacological basis of therapeutics, 11th Ed. Laurence L. Brunton, New York u.a.: McGraw-Hill, 2006, p. 61
5. Pirmohamed M, James S, Meakin S, Green C, Scott AK, Walley TJ, Farrar K, Park BK, Breckenridge AM. Adverse drug reactions as cause of admission to hospital: prospective analysis of 18,820 patients. Br Med J. 2004 Jul 3;329(7456):15–9.
6. Scott-Evans R, Lloyd JF, Stoddard GJ, Nebeker JR, Samore MH. Risk factors for adverse drug events: a 10-year analysis. Ann Pharmacother 2005;39.
7. WHO (2002) The importance of pharmacovigilance, WHO, Geneva; http://www.who.int/mediacentre/factsheets/fs293/en/index.html

2.2 Male Sexual Health and Drugs

The descriptions of the effects of ADEs on male sexual function are generally scarce and restricted to few topics. Any intervention which influences the sexual hormone system obviously also influences male sexual functions, e.g. antiandrogenic compounds, which depress sexual libido and other sexual functions. In some circumstances, it may be questionable as to whether the effect of a drug on male sexual functions is a desired therapeutic effect, or whether it is an untoward effect. For example, the depression of pituitary hormone secretion by the gonadotropin-releasing hormone (GnRH) analogues in the treatment of prostate carcinoma is important in order to achieve androgen deprivation and prolong the remission of the disease. On the other hand, the depression of gonadotropin secretion in these men by GnRH leads to impotence and infertility, which is definitely an untoward effect.

Some sexual ADEs which occur during treatment of other diseases are broadly recognized, e.g. erectile dysfunction as an ADE of β-blockers, which seems to be an unavoidable consequence of treating hypertension. It appears to be well explainable from the pathophysiology, although the clinical database is not so clear, as suggested in lay media. Other ADEs mentioned in the literature become clear only with expanded insight into the pharmacodynamics of the drug concerned, e.g. the unexpected antiandrogenic effect of ketoconazole, an antifungal drug.

The ADEs on sexual functions are usually mild or moderate. They rarely prompt hospital admissions, which are classified as resulting from severe ADEs. This fact may explain why standard textbooks of pharmacology note sexual side effects of drugs only marginally. Entries of the 11th edition (2005) of standard textbook *Goodman & Gilman's Pharmacological Basis of Therapeutics* can be quoted as examples of the unsatisfactory consequences of sexual side effects. Concerning the interaction of β-receptor antagonists with erectile function, which is considered an important cause of sexual dysfunction in elderly men, the textbook contains only two sentences: "The incidence of sexual dysfunction in men with hypertension who are treated with β-adrenoreceptor antagonists is not clearly defined. Although experience with the use of β-adrenoreceptor antagonists in pregnancy is increasing, information about the safety of those drugs during pregnancy is still limited [Widerhorn et al., 1987]". Specific serotonin reuptake inhibitors (SSRI), which delay ejaculation as an important sexual side effect, and thus are also used in the treatment of premature ejaculation, are considered also with only one sentence: "The SSRIs, as a group, have a high risk of nausea and vomiting, headache, and sexual dysfunction, including inhibited ejaculation in men and impaired orgasm in women." The chapter "Contraceptives" contains only 15 lines on the topic "Contraception, male". In the index, the entry "sexual function" is associated with the sub-entries "β-adrenoreceptor blockers, amylnitrite, androgens, antidepressants, antipsychotics, clonidine, cocaine, ethanol, guanandrel, PDE 5-inhibitors, phenoxylamin, phentolamin, prostaglandin, yohimbine". The entry "impotence" is associated with the sub-entries "β-adrenoreceptor blockers, alprostadil, ethanol, phentoalmin, PDE 5-inhibitors, prolactin, 5-α-reductase inhibitors, thiazide, yohimbine". The entries "sperm" or "spermatogenesis" are not included.

The standard textbook of drug side effects, *Meyler's side effects of drugs*, in its 13th edition, contains a list of side effects on organs and systems, which includes "sexual functions" but not "fertility" (Dukes et al. 1996).

Although ADEs on sexual functions undoubtedly may impair the quality of life, it becomes evident that sexuality is among the less important spheres of quality of life. In a survey, all people interviewed (men, women, young people, elderly people) placed sexual life at position 25 of 25 life spheres concerning importance (Angermeyer et al. 2000).

Only a small number of drugs have been developed to improve male sexual health up to now, e.g. phosphodiesterase-5 inhibitors, in order to treat insufficient erectile function. These drugs compromise male sexual health owing to their adverse effects in other organ systems. As an example, the reports in the international press on heart attacks in patients using Viagra may be considered, which prompted many impotent patients to abstain from this drug. Today we know that Viagra, on the contrary, exerts favourable effects in coronary heart disease and pulmonary hypertension.

The description of sexual side effects of specific drugs, however, does not allow definitive statements on the cause of sexual dysfunction by drugs in a individual patient. There are only a few published articles which report the incidence of drug use in patients with sexual dysfunction. They describe the frequency with which men with erectile dysfunction use a drug and the extent of sexual dysfunction. The Massachusetts Male Aging Study conducted by the New England Research Institute identified a number of drugs used in ageing men for different purposes, which was associated with sexual dysfunction, but the question remained unanswered as to whether these associations are independent of the underlying health conditions (Derby et al. 2001). The answer to this question is complex and may be facilitated by a comprehensive database on sexual side effects of distinct drugs.

References

1. Angermeyer MC, Kilian R, Matschinger H. WHOQOL – 100 und WHOQOL – BREF: Handbuch für die deutschsprachige Version der WHO-Instrumente zur Erfassung von Lebensqualität . Göttingen, Hogrefe, 2000
2. Dukes MNG et al. (Eds) Meyler's side effects of drugs, 13th Ed. Elsevier, Amsterdam, 1996
3. Derby CA, Barbour MM, Hume AL, McKinlay JB. Drug therapy and prevalence of erectile dysfunction in the Massachusetts Male Aging Study cohort. Pharmacotherapy. 2001 Jun;21(6):676–83.
4. Goodman and Gilman. The pharmacological basis of therapeutics, 11th Ed. Laurence L. Brunton, New York u.a.: McGraw-Hill, 2006

2.3 Drugs Which Compromise Testicular Function

A02 Drugs for Acid-Related Disorders

Cimetidine is effective on Ca2+ influx into sperm cells in vitro. In vivo, it exerts an antiandrogenic effect. During treatment of peptic ulcer and in healthy men, testosterone levels decreased, gonadotropin levels increased and sperm count decreased in a considerable number of men. In contrast, ranitidine, famotidine, pantoprazole and lansoprazole did not demonstrate this effect.

Overall level of evidence of adverse effects: B

Compound	Drugs for peptic ulcer and gastro-oesophageal reflux disease (A02B)
Disease treated	Gastrointestinal complaints
Quantification of adverse effects	Semen
No. of patients treated	92; 73
Age group	34.4 (mean)
Treatment period	Various
Dose	Various
Treatment consequences	Prevalence of oligozoospermia as compared with healthy men
Efficacy	OR 6.2 (95% CI 1.4–26.8)
Randomization of patients	No
Study quality	**2–**
Reference	2177: Wong WY, Zielhuis GA, Thomas CM, Merkus HM, Steegers-Theunissen RP. New evidence of the influence of exogenous and endogenous factors on sperm count in man. Eur J Obstet Gynecol Reprod Biol. 2003 Sep 10;110(1):49–54.
Language	English

Compound	Histamin-2 receptor antagonists (A02BA)
Disease treated	Spermatozoa in vitro
Quantification of adverse effects	Ca2+ influx

Age group	Young
Treatment period	In vitro
Treatment consequences	Sperm cells, rise of Ca2+
Efficacy	Faster with addition of H2 receptor antagonists
Study quality	**2+**
Reference	803: Gupta A, Gupta S, Tiwary AK. Spermicidal efficacy of H2-receptor antagonists and potentiation with 2′, 4′-dichlorobenzamil hydrochloride: role of intrasperm $Ca2^{+}$. Contraception. 2003 Jul;68(1):61–4.
Language	English

Compound	Cimetidine (A02BA01)
Disease treated	Healthy
Quantification of adverse effects	Sperm count, hormones
No. of patients treated	7
Age group	Young
Treatment period	9 weeks
Dose	1200 mg/day
Treatment consequences	Sperm count, decrease; testosterone level, decrease
Efficacy	By 43%
Randomization of patients	No
Study quality	**3**
Reference	804: Van Thiel DH, Gavaler JS, Smith WI Jr, Paul G. Hypothalamic–pituitary–gonadal dysfunction in men using cimetidine. N Engl J Med. 1979 May 3;300(18):1012–5.
Language	English

Compound	Cimetidine (A02BA01)
Disease treated	Peptic ulcer
Quantification of adverse effects	Hormones
No. of patients treated	n.g.
Age group	Young
Treatment period	6 months
Dose	400 mg/days
Treatment consequences	Gonadotropin levels, increase
Efficacy	Significant

Randomization of patients	No
Study quality	**3**
Reference	889: Knigge U, Dejgaard A, Wollesen F, Ingerslev O, Bennett P, Christiansen PM. The acute and long term effect of the H2-receptor antagonists cimetidine and ranitidine on the pituitary–gonadal axis in men. Clin Endocrinol (Oxf). 1983 Mar;18(3):307–13.
Language	English

Compound	Ranitidine (A02BA02)
Disease treated	Peptic ulcer
Quantification of adverse effects	Semen, hormones
No. of patients treated	20
Age group	Young
Treatment period	3 months
Dose	300 mg/days
Treatment consequences	Sperm parameters, gonadotropin levels, testosterone level, alteration
Efficacy	No difference between exposed and control men
Randomization of patients	No
Dose arms 1–3	Ranitidine; placebo
Study quality	**2–**
Reference	888: Wang C, Wong KL, Lam KC, Lai CL. Ranitidine does not affect gonadal function in man. Br J Clin Pharmacol. 1983 Oct;16(4):430–2.
Language	English

Compound	Famotidine (A02BA03)
Disease treated	Peptic ulcer
Quantification of adverse effects	Semen
No. of patients treated	8
Age group	Young
Treatment period	4 weeks
Dose	40 mg
Treatment consequences	Sperm parameters, impairment
Efficacy	None

2

Randomization of patients	No
Study quality	**3**
Reference	369: Savarino V, Giusti M, Scalabrini P, Bessarione D, Magnolia MR, Percario G, Celle G. Famotidine has no significant effect on gonadal function in man. Gastroenterol Clin Biol. 1988 Jan;12(1):19–22.
Language	English

Compound	Omeprazole (A02BC01)
Disease treated	Gastric hypersecretion
Quantification of adverse effects	Clinical reports
No. of patients treated	30
Age group	52 (mean)
Treatment period	>8 months
Dose	20–40 mg/days
Treatment consequences	Notifications of problems with male reproductive system
Efficacy	Impotence 15 men; gynaecomastia 15 men
Randomization of patients	No
Study quality	**3**
Reference	2143: Lindquist M, Edwards IR. Endocrine adverse effects of omeprazole. Br Med J. 1992 Aug 22;305(6851):451–2
Language	English

Compound	Pantoprazole (A02BC02)
Disease treated	Healthy
Quantification of adverse effects	Hormones
No. of patients treated	12
Age group	Young
Treatment period	2 weeks
Dose	40 mg/days
Treatment consequences	Testosterone level and response to hCG, alteration
Efficacy	No difference between groups
Randomization of patients	Yes
Dose arms 1–3	Pantoprazole; placebo
Study quality	**1–**

Reference	872: Dammann HG, Bethke T, Burkhardt F, Wolf N, Khalil H, Luehmann R. Effects of pantoprazole on endocrine function in healthy male volunteers. Aliment Pharmacol Ther. 1994 Oct;8(5):549–54.
Language	English

Compound	Lansoprazole (A02BC03)
Disease treated	Healthy
Quantification of adverse effects	Hormones
No. of patients treated	11
Age group	Young
Treatment period	3 weeks
Dose	30 mg/day
Treatment consequences	LH pulsatility, alteration
Efficacy	No difference between groups
Randomization of patients	Yes
Dose arms 1–3	Lansoprazole; placebo
Study quality	**1–**
Reference	870: Adler ID, Schmid TE, Baumgartner A. Induction of aneuploidy in male mouse germ cells detected by the sperm-FISH assay: a review of the present database. Mutat Res. 2002 Jul 25;504(1–2):173–82.
Language	English

A03 Drugs for Functional Gastrointestinal Disorders

There are a number of older, non-randomized studies on the gonadal effects of metoclopramide. A decrease of testosterone levels, an improvement of sperm morphology and an enhanced response of prolactin secretion to metoclopramide have been described. In summary, effects of metoclopramide on testicular function are questionable.

Overall level of evidence of adverse effects: C

Compound	Metoclopramide (A03FA01)
Disease treated	Healthy
Quantification of adverse effects	Sperm parameters, hormones
No. of patients treated	24

Age group	Young
Treatment period	7 weeks
Dose	10 mg/4 times/day
Treatment consequences	Sperm parameters, alteration
Efficacy	No alteration
Randomization of patients	Yes
Dose arms 1–3	Metoclopramide; placebo
Study quality	**1–**
Reference	786: Graf KJ, Schmidt-Gollwitzer M, Horowski R, Dorow R. Effect of metoclopramide and lisuride on hypophyseal and gonadal function in men. Clin Endocrinol (Oxf). 1982 Sep;17(3):243–51.
Language	English

Compound	Metoclopramide (A03FA01)
Disease treated	Infertility
Quantification of dysfunction	Sperm parameters
No. of patients treated	20
Age group	Young
Treatment period	16 weeks
Dose	10 mg/days
Treatment consequences	Sperm morphology, improvement
Efficacy	Abnormal sperm from 66.75 to 24.7% (prolactin) and 31% (metoclopramide)
Randomization of patients	No
Dose arms 1–3	Metoclopramide, prolactin
Study quality	**2–**
Reference	849: Ufearo CS, Orisakwe OE. Restoration of normal sperm characteristics in hypoprolactinemic infertile men treated with metoclopramide and exogenous human prolactin. Clin Pharmacol Ther. 1995 Sep;58(3):354–9.
Language	English

Compound	Metoclopramide (A03FA01)
Disease treated	Infertility
Quantification of dysfunction	Hormones

No. of patients treated	17
Age group	Young
Treatment period	Single dose
Dose	10 mg
Treatment consequences	Prolactin response to metoclopramide
Efficacy	Enhanced in low sperm count
Randomization of patients	No
Study quality	**3**
Reference	852: Spitz IM, Halperin Y, Zylber-Haran E, Shilo S, Leroith D, Liel Y, Livshin J, Laufer N, Schenker J. Prolactin response to metoclopramide and chlorpromazine in primary testicular failure and isolated gonadotrophin deficiency. Clin Endocrinol (Oxf). 1981 Apr;14(4):375–80.
Language	English

Compound	Metoclopramide (A03FA01)
Disease treated	Infertility
Quantification of dysfunction	Hormones
No. of patients treated	13
Age group	21–34 years
Treatment period	Single dose
Dose	10 mg
Treatment consequences	Prolactin response to metoclopramide
Efficacy	Enhanced in low sperm count
Randomization of patients	No
Study quality	**2–**
Reference	851: Baranowska B, Jeske W, Niewiadomska A, Rozbicka G, Walczak L, Zgliczynski S. Enhanced serum prolactin concentration after metoclopramide stimulation in idiopathic oligozoospermia and azoospermia. Andrologia. 1983;15 Spec No:554–9.
Language	English

Compound	Metoclopramide (A03FA01)
Disease treated	Healthy
Quantification of adverse effects	Sperm count

2

No. of patients treated	9
Age group	Young
Treatment period	4 weeks
Dose	10 mg/days
Treatment consequences	Sperm count and prolactin levels, increase
Efficacy	Twofold
Randomization of patients	No
Study quality	**3**
Reference	787: Jecht E, Kleissl HP, Pache U. Short-term increase of sperm output under metoclopramide administration. Int J Androl. 1981 Feb;4(1):49–54.
Language	English

Compound	Metoclopramide (A03FA01)+baclofen
Disease treated	Healthy
Quantification of adverse effects	Hormones
No. of patients treated	6
Age group	Young
Treatment period	Single dose
Dose	10 mg
Treatment consequences	GnRH-induced LH release
Efficacy	Blunted in the baclofen group
Randomization of patients	Subsequent treatment
Study quality	**2–**
Reference	850: Elias AN, Szekeres AV, Stone S, Valenta LJ, Haw T, Ascher MS. GABA-ergic and dopaminergic mechanisms in gonadotrophin secretion in males: effects of baclofen and metoclopramide. Acta Endocrinol (Copenh). 1983 Aug;103(4):451–6.
Language	English

Compound	Metoclopramide (A03FA01)
Disease treated	Healthy
Quantification of adverse effects	Sperm parameters
No. of patients treated	5

Age group	Young
Treatment period	4 weeks
Dose	10 mg
Treatment consequences	Sperm count, seminal volume decrease
Efficacy	In all participants
Randomization of patients	No
Study quality	**3**
Reference	788: Falaschi P, Frajese G, Sciarra F, Rocco A, Conti C. Influence of hyperprolactinaemia due to metoclopramide on gonadal function in men. Clin Endocrinol (Oxf). 1978 May;8(5):427–33.
Language	English

Compound	Metoclopramide (A03FA01)
Disease treated	Healthy
Quantification of adverse effects	Hormones
No. of patients treated	n.g.
Age group	Young
Treatment period	3 days
Dose	10 mg/day
Treatment consequences	Testosterone level and response to hCG, decrease
Efficacy	Significant
Randomization of patients	No
Study quality	**3**
Reference	896: Nakagawa K, Obara T, Matsubara M, Kubo M. Relationship of changes in serum concentrations of prolactin and testosterone during dopaminergic modulation in males. Clin Endocrinol (Oxf). 1982 Oct;17(4):345–52.
Language	English

A07 Antidiarrheals, Intestinal Antiinflammatory/Antiinfective Agents

Following the first report by Levi et al. (1979) on oligozoospermia during treatment with sulfosalazine, and the recovery after cessation treatment, a number of studies stated limited or no impairment of spermatogenesis in treated men, while 5-amino salicylic acid was suggested to lack this effect completely. There are, however, no RCTs which demonstrate this effect without doubt. An interesting explanation of the contrasting results was given by Niederberger (2002), who suggested that the deleterious effect of sulphasalazine might take place only after ejaculation and result in asthenozoospermia.

Overall level of evidence of adverse effects: C

Compound	Sulphasalazine (A07EC01)
Disease treated	Inflammatory bowel disease
Quantification of adverse effects	Semen
No. of patients treated	28
Age group	Young
Treatment period	1 month
Dose	2–4 g/day
Treatment consequences	Sperm parameters, impairment
Efficacy	Abnormalities in 18 of 28 patients. Improvement after discontinuation, ten pregnancies reported
Randomization of patients	No
Dose arms 1–3	Sulphasalazine
Study quality	**3**
Reference	2141: Toovey S, Hudson E, Hendry WF, Levi AJ. Sulphasalazine and male infertility: reversibility and possible mechanism. Gut. 1981 Jun;22(6):445–51
Language	English

Compound	Sulphasalazine (A07EC01)
Disease treated	Inflammatory bowel disease
Quantification of adverse effects	Semen
No. of patients treated	27

Age group	Young
Treatment period	Continuous
Dose	n.g.
Treatment consequences	Spermatogenesis, impairment
Efficacy	Few patients
Randomization of patients	No
Dose arms 1–3	Sulphasalazine; sulphasalazine+cortisone; untreated
Study quality	**2–**
Reference	533: Karbach U, Ewe K, Schramm P. Quality of semen in patients with Crohn's disease. Z Gastroenterol. 1982 Jun;20(6):314–20.
Language	German

Compound	Sulphasalazine (A07EC01)
Disease treated	Inflammatory bowel disease
Quantification of adverse effects	Semen
No. of patients treated	17
Age group	Young
Treatment period	Continuous
Dose	n.g.
Treatment consequences	Spermatogenesis, impairment
Efficacy	In most men
Randomization of patients	No
Dose arms 1–3	Sulphasalazine; no sulphasalazine
Study quality	**2–**
Reference	548: Freeman JG, Reece VA, Venables CW. Sulphasalazine and spermatogenesis. Digestion. 1982;23(1):68–71.
Language	English

Compound	Sulphasalazine (A07EC01)
Disease treated	Inflammatory bowel disease
Quantification of adverse effects	Semen
No. of patients treated	4
Age group	Young

Treatment period	Continuous
Dose	n.g.
Treatment consequences	Spermatogenesis, recovery
Efficacy	After withdrawal in three of four, three pregnancies
Randomization of patients	No
Study quality	**3**
Reference	615: Levi AJ, Fisher AM, Hughes L, Hendry WF. Male infertility due to sulphasalazine. Lancet. 1979 Aug 11;2(8137):276–8.
Language	English

Compound	Sulphasalazine (A07EC01)
Disease treated	Spermatogenic dysfunction
Quantification of adverse effects	Semen
Age group	Young
Treatment consequences	Spermatogenesis, impairment
Efficacy	None
Study quality	**4 (review)**
Reference	458: Steeno OP. Side-effects of salazopyrin on male fertility. Eur J Obstet Gynecol Reprod Biol. 1984 Dec;18(5–6):361–4.
Language	English

Compound	Sulphasalazine (A07EC01)
Disease treated	Inflammatory bowel disease
Quantification of adverse effects	Semen
Age group	Young
Treatment period	Continuous
Dose	n.g.
Treatment consequences	Spermatogenesis, impairment
Efficacy	None
Randomization of patients	No
Remarks	Sulfosalazine seems to exert no direct effect on spermatogenesis. The deleterious effect might therefore occur only after ejaculation and result in asthenozoospermia

Study quality	**4 (review)**
Reference	79: Niederberger C. The adverse effect of sulphasalazine on spermatogenesis and male reproductive potential. J Androl. 2002 Mar–Apr;23(2):180.
Language	English

Compound	5-amino salicylic acid (A07EC02) after sulphasalazine
Disease treated	Inflammatory bowel disease
Quantification of adverse effects	Sperm parameters
No. of patients treated	16
Age group	Young
Treatment period	4 months
Dose	n.g.
Treatment consequences	Sperm parameters, improvement
Efficacy	3 months after discontinuation of sulfosalazine, four pregnancies
Randomization of patients	No
Study quality	**3**
Reference	846: Riley SA, Lecarpentier J, Mani V, Goodman MJ, Mandal BK, Turnberg LA. Sulphasalazine induced seminal abnormalities in ulcerative colitis: results of mesalazine substitution. Gut. 1987 Aug;28(8):1008–12.
Language	English

Compound	5-amino salicylic acid (A07EC02) after sulphasalazine
Disease treated	Inflammatory bowel disease
Quantification of adverse effects	Sperm parameters
No. of patients treated	11
Age group	Young
Treatment period	4 months
Dose	n.g.
Treatment consequences	Sperm parameters, improvement
Efficacy	5 months after discontinuation of sulfosalazine, three pregnancies
Randomization of patients	No
Study quality	**3**

2

Reference	845: Zelissen PM, van Hattum J, Poen H, Scholten P, Gerritse R, te Velde ER. Influence of salazosulphapyridine and 5-aminosalicylic acid on seminal qualities and male sex hormones. Scand J Gastroenterol. 1988 Nov;23(9):1100–4.
Language	English

Compound	5-amino salicylic acid (A07EC02) after sulphasalazine
Disease treated	Inflammatory bowel disease
Quantification of adverse effects	Sperm parameters
No. of patients treated	6
Age group	Young
Treatment period	16 weeks
Dose	n.g.
Treatment consequences	Sperm parameters, improvement
Efficacy	No change in ROS activity
Randomization of patients	No
Study quality	**3**
Reference	843: Wu FC, Aitken RJ, Ferguson A. Inflammatory bowel disease and male infertility: effects of sulphasalazine and 5-aminosalicylic acid on sperm-fertilizing capacity and reactive oxygen species generation. Fertil Steril. 1989 Nov;52(5):842–5.
Language	English

Compound	5-amino salicylic acid (A07EC02) after sulphasalazine
Disease treated	Inflammatory bowel disease
Quantification of adverse effects	Sperm parameters
No. of patients treated	1
Age group	Young
Treatment period	3 months
Dose	No
Treatment consequences	Sperm parameters, improvement; pregnancy in the female partner
Efficacy	3 months after discontinuation of sulfosalazine
Study quality	**3**
Reference	844: Delaere KP, Strijbos WE, Meuleman EJ. Sulphasalazine-induced reversible male infertility. Acta Urol Belg. 1989;57(1):29–33.

Language	English

Compound	5-amino salicylic acid (A07EC02) after sulphasalazine
Disease treated	Inflammatory bowel disease
Quantification of adverse effects	Semen
No. of patients treated	1
Age group	33
Treatment period	12 months
Dose	3×1 g/day
Treatment consequences	Semen parameters, improvement
Efficacy	After change from sulphasalazine to 5-ASA
Study quality	**3**
Reference	2140: Cann PA, Holdsworth CD. Reversal of male infertility on changing treatment from sulphasalazine to 5-amino-salicylic acid. Lancet. 1984 May 19;1(8386):1119.
Language	English

A08 Antiobesity Preparations

A case-control study demonstrated a negative association of semen parameters and obesity. The possible influence of drug treatment was not mentioned.

Overall level of evidence for adverse effects: B

Compound	Antiobesity preparations (A08)
Disease treated	Obesity
Quantification of adverse effects	Semen
No. of patients treated	2111
Age group	Young
Treatment period	No treatment
Treatment consequences	Infertility associated with obesity
Efficacy	A 3-unit change in body mass index was associated with adjusted ORs of 1.11–1.12
Randomization of patients	No

2

Study quality	**2+**
Reference	2170: Sallmen M, Sandler DP, Hoppin JA, Blair A, Baird DD. Reduced fertility among overweight and obese men. Epidemiology. 2006 Sep;17(5):520–3.
Language	English

A10	**Drugs Used in Diabetes**
	Metformin may result in a decline of testosterone levels in diabetic men, similar to its effects in the treatment of polycystic ovary syndrome in women. **Overall level of evidence of adverse effects: C**

Compound	Metformin (A10BA02)
Disease treated	Obesity and type-2 diabetes
Quantification of adverse effects	Hormones
No. of patients treated	40
Age group	Middle-aged
Treatment period	3 months
Dose	1700 mg/day
Treatment consequences	Sex steroid hormones, decrease
Efficacy	Significant in diabetic group
Randomization of patients	No
Study quality	**2–**
Reference	847: Ozata M, Oktenli C, Bingol N, Ozdemir IC. The effects of metformin and diet on plasma testosterone and leptin levels in obese men. Obes Res. 2001 Nov;9(11):662–7.
Language	English

A11	Vitamins
	There is an uncontrolled study which describes an increase of sperm count following treatment with vitamin C.
	Overall level of evidence of adverse effects: D

Compound	Vitamin C (A11GA01)
Disease treated	Infertility
Quantification of dysfunction	Semen
No. of patients treated	13
Age group	25–35
Treatment period	2 months
Dose	2000 mg/day
Treatment consequences	Sperm count, increase
Efficacy	From 14×10^6 to 32×10^6
Randomization of patients	No
Study quality	**3**
Reference	29. Akmal M, Qadri JQ, Al-Waili NS, Thangal S, Haq A, Saloom KY. Improvement in human semen quality after oral supplementation of vitamin C. J Med Food. 2006 Fall;9(3):440–2.
Language	English

A12	Mineral Supplements
	Work-place exposition to fluorides impairs sperm parameters at a higher dose. Zinc is a normal component of seminal fluid; it is secreted by the prostate gland. A number of investigations have studied the association of zinc levels and sperm parameters. Since some reports describe higher seminal zinc levels in normozoospermia, supplementation is often recommended in patients with oligozoospermia in order to improve seminal parameters. There are no RCTs available that use zinc alone. The largest controlled study in 87 patients did not describe an improvement in seminal parameters, but instead a disappearance of a correlation between sperm count and zinc levels. A study in five healthy men reported impairment of spermatogenesis as a consequence of dietary zinc restriction.
	Overall level of evidence of adverse effects: C

Compound	Fluorides (A12CD)
Disease treated	Fluoride exposition
Quantification of adverse effects	Semen
No. of patients treated	n.g.
Age group	Young
Treatment period	Continuous
Dose	3–27 mg/day
Treatment consequences	Sperm count, alteration
Efficacy	No difference to lower exposition
Randomization of patients	No
Study quality	**2–**
Reference	995. Ortiz-Perez D, Rodriguez-Martinez M, Martinez F, Borja-Aburto VH, Castelo J, Grimaldo JI, Cruz E de la, Carrizales L, Diaz-Barriga F. Fluoride-induced disruption of reproductive hormones in men. Environ Res. 2003 Sep;93(1):20–30.
Language	English

Compound	Zinc (A12CB)
Disease treated	Infertility
Quantification of adverse effects	Semen
No. of patients treated	210
Age group	Young
Treatment period	No treatment
Treatment consequences	Concentrations of calcium, magnesium, zinc, and copper in blood and seminal plasma
Efficacy	Not different between the subfertile and fertile men. Weak correlations between blood plasma zinc concentrations and sperm count, sperm motility, abnormal sperm morphology
Randomization of patients	No
Study quality	**2–**
Reference	2301: Wong WY, Flik G, Groenen PM, Swinkels DW, Thomas CM, Copius-Peereboom JH, Merkus HM, Steegers-Theunissen RP. The impact of calcium, magnesium, zinc, and copper in blood and seminal plasma on semen parameters in men. Reprod Toxicol. 2001 Mar–Apr;15(2):131–6.
Language	English

Compound	Zinc (A12CB)
Disease treated	Infertility
Quantification of adverse effects	Semen
No. of patients treated	210
Age group	Young
Treatment period	No treatment
Treatment consequences	Zinc concentration in blood
Efficacy	No significant differences in the geometric means between the fertile and infertile men
Randomization of patients	No
Study quality	**2–**
Reference	2302: Chia SE, Ong CN, Chua LH, Ho LM, Tay SK. Comparison of zinc concentrations in blood and seminal plasma and the various sperm parameters between fertile and infertile men. J Androl. 2000 Jan–Feb;21(1):53–7.
Language	English

Compound	Zinc sulphate+folic acid (A12CB)
Disease treated	Infertility
Quantification of adverse effects	Semen
No. of patients treated	87
Age group	Young
Treatment period	26 weeks
Dose	66 mg/day
Treatment consequences	Positive correlation between zinc levels and sperm count
Efficacy	Disappearance after intervention
Side effects	Not mentioned
Randomization of patients	Yes
Dose arms 1–3	Zinc+folic acid; placebo
Study quality	**1–**
Reference	2199: Ebisch IM, Pierik FH, DE Jong FH, Thomas CM, Steegers-Theunissen RP. Does folic acid and zinc sulphate intervention affect endocrine parameters and sperm characteristics in men? Int J Androl. 2006 Apr;29(2):339–45.
Language	English

Compound	Zinc (A12CB)
Disease treated	Infertility
Quantification of adverse effects	Semen
No. of patients treated	75
Age group	Young
Treatment period	No treatment
Treatment consequences	Zinc concentration in blood
Efficacy	Significantly lower in infertile than in fertile men
Randomization of patients	No
Study quality	**2–**
Reference	2303: Mohan H, Verma J, Singh I, Mohan P, Marwah S, Singh P. Inter-relationship of zinc levels in serum and semen in oligospermic infertile patients and fertile males. Indian J Pathol Microbiol. 1997 Oct;40(4):451–5.
Language	English

Compound	Zinc (A12CB)
Disease treated	Infertility
Quantification of adverse effects	Semen
No. of patients treated	58
Age group	20–40 years
Treatment period	No treatment
Treatment consequences	Zinc serum levels
Efficacy	Lower in men with oligozoospermia than with normozoospermia
Randomization of patients	No
Study quality	**2–**
Reference	2300: Ali H, Baig M, Rana MF, Ali M, Qasim R, Khem AK. Relationship of serum and seminal plasma zinc levels and serum testosterone in oligospermic and azoospermic infertile men. J Coll Phys Surg Pak. 2005 Nov;15(11):671–3.
Language	English

Compound	Zinc (A12CB)
Disease treated	Infertility
Quantification of adverse effects	Semen
No. of patients treated	33
Age group	Young
Treatment period	n.g.
Dose	n.g.
Treatment consequences	Sperm motility
Efficacy	Increase after application
Randomization of patients	No
Study quality	**1–**
Reference	2305: Kynaston HG, Lewis-Jones DI, Lynch RV, Desmond AD. Changes in seminal quality following oral zinc therapy. Andrologia. 1988 Jan–Feb;20(1):21–2.
Language	English

Compound	Zinc (A12CB)
Disease treated	Infertility
Quantification of adverse effects	Semen
No. of patients treated	14
Age group	24–45 years
Treatment period	4 months
Dose	220 mg/day
Treatment consequences	Sperm count, sperm motility
Efficacy	Significantly increased
Side effects	Not mentioned
Randomization of patients	No
Study quality	**1–**
Reference	2306: Tikkiwal M, Ajmera RL, Mathur NK. Effect of zinc administration on seminal zinc and fertility of oligospermic males. Indian J Physiol Pharmacol. 1987 Jan–Mar;31(1):30–4.
Language	English

Compound	Zinc (A12CB)
Disease treated	Healthy
Quantification of adverse effects	Semen, hormones
No. of patients treated	11
Age group	Young
Treatment period	63
Dose	0.4, 2.5, 3.4, 4.4 or 10.4 mg/day
Treatment consequences	T levels, seminal volume
Efficacy	Sensitive to zinc loss
Side effects	Not mentioned
Randomization of patients	No
Study quality	**1–**
Reference	2304: Hunt CD, Johnson PE, Herbel J, Mullen LK. Effects of dietary zinc depletion on seminal volume and zinc loss, serum testosterone concentrations, and sperm morphology in young men. Am J Clin Nutr. 1992 Jul;56(1):148–57.
Language	English

Compound	Zinc restriction (A12CB)
Disease treated	Healthy
Quantification of adverse effects	Semen
No. of patients treated	5
Age group	51–65 years
Treatment period	40 weeks
Treatment consequences	Spermatogenesis, impairment
Efficacy	All
Randomization of patients	No
Study quality	**3**
Reference	632: Abbasi AA, Prasad AS, Rabbani PR. Experimental zinc deficiency in man: effect on spermatogenesis. Trans Assoc Am Phys. 1979;92:292–302.
Language	English

A14 Anabolic Agents for Systemic Use

High doses of anabolic steroids are frequently used by bodybuilders; about half of these use anabolic steroids. The drugs impair spermatogenesis due to their androgenic effects in about half of the (ab-)users. The strength of the effect may vary between induction of asthenozoospermia and azoospermia with resulting infertility. Cessation of abuse allows improvement of spermatogenesis.

Overall level of evidence of adverse effects: B

Compound	Anabolic steroids (A14A)
Disease treated	Anabolic steroid abuse
Quantification of adverse effects	Abuse in bodybuilders
No. of patients treated	500
Age group	Young
Treatment period	Continuous
Treatment consequences	Anabolic steroids, abuse
Efficacy	99.2% of bodybuilders
Randomization of patients	No
Study quality	**2–**
Reference	9: Parkinson AB, Evans NA. Anabolic androgenic steroids: a survey of 500 users. Med Sci Sports Exerc. 2006 Apr;38(4):644–51.
Language	English

Compound	Anabolic steroids, cessation (A14A)
Disease treated	Anabolic steroid abuse
Quantification of adverse effects	Semen
No. of patients treated	41; 41
Age group	26.7 (mean)
Treatment period	Continuous
Dose	Various
Treatment consequences	Sperm count, depression
Efficacy	24 of 41 in abuse, 5 of 41 in normal controls
Randomization of patients	No

2

Dose arms 1–3	Anabolic steroids; normal volunteers
Study quality	**2+**
Reference	986: Knuth UA, Maniera H, Nieschlag E. Anabolic steroids and semen parameters in bodybuilders. Fertil Steril. 1989 Dec;52(6):1041–7.
Language	English

Compound	**Anabolic steroids, cessation (A14A)**
Disease treated	Anabolic steroid abuse
Quantification of adverse effects	Semen
No. of patients treated	15; 15
Age group	26 (mean)
Treatment period	Continuous
Dose	Various
Treatment consequences	Spermatogenesis, impairment
Efficacy	Three men had azoospermia
Randomization of patients	No
Dose arms 1–3	Anabolic steroids; no anabolic steroids
Study quality	**2–**
Reference	985: Torres-Calleja J, Gonzalez-Unzaga M, DeCelis-Carrillo R, Calzada-Sanchez L, Pedron N. Effect of androgenic anabolic steroids on sperm quality and serum hormone levels in adult male bodybuilders. Life Sci. 2001 Mar 2;68(15):1769–74.
Language	English

Compound	**Anabolic steroids, cessation (A14A)**
Disease treated	Anabolic steroid abuse
Quantification of adverse effects	Semen
No. of patients treated	18
Age group	Young
Treatment period	n.g.
Dose	Various
Treatment consequences	Spermatogenesis, improvement
Efficacy	In 18 patients
Randomization of patients	No

Dose arms 1–3	Anabolic steroids; anabolic steroids+hCG
Study quality	**2–**
Reference	21: Karila T, Hovatta O, Seppala T. Concomitant abuse of anabolic androgenic steroids and human chorionic gonadotrophin impairs spermatogenesis in power athletes. Int J Sports Med. 2004 May;25(4):257–63.
Language	English

Compound	Anabolic steroids (A14A)
Disease treated	Gynaecomastia
Quantification of adverse effects	Receptor status
No. of patients treated	8
Age group	21–45 years
Treatment period	Continuous
Dose	Various
Treatment consequences	Receptor density
Efficacy	Significantly higher than in non-anabolic-induced gynaecomastia
Randomization of patients	No
Study quality	**2–**
Reference	999: Salazar EL, Torres JA, Avila A, Andrade A. Hyperplastic changes and receptor status in the breast tissue of bodybuilders under anabolic–androgenic steroid stimulation. Arch Androl. 2000 Jul–Aug;45(1):1–7.
Language	English

Compound	Anabolic steroids, cessation (A14A)
Disease treated	Anabolic steroid abuse
Quantification of adverse effects	Semen
No. of patients treated	4
Age group	27–33 years
Treatment period	5 years
Dose	Various
Treatment consequences	Azoospermia, reversal after cessation
Efficacy	Spontaneously within 12 months
Randomization of patients	No

Study quality	**3**
Reference	33: Gazvani MR, Buckett W, Luckas MJ, Aird IA, Hipkin LJ, Lewis-Jones DI. Conservative management of azoospermia following steroid abuse. Hum Reprod. 1997 Aug;12(8):1706–8.
Language	English

Compound	Anabolic steroids (A14A)
Disease treated	Anabolic steroid abuse
Quantification of adverse effects	Abuse in bodybuilders
No. of patients treated	n.g.
Age group	Young
Treatment period	Continuous
Dose	Various
Treatment consequences	Anabolic steroids, abuse
Efficacy	In 54% of bodybuilders
Randomization of patients	No
Study quality	**2–**
Reference	994: Tricker R, O'Neill MR, Cook D. The incidence of anabolic steroid use among competitive bodybuilders. J Drug Educ. 1989;19(4):313–25.
Language	English

Compound	Metandienone (A14AA03)
Disease treated	Anabolic steroid abuse
Quantification of adverse effects	Semen
No. of patients treated	15
Age group	Young
Treatment period	2 months
Dose	15 mg/day
Treatment consequences	Sperm parameters, impairment
Efficacy	Decrease of motility
Randomization of patients	No
Study quality	**3**

Reference	676: Holma PK. Effects of an anabolic steroid (metandienone) on spermatogenesis. Contraception. 1977 Feb;15(2):151–62.
Language	English

C01 Cardiac Therapy

Amiodarone was suggested to cause gynaecomastia. A report in 44 men described marginal alterations of hormone levels.

Compound	Amiodarone (C01BD01)
Disease treated	Cardiac disease
Quantification of adverse effects	Hormones
No. of patients treated	44
Age group	Old
Treatment period	Continuous
Dose	n.g.
Treatment consequences	Gonadotropin levels, increase; testosterone level, alteration
Efficacy	No effects
Randomization of patients	No
Study quality	**3**
Reference	918: Dobs AS, Sarma PS, Guarnieri T, Griffith L. Testicular dysfunction with amiodarone use. J Am Coll Cardiol. 1991 Nov 1;18(5):1328–32.
Language	English

2

C04	Peripheral Vasodilators
	Pentoxifylline enhances the intracellular cyclic adenosine monophosphate (cAMP) concentration in spermatozoa. In vitro, the addition of pentoxyfylline improves sperm motility parameters and the acrosome reaction. On the basis of these observations, the use of pentoxyfylline was studied in order to improve fertility rate under certain conditions; however, the results were disappointing. Although some uncontrolled studies describe an improvement of sperm parameters after oral application of the drug, this could not be proven in controlled studies. The treatment, on the other hand, did not induce side effects. In-vitro application of the drug to spermatozoa prior to in-vitro fertilization procedures was not able to improve the fertilization rates. No adverse effects were reported. **Overall level of evidence of positive effects: B** **Overall level of evidence of adverse effects compromising effectiveness: D**

Compound	Pentoxifylline (C04AD03)
Disease treated	Infertility
Quantification of dysfunction	Sperm motility
No. of patients treated	77 cycles
Age group	Young
Treatment period	In vitro
Dose	1.76 mmol
Treatment consequences	Motility of frozen sperm, improvement; pregnancy rate, improvement
Efficacy	95%; no alteration
Randomization of patients	No
Dose arms 1–3	Pentoxifylline; no additive in vitro
Study quality	**2–**
Reference	55: Kovacic B, Vlaisavljevic V, Reljic M. Clinical use of pentoxifylline for activation of immotile testicular sperm before ICSI in patients with azoospermia. J Androl. 2006 Jan–Feb;27(1):45–52.
Language	English

Compound	Pentoxifylline (C04AD03)
Disease treated	Infertility
Quantification of dysfunction	Sperm motility
No. of patients treated	64 cycles
Age group	Young
Treatment period	In vitro
Dose	1.5 mmol
Treatment consequences	Motility of frozen sperm, improvement
Efficacy	54% fertilization rate
Randomization of patients	No
Study quality	**2–**
Reference	51: Griveau JF, Lobel B, Laurent MC, Michardiere L, Le Lannou D. Interest of pentoxifylline in ICSI with frozen-thawed testicular spermatozoa from patients with non-obstructive azoospermia. Reprod Biomed Online. 2006 Jan;12(1):14–8.
Language	English

Compound	Pentoxifylline (C04AD03)
Disease treated	Spermatogenic dysfunction
Quantification of dysfunction	Semen
No. of patients treated	65
Dose	1.2 g/day
Age group	Young
Treatment consequences	Alteration of sperm parameters, conception rate
Efficacy	Conception rate in the asthenozoospermic group 37%. In oligozoospermic group no alteration of sperm parameters, conception rate 17%
Randomization of patients	No
Study quality	**3**
Reference	536: Schill WB. Therapy of idiopathic astheno- and oligozoospermia with pentoxifylline. Fortschr Med. 1982 Apr 22;100(15):696–700.
Language	German

Compound	Pentoxifylline (C04AD03)
Disease treated	Infertility
Quantification of dysfunction	IVF outcome
No. of patients treated	51
Age group	Young
Treatment period	In vitro
Dose	3.6 mmol
Treatment consequences	IVF outcome, improvement
Efficacy	Parallel to increase of acrosome reaction
Side effects	None
Randomization of patients	No
Dose arms 1–3	Pentoxifylline; no additive in vitro
Study quality	**2–**
Reference	101: Tasdemir M, Tasdemir I, Kodama H, Tanaka T. Pentoxifylline-enhanced acrosome reaction correlates with fertilization in vitro. Hum Reprod. 1993 Dec;8(12):2102–7.
Language	English

Compound	Pentoxifylline (C04AD03)
Disease treated	Spinal cord injury
Quantification of dysfunction	Sperm motility
No. of patients treated	36
Age group	Young
Treatment period	In vitro
Dose	3.6 mmol
Treatment consequences	Motility of frozen sperm, improvement
Efficacy	No significant effect
Side effects	n.g.
Randomization of patients	No
Dose arms 1–3	Pentoxifylline; no additive in vitro
Study quality	**2–**
Reference	78: Kolon TF, Philips KA, Buch JP. Pentoxifylline enhancement of post-thaw motility in cryopreserved semen of spinal cord-injured men. Int J Fertil Menopausal Stud. 1995 May–Jun;40(3):156–60.
Language	English

Compound	Pentoxifylline (C04AD03)
Disease treated	Immune infertility
Quantification of dysfunction	Sperm motility
No. of patients treated	28
Age group	Young
Treatment period	In vitro
Dose	3.6 mmol
Treatment consequences	Motility of frozen sperm, improvement; ICSI outcome, improvement
Efficacy	No alteration
Randomization of patients	Yes
Dose arms 1–3	Pentoxifylline; no additive in vitro
Study quality	**1+**
Reference	80: Verheyen G, Tournaye H, Janssenswillen C, Henderix P, Devroey P, Van Steirteghem A. The effect of pentoxifylline on in-vitro fertilization in the presence of antisperm antibodies. J Reprod Immunol. 1994 Dec;27(3):187–97.
Language	English

Compound	Pentoxifylline (C04AD03)
Disease treated	Infertility
Quantification of dysfunction	Sperm parameters
No. of patients treated	25
Age group	Young
Treatment period	3 months
Dose	1200 mg/day
Treatment consequences	Sperm parameters, improvement
Efficacy	No alteration
Randomization of patients	No
Study quality	**3**
Reference	93: Maier U, Szabo N, Ludvik G. Oral pentoxifylline in therapy-resistant idiopathic OAT syndrome. Arch Androl. 1994 Jul–Aug;33(1):59–62.
Language	English

2

Compound	Pentoxifylline (C04AD03)
Disease treated	Infertility
Quantification of dysfunction	Sperm parameters
No. of patients treated	22
Age group	Young
Treatment period	6 months
Dose	1200 mg/day
Treatment consequences	Sperm parameters, improvement
Efficacy	Sperm count increased twofold, sperm motility increased 2.8-fold
Side effects compromising effectiveness	Not mentioned
Randomization of patients	No
Study quality	**3**
Reference	104: Marrama P, Baraghini GF, Carani C, Celani MF, Giovenco P, Grandi F, Montanini V. Further studies on the effects of pentoxifylline on sperm count and sperm motility in patients with idiopathic oligo-asthenozoospermia. Andrologia. 1985 Nov–Dec;17(6):612–6.
Language	English

Compound	Pentoxifylline (C04AD03)
Disease treated	Infertility
Quantification of dysfunction	Sperm parameters
No. of patients treated	15
Age group	Young
Treatment period	6 months
Dose	1200 mg/day
Treatment consequences	Sperm parameters, improvement
Efficacy	Forward progressive spermatozoa and of live and motile spermatozoa
Side effects compromising effectiveness	Not mentioned
Randomization of patients	No
Study quality	3

Reference	105: Aparicio NJ, Schwarzstein L, de Turner EA. Pentoxifylline (BL 191) by oral administration in the treatment of asthenozoospermia. Andrologia. 1980 May–Jun;12(3):228–31.
Language	English

Compound	Pentoxifylline (C04AD03)
Disease treated	Infertility
Quantification of dysfunction	Sperm parameters
No. of patients treated	14
Age group	Young
Treatment period	n.g.
Dose	1200 mg/day
Treatment consequences	Sperm parameters, improvement
Efficacy	Slight improvement of sperm count and motility
Randomization of patients	No
Study quality	**3**
Reference	82: Faka B, Api M, Ficicioglu C, Gurbuz A, Oral O. Pentoxifylline in male-factor infertility: its therapeutic efficacy after oral administration. Acta Eur Fertil. 1994 Nov–Dec;25(6):351–3.
Language	English

Compound	Pentoxifylline (C04AD03)
Disease treated	Infertility
Quantification of dysfunction	Sperm motility
No. of patients treated	10
Age group	Young
Treatment period	In vitro
Dose	3.6 mmol
Treatment consequences	Motility of frozen sperm, improvement; ICSI outcome, improvement
Efficacy	No alteraton
Randomization of patients	No
Dose arms 1–3	Pentoxifylline; no addition in vitro
Study quality	**2–**

Reference	70: Terriou P, Hans E, Giorgetti C, Spach JL, Salzmann J, Urrutia V, Roulier R. Pentoxifylline initiates motility in spontaneously immotile epididymal and testicular spermatozoa and allows normal fertilization, pregnancy, and birth after intracytoplasmic sperm injection. J Assist Reprod Genet. 2000 Apr;17(4):194–9.
Language	English

Compound	Pentoxifylline (C04AD03)
Disease treated	Infertility
Quantification of dysfunction	IVF outcome
No. of patients treated	n.g.
Age group	Young
Treatment period	In vitro
Dose	3.6 mmol
Treatment consequences	IVF outcome, improvement
Efficacy	No alteration
Randomization of patients	Yes
Dose arms 1–3	Pentoxifylline; no addition in vitro
Study quality	**1+**
Reference	103: Tournaye H, Janssens R, Camus M, Staessen C, Devroey P, Van Steirteghem A. Pentoxifylline is not useful in enhancing sperm function in cases with previous in vitro fertilization failure. Fertil Steril. 1993 Jan;59(1):210–5.
Language	English

C07 Beta-blocking Agents

Beta-blocking agents may inhibit sperm motility in vitro; however, no studies are available which show this effect in vivo or a reduction of male fertility.

Overall level of evidence of adverse effects: B

Compound	Propranolol (C07AA05)
Disease treated	Hypertension
Quantification of adverse effects	Hormones

No. of patients treated	34
Age group	Middle-aged
Treatment period	Continuous
Dose	Various
Treatment consequences	Gonadotropin and testosterone levels
Efficacy	No difference between exposed and untreated men
Randomization of patients	No
Study quality	**2–**
Reference	886: Taylor RG, Crisp AJ, Hoffbrand BI, Maguire A, Jacobs HS. Plasma sex hormone concentrations in men with hypertension treated with methyldopa and/or propranolol. Postgrad Med J. 1981 Jul;57(669):425–6.
Language	English

Compound	Propranolol (C07AA05)
Disease treated	Healthy
Quantification of adverse effects	Sperm motility
No. of patients treated	n.g.
Age group	Sperm in vitro
Treatment period	In vitro
Dose	n.g.
Treatment consequences	Sperm motility, impairment
Efficacy	Complete immobilization, not based on $Ca2+$ influx
Randomization of patients	Yes
Study quality	**1–**
Reference	885: White DR, Clarkson JS, Ratnasooriya WD, Aitken RJ. Complementary effects of propranolol and nonoxynol-9 upon human sperm motility. Contraception. 1995 Oct;52(4):241–7.
Language	English

2

C08 Calcium Channel Blockers

A case report discussed the possibility that the cessation of nifedipine medication abandoned a period of male infertility (Hershlag et al. 1995). In vitro, nifedipine inhibited sperm motility and acrosome reaction. This effect was assumed to be a "unique target for the design of new male contraceptive agents" (Goodwin et al. 1997).

Overall level of evidence of adverse effects: B

Compound	Nifedipine (C08CA05)
Disease treated	Infertility
Quantification of adverse effects	Conception rate
No. of patients treated	1
Age group	30
Treatment period	Continuous
Dose	Not mentioned
Treatment consequences	Conception
Efficacy	3 months after cessation of medication
Study quality	**3**
Reference	867: Hershlag A, Cooper GW, Benoff S. Pregnancy following discontinuation of a calcium channel blocker in the male partner. Hum Reprod. 1995 Mar;10(3):599–606.
Language	English

Compound	Nifedipine (C08CA05)
Disease treated	Healthy
Quantification of adverse effects	Ca2+ influx
Age group	Sperm in vitro
Treatment period	In vitro
Dose	n.g.
Treatment consequences	Acrosome reaction, inhibition
Efficacy	No influence of progesterone-induced Ca2+ influx
Study quality	**1–**
Reference	862: Kirkman-Brown JC, Barratt CL, Publicover SJ. Nifedipine reveals the existence of two discrete components of the progesterone-induced [Ca2+]i transient in human spermatozoa. Dev Biol. 2003 Jul 1;259(1):718–2.

Language	English

Compound	**Nifedipine (C08CA05)**
Disease treated	Healthy
Quantification of adverse effects	Progesterone-stimulated acrosome reaction
Age group	Sperm in vitro
Treatment period	In vitro
Dose	n.g.
Treatment consequences	Calcium channel, voltage dependent, protein binding
Efficacy	Inhibition of acrosome reaction by inhibition of Ca2+ influx
Remarks	Unique target for the design of new male contraceptive agents
Study quality	**1–**
Reference	865: Goodwin LO, Leeds NB, Hurley I, Mandel FS, Pergolizzi RG, Benoff S. Isolation and characterization of the primary structure of testis-specific L-type calcium channel: implications for contraception. Mol Hum Reprod. 1997 Mar;3(3):255–68.
Language	English

Compound	**Nifedipine (C08CA05)**
Disease treated	Healthy
Quantification of adverse effects	Sperm motility
No. of patients treated	n.g.
Age group	Sperm in vitro
Treatment period	In vitro
Treatment consequences	Sperm motility
Efficacy	Dose-dependent influence
Study quality	**1–**
Reference	868: Kanwar U, Anand RJ, Sanyal SN. The effect of nifedipine, a calcium channel blocker, on human spermatozoal functions. Contraception. 1993 Nov;48(5):453–70.
Language	English

Compound	Verapamil (C08DA01)
Disease treated	Sperm in vitro
Quantification of adverse effects	Motility, Ca2+ influx
No. of patients treated	n.g.
Age group	Young
Treatment period	In vitro
Dose	50 μmol
Treatment consequences	Sperm motility, inhibition; Ca2+ influx, inhibition
Efficacy	Significant
Study quality	**1–**
Reference	907: Anand RJ, Kanwar U, Sanyal SN. Calcium channel antagonist verapamil modulates human spermatozoal functions. Res Exp Med (Berl). 1994;194(3):165–78.
Language	English

Compound	Verapamil (C08DA01)
Disease treated	Sperm in vitro
Quantification of adverse effects	Hamster oocyte penetration
No. of patients treated	n.g.
Age group	Young
Treatment period	In vitro
Dose	100 μmol
Treatment consequences	Zona-free hamster oocyte test
Efficacy	Increase by an acceleration of the acrosome reaction
Study quality	**1–**
Reference	909: Roldan ER, Wramsby H, Yanagimachi R. Verapamil, a $Ca2^{+}$ channel antagonist, accelerates the in vitro penetration of zona-free hamster eggs by human spermatozoa. Clin Reprod Fertil. 1987 Feb–Apr;5(1–2):1–4.
Language	English

C09	Agents Which Act on the Renin–Angiotensin System
	Although the existence of angiotensin receptors in spermatozoa has been demonstrated, and sperm functions may be altered by in-vitro incubation with these drugs, in-vivo effects of these drug groups on testicular function have not yet been described. **Overall level of evidence of adverse effects: C**

Compound	Captopril (C09AA01)
Disease treated	Infertility
Quantification of adverse effects	Sperm functions
No. of patients treated	35
Age group	Sperm in vitro
Treatment period	In vitro
Dose	100 μmol
Treatment consequences	Acrosome reaction, induction; oolemma binding, inhibition
Efficacy	Not affected by incubation with captopril; significant inhibition
Randomization of patients	Yes
Dose arms 1–3	Captopril; placebo
Study quality	**1–**
Reference	859: Kohn FM, Muller C, Drescher D, Neukamm C, el Mulla KF, Henkel R, Hagele W, Hinsch E, Habenicht UF, Schill WB. Effect of angiotensin converting enzyme (ACE) and angiotensins on human sperm functions. Andrologia. 1998 Aug–Sep;30(4–5):207–15.

Compound	Captopril (C09AA01)
Disease treated	Healthy
Quantification of adverse effects	Sperm paramters
Age group	Sperm in vitro
Treatment period	In vitro
Dose	100 nmol
Treatment consequences	Acrosome reaction, inhibition; hypoosmotic swelling test, reduction
Efficacy	Significant
Study quality	**1–**

Reference	925: Foresta C, Mioni R, Rossato M, Varotto A, Zorzi M. Evidence for the involvement of sperm angiotensin converting enzyme in fertilization. Int J Androl. 1991 Oct;14(5):333–9.
Language	English

Compound	Lisinopril (C09AA03)
Disease treated	Hypertension
Quantification of adverse effects	Hormones
No. of patients treated	20
Age group	Young
Treatment period	6 months
Dose	5–20 mg
Treatment consequences	Testosterone level, alteration; free testosterone, decrease
Efficacy	Insignificant
Randomization of patients	No
Study quality	**3**
Reference	834: Koshida H, Takeda R, Miyamori I. Lisinopril decreases plasma free testosterone in male hypertensive patients and increases sex hormone binding globulin in female hypertensive patients. Hypertens Res. 1998 Dec;21(4):279–82.
Language	English

Compound	Angiotensin II (not listed)
Disease treated	Infertility
Quantification of dysfunction	Sperm functions in vitro
Age group	Young
Treatment period	In vitro
Treatment consequences	Sperm motility, CASA parameters, alteration
Efficacy	Several parameters
Study quality	**2–**
Reference	860: Vinson GP, Mehta J, Evans S, Matthews S, Puddefoot JR, Saridogan E, Holt WV, Djahanbakhch O. Angiotensin II stimulates sperm motility. Regul Pept. 1996 Dec 3;67(2):131–5.
Language	English

C10	Lipid-Modifying Agents
	There is no evidence for an effect on testosterone synthesis and spermatogenesis by statins (hydroxymethylglutaryl-CoA reductase inhibitors), also in RCT. **Overall level of evidence of adverse effects: A**

Compound	Simvastatin (C10AA01), pravastatin
Disease treated	Hypercholesterinaemia
Quantification of adverse effects	Lipids in serum
No. of patients treated	159
Age group	29–55 years
Treatment period	Continuous
Treatment consequences	Testosterone level, decline
Efficacy	No alteration
Randomization of patients	Yes
Dose arms 1–3	Simvastatin 20 mg/day; simvastatin 40 mg/day; pravastatin 40 mg/day
Study quality	**1++**
Reference	125: Dobs AS, Miller S, Neri G, Weiss S, Tate AC, Shapiro DR, Musliner TA. Effects of simvastatin and pravastatin on gonadal function in male hypercholesterolemic patients. Metabolism. 2000 Jan;49(1):115–21.
Language	English

Compound	Simvastatin (C10AA01)
Disease treated	Familial hypercholesterolaemia
Quantification of adverse effects	Hormones
No. of patients treated	19
Age group	Young
Treatment period	14 weeks
Dose	40 mg/day
Treatment consequences	Testosterone level, semen parameters, alteration
Efficacy	No change during treatment
Randomization of patients	No

Study quality	**3**
Reference	840: Purvis K, Tollefsrud A, Rui H, Haug E, Norseth J, Viksmoen L, Ose L, Lund H. Short-term effects of treatment with simvastatin on testicular function in patients with heterozygous familial hypercholesterolaemia. Eur J Clin Pharmacol. 1992;42(1):61–4.
Language	English

Compound	Simvastatin (C10AA01)
Disease treated	Hypercholesterolaemia
Quantification of adverse effects	Hormones
No. of patients treated	8
Age group	Middle-aged
Treatment period	Continuous
Dose	20 mg/day
Treatment consequences	Testosterone level and response to hCG
Efficacy	No change during treatment
Randomization of patients	No
Study quality	**3**
Reference	837: Azzarito C, Boiardi L, Vergoni W, Zini M, Portioli I. Testicular function in hypercholesterolemic male patients during prolonged simvastatin treatment. Horm Metab Res. 1996 Apr;28(4):193–8.
Language	English

Compound	Lovastatin (C10AA02)
Disease treated	Familial hypercholesterolaemia
Quantification of adverse effects	Hormones
No. of patients treated	32
Age group	40–45 years
Treatment period	4 weeks
Dose	40 mg/day
Treatment consequences	Testosterone level, alteration
Efficacy	No change during treatment with lovastatin, but decrease with clofibrate
Randomization of patients	Yes

Dose arms 1–3	Lovastatin; clofibrate
Study quality	**1+**
Reference	842: Mastroberardino G, Costa C, Gavelli MS, VItaliano E, Rossi F, Catalano A, Barletta R, Guarini G. Plasma cortisol and testosterone in hypercholesterolaemia treated with clofibrate and lovastatin. J Int Med Res. 1989 Jul–Aug;17(4):388–94.
Language	English

Compound	Lovastatin (C10AA02)
Disease treated	Renal insufficiency
Quantification of adverse effects	Hormones
No. of patients treated	25
Age group	Middle-aged
Treatment period	Continuous
Dose	n.g.
Treatment consequences	Testosterone level and GnRH stimulation, alteration
Efficacy	No alteration
Randomization of patients	No
Study quality	**2–**
Reference	838: Segarra A, Chacon P, Vilardell M, Piera LL. Prospective case control study to determine the effect of lovastatin on serum testosterone and cortisol concentrations in hyperlipidemic nephrotic patients with chronic renal failure. Nephron. 1996;73(2):186–90.
Language	English

Compound	Pravastatin (C10AA03)
Disease treated	Hyperlipidaemia
Quantification of adverse effects	Hormones
No. of patients treated	15
Age group	Young
Treatment period	Continuous
Dose	40 mg/day
Treatment consequences	Steroid hormone levels, alteration
Efficacy	No alteration

Randomization of patients	Yes
Dose arms 1–3	Pravastatin; placebo
Study quality	**1+**
Reference	883: Bohm M, Herrmann W, Wassmann S, Laufs U, Nickenig G. Does statin therapy influence steroid hormone synthesis? Z Kardiol. 2004 Jan;93(1):43–8.
Language	English

Compound	Pravastatin (C10AA03)
Disease treated	Hypercholesterinaemia
Quantification of adverse effects	Semen, hormones
No. of patients treated	8
Age group	Middle-aged
Treatment period	26 weeks
Dose	20 mg/day
Treatment consequences	Spermatogenesis, alteration
Efficacy	8 of 8 unaltered
Side effects	None
Randomization of patients	No
Study quality	**2–**
Reference	153: Bernini GP, Brogi G, Argenio GF, Moretti A, Salvetti A. Effects of long-term pravastatin treatment on spermatogenesis and on adrenal and testicular steroidogenesis in male hypercholesterolemic patients. J Endocrinol Invest. 1998 May;21(5):310–7.
Language	English

D05	**Antipsoriatics**
D10	*Antiacne Preparations*

Some experts suggested that etretinate might have also gonadotoxic effects, similar to those seen in methotrexate, another antipsoriatic drug. There is, however, no evidence from uncontrolled studies. The same statement holds true for isotretinoin.

Overall level of evidence of adverse effects: D

Compound	Etretinate, isotretinoin (D05BB01)
Disease treated	Acne
Quantification of adverse effects	Sperm parameters
No. of patients treated	28
Age group	Young
Treatment period	16 weeks
Dose	n.g.
Treatment consequences	Sperm parameters, alteration
Efficacy	Unaltered during treatment
Randomization of patients	No
Study quality	**3**
Reference	824: Torok L, Kadar L, Kasa M. Spermatological investigations in patients treated with etretinate and isotretinoin. Andrologia. 1987 Nov–Dec;19(6):629–33.
Language	English

Compound	Isotretinoin (D10AD04)
Disease treated	Acne
Quantification of adverse effects	Clinical reports
No. of patients treated	150
Age group	Young
Treatment period	6 months
Dose	Various
Treatment consequences	Notifications of problems with male reproductive system:
Efficacy	gynaecomastia 48; discomfort 38; impotence 32; reduced fertility 12; ejaculatory faiilure 2; others 20
Randomization of patients	No
Study quality	**3**
Reference	2142: Coleman R, MacDonald D. Effects of isotretinoin on male reproductive system. Lancet. 1994 Jul 16;344(8916):198.
Language	English

Compound	Isotretinoin (D10AD04)
Disease treated	Acne
Quantification of adverse effects	Semen
No. of patients treated	20
Age group	Young
Treatment period	12 months
Dose	1 mg/kg day^{-1}
Treatment consequences	Spermatogenesis, impairment
Efficacy	None
Randomization of patients	No
Study quality	**3**
Reference	276: Hoting VE, Schutte B, Schirren C. Isotretinoin treatment of acne conglobata. Andrologic follow-up Fortschr Med. 1992 Aug 20;110(23):427–30.
Language	German

Compound	Isotretinoin (D10AD04)
Disease treated	Acne
Quantification of adverse effects	Semen
No. of patients treated	20
Age group	Young
Treatment period	12 weeks
Dose	1 mg/kg day^{-1}
Treatment consequences	Spermatogenesis, impairment
Efficacy	None
Randomization of patients	No
Study quality	**3**
Reference	448: Vogt HJ, Ewers R. 13-cis-Retinoic acid and spermatogenesis. spermatological and impulse cytophotometric studies. Hautarzt. 1985 May;36(5):281–6.
Language	German

Compound	Isotretinoin (D10AD04)
Disease treated	Infertility
Quantification of adverse effects	Semen

No. of patients treated	10
Age group	Young
Treatment period	3 month
Dose	1 mg/kg day^{-1}
Treatment consequences	Spermatogenesis, impairment
Efficacy	None
Randomization of patients	No
Study quality	**3**
Reference	311: Parsch EM, Ruzicka T, Przybilla B, Schill WB. Andrological investigations in men treated with acitretin (Ro 10-1670). Andrologia. 1990 Sep–Oct;22(5):479–82.
Language	English

G02 Gynaecologicals – Prolactin Inhibitors

The application of quinagolide together with testosterone is assumed to depress spermatogenesis. That observation has not been confirmed by other studies. Other observations concerning prolactin inhibitors, in particular bromocriptine, are listed in the chapter "AntiParkinson drugs (N04)".

Overall level of evidence of adverse effects: B

Compound	Quinagolide (G02CB04)
Disease treated	Contraception
Quantification of dysfunction	Semen, hormones
No. of patients treated	46
Age group	Young
Treatment period	24 weeks
Dose	75 µg/day
Treatment consequences	Azoospermia, induction
Efficacy	Group 1: 11 of 13; group 2: 11 of 12; group 3: 8 of 13
Randomization of patients	Yes
Dose arms 1–3	T 1200 mg/month+75 µg/day quinagolide; T 800 mg/month+75 µg/day quinagolide; T+placebo
Remarks	No other studies including this compound are available

Study quality	**1–**
Reference	50: Hair WM, Wu FC, Lincoln GA. An investigation of the effectiveness of testosterone implants in combination with the prolactin inhibitor quinagolide in the suppression of spermatogenesis in men. Hum Reprod. 2003 Apr;18(4):749–55.
Language	English

G03	**Sex Hormones and Modulators of the Genital System**
G03A	*Hormonal Contraceptives for Systemic Use – Progestogens*

Progestogens depress testicular function; thus, a variety of progestogens, in particular, levonorgestrel (LNG), medroxyprogesterone (MPA), etenogestrel, and desogestrel (DSG), which are established as part of female contraceptives, have been suggested to act also as male contraceptives. Since they do not only suppress spermatogenic activity, but also testosterone secretion by the Leydig cells, in most trials a combination with testosterone was applied. Randomized trials included only a limited number of volunteers (<100), and the usual effect expected was the induction of azoospermia or at least of severe oligozoospermia. This aim was achieved in up to 93% of the volunteers; however, frequently the rate was significantly lower.

The overall result of the trials is that these drugs and combinations are not suitable for male contraception, since male infertility is suggested only when complete azoospermia is present. Only few studies give the number of pregnancies which occurred in the female partners of the study participants; there is indeed an unacceptable high rate.

Overall level of evidence of positive effects: B
Overall level of evidence of adverse effects compromising effectiveness: B

Compound	Norethisterone enanthate (NETE) (G03AC01)
Disease treated	Contraception
Quantification of dysfunction	Semen
No. of patients treated	40
Age group	Young
Treatment period	48 weeks
Dose	200 mg/week plus T 1000 mg/12 weeks

Treatment consequences	Azoospermia, induction
Efficacy	90% verum, 37% placebo
Side effects compromising effectiveness	Not mentioned
Randomization of patients	Yes
Dose arms 1–3	NETE+T; NETE+placebo
Study quality	**1–**
Reference	7: Meriggiola MC, Costantino A, Saad F, D'Emidio L, Morselli Labate AM, Bertaccini A, Bremner WJ, Rudolph I, Ernst M, Kirsch B, Martorana G, Pelusi G. Norethisterone enanthate plus testosterone undecanoate for male contraception: effects of various injection intervals on spermatogenesis, reproductive hormones, testis, and prostate. J Clin Endocrinol Metab. 2005 Apr;90(4): 2005–14.
Language	English

Compound	Levonorgestrel (G03AC03)
Disease treated	Contraception
Quantification of dysfunction	Semen
No. of patients treated	54
Age group	Young
Treatment period	6 months
Dose	
Treatment consequences	Azoospermia, induction
Efficacy	Severe oligoazoospermia in 89% of the LNG 125, 89% of the LNG 250, and 78% of the LNG 500 groups vs 56% of the men in no LNG.
Randomization of patients	Yes
Dose arms 1–3	125 mg/day LNG+T 100 mg/week; 250 mg/day LNG+T 100 mg/week
Study quality	**1–**
Reference	137: Anawalt BD, Bebb RA, Bremner WJ, Matsumoto AM. A lower dosage levonorgestrel and testosterone combination effectively suppresses spermatogenesis and circulating gonadotropin levels with fewer metabolic effects than higher dosage combinations. J Androl. 1999 May–Jun;20(3):407–14.
Language	English

Compound	Levonorgestrel implants (G03AC03)
Disease treated	Contraception
Quantification of dysfunction	Semen, hormones
No. of patients treated	52
Age group	Young
Treatment period	24 week
Dose	300 mg implant
Treatment consequences	Azoospermia, induction
Efficacy	62%
Side effects compromising effectiveness	Not mentioned
Randomization of patients	Yes
Dose arms 1–3	T 500 mg/8 week+LNG; T 500 mg/8 week; T 1000 mg/8 week
Study quality	**1–**
Reference	18: Gui YL, He CH, Amory JK, Bremner WJ, Zheng EX, Yang J, Yang PJ, Gao ES. Male hormonal contraception: suppression of spermatogenesis by injectable testosterone undecanoate alone or with levonorgestrel implants in chinese men. J Androl. 2004 Sep–Oct;25(5):720–7.
Language	English

Compound	Levonorgestrel implants (G03AC03)
Disease treated	Contraception
Quantification of dysfunction	Semen
No. of patients treated	68
Age group	20–45 years
Treatment period	34 weeks
Dose	125 mg/day
Treatment consequences	Azoospermia, induction
Efficacy	24, 35, 33, 93% dependent on dose of LNG
Side effects compromising effectiveness	None
Randomization of patients	Yes

Dose arms 1–3	T patch; LNG, 4 implants+T patch; LNG 125 mg/day+T patch; LNG, four implants+T 100 mg/weeks
Study quality	**1–**
Reference	67: Gonzalo IT, Swerdloff RS, Nelson AL, Clevenger B, Garcia R, Berman N, Wang C. Levonorgestrel implants (Norplant II) for male contraception clinical trials: combination with transdermal and injectable testosterone. J Clin Endocrinol Metab. 2002 Aug;87(8):3562–72.
Language	English

Compound	Levonorgestrel (G03AC03)
Disease treated	Contraception
Quantification of dysfunction	Semen
No. of patients treated	36
Age group	20–42 years
Treatment period	6 months
Dose	500 mg/day
Treatment consequences	Azoospermia, induction
Efficacy	33 and 67%
Side effects compromising effectiveness	None serious
Randomization of patients	Yes
Dose arms 1–3	LNG+T 100 mg/week; T 100 mg/week alone
Study quality	**1–**
Reference	205: Bebb RA, Anawalt BD, Christensen RB, Paulsen CA, Bremner WJ, Matsumoto AM. Combined administration of levonorgestrel and testosterone induces more rapid and effective suppression of spermatogenesis than testosterone alone: a promising male contraceptive approach. J Clin Endocrinol Metab. 1996 Feb;81(2):757–62.
Language	English

Compound	Levonorgestrel (G03AC03)
Disease treated	Contraception
Quantification of dysfunction	Semen
No. of patients treated	28
Age group	Young

Treatment period	24 weeks
Treatment consequences	Azoospermia, induction
Efficacy	8 of 14; 7 of 14
Side effects compromising effectiveness	Decrease of high-density lipoprotein (HDL) levels
Randomization of patients	Yes
Dose arms 1–3	250 mg/day LNG+T 1000 mg/12 weeks; placebo T+1000 mg/12
Study quality	**1–**
Reference	112: Kamischke A, Ploger D, Venherm S, von Eckardstein S, von Eckardstein A, Nieschlag E. Intramuscular testosterone undecanoate with or without oral levonorgestrel: a randomized placebo-controlled feasibility study for male contraception. Clin Endocrinol (Oxf). 2000 Jul;53(1):43–52.
Language	English

Compound	Levonorgestrel (G03AC03)+dutasteride
Disease treated	Contraception
Quantification of dysfunction	Semen, hormones
No. of patients treated	22
Age group	Young
Treatment period	8 weeks
Dose	100 mg/week T
Treatment consequences	Spermatogenesis, impairment
Efficacy	20 of 22, no improvement by dutasteride
Side effects compromising effectiveness	Not mentioned
Randomization of patients	Yes
Dose arms 1–3	125 mg/week LNG+T 100 mg/week T; 125 mg/week LNG+0.5 mg/day dutasteride+100 mg/week T
Study quality	**1–**
Reference	15: Matthiesson KL, Amory JK, Berger R, Ugoni A, McLachlan RI, Bremner WJ. Novel male hormonal contraceptive combinations: the hormonal and spermatogenic effects of testosterone and levonorgestrel combined with a 5-alpha-reductase inhibitor or gonadotropin-releasing hormone antagonist. J Clin Endocrinol Metab. 2005 Jan;90(1):91–7.

Language	English

Compound	Levonorgestrel (G03AC03)
Disease treated	Contraception
Quantification of dysfunction	Semen
No. of patients treated	16
Age group	Young
Treatment period	18 weeks
Dose	LNG implants
Treatment consequences	Azoospermia, induction
Efficacy	6 of 16
Side effects compromising effectiveness	Not mentioned
Randomization of patients	No
Study quality	**3**
Reference	26: Liu ST, Gui YL, Lin CH, He CH. Hormonal contraception in Chinese men: variations in suppression of spermatogenesis with injectable testosterone undecanoate and levonorgestrel implants. Asian J Androl. 2004 Mar;6(1):41–6.
Language	English

Compound	Levonorgestrel (G03AC03)
Disease treated	Contraception
Quantification of dysfunction	Semen
No. of patients treated	12
Age group	Young
Treatment period	6 months
Dose	250 mg
Treatment consequences	Spermatogenesis, impairment
Efficacy	All
Side effects compromising effectiveness	None
Randomization of patients	Yes

Dose arms 1–3	250 mg/day LNG+T; 500 mg/day LNG+T
Study quality	**1–**
Reference	579: Fogh M, Corker CS, McLean H, Hunter WM, Petersen IB, Philip J, Schou G, Skakkebaek NE. Clinical trial with levonorgestrel and testosterone oenanthate for male fertility control. Acta Endocrinol (Copenh). 1980 Oct;95(2):251–7.
Language	English

Compound	Levonorgestrel (G03AC03)
Disease treated	Healthy
Quantification of dysfunction	T concentration in intratesticular fluid (ITT)
No. of patients treated	7
Age group	Young
Treatment period	6 months
Treatment consequences	Intratesticular T levels (ITT), decline
Efficacy	ITT (822±136 nmol/l) was approximately 40× higher than serum T at baseline. It was suppressed by 98% to 13.1×4.5 nmol/l.
Side effects compromising effectiveness	Not mentioned
Randomization of patients	No
Dose arms 1–3	61 mg/day LNG+100 mg/week T; 31 mg/day LNG+100 mg/week T
Study quality	**1–**
Reference	16: Coviello AD, Bremner WJ, Matsumoto AM, Herbst KL, Amory JK, Anawalt BD, Yan X, Brown TR, Wright WW, Zirkin BR, Jarow JP. Intratesticular testosterone concentrations comparable with serum levels are not sufficient to maintain normal sperm production in men receiving a hormonal contraceptive regimen. J Androl. 2004 Nov–Dec;25(6):931–8.
Language	English

Compound	Levonorgestrel (G03AC03), oestrone
Disease treated	Contraception
Quantification of dysfunction	Semen
No. of patients treated	7
Age group	Young

Treatment period	3 months
Dose	Six implants
Treatment consequences	Sperm count, depression
Efficacy	In all men to $<1\times10^6$
Randomization of patients	No
Study quality	**3**
Reference	532: Brache V, Alvarez-Sanchez F, Leon P, Schmidt F, Faundes A. The effect of levonorgestrel and estrone rods on male reproductive function. Contraception. 1982 Jun;25(6):591–603.
Language	English

Compound	Levonorgestrel (G03AC03)
Disease treated	Contraception
Quantification of dysfunction	Hormones
No. of patients treated	4
Age group	Young
Treatment period	9 months
Dose	250 mg/day LNG+400 mg T
Treatment consequences	Spermatogenesis, impairment
Efficacy	Most
Side effects compromising effectiveness	Hypercholesterinaemia
Randomization of patients	No
Study quality	**3**
Reference	591: Foegh M, Damgaard-Pedersen F, Gormsen J, Knudsen JB, Schou G. Oral levo-norgestrel – testosterone effects on spermatogenesis, hormone levels, coagulation factors and lipoproteins in normal men. Contraception. 1980 Apr;21(4):381–91.
Language	English

Compound	Levonorgestrel (G03AC03), cyproterone, desogestrel
Disease treated	Contraception
Quantification of dysfunction	Hormones

No. of patients treated	128
Age group	Young
Treatment period	up to 48 weeks
Dose	progestin+T 100–200 mg/week
Treatment consequences	Spermatogenesis, impairment
Efficacy	Via depression of gonadotropins
Randomization of patients	Yes
Dose arms 1–3	LNG+T; CPA+T; DSG+T
Study quality	**1+**
Reference	34: McLachlan RI, Robertson DM, Pruysers E, Ugoni A, Matsumoto AM, Anawalt BD, Bremner WJ, Meriggiola C. Relationship between serum gonadotropins and spermatogenic suppression in men undergoing steroidal contraceptive treatment. J Clin Endocrinol Metab. 2004 Jan;89(1):142–9.
Language	English

Compound	Medroxyprogesterone acetate (G03AC06)+T
Disease treated	Contraception
Quantification of dysfunction	Semen
No. of patients treated	30
Age group	Young
Treatment period	60 weeks
Treatment consequences	Spermatogenesis, impairment
Efficacy	100%
Side effects compromising effectiveness	None
Randomization of patients	Yes
Dose arms 1–3	15 mg/day MPA+T 1000 mg/12; 30 mg/day MPA+T 1000 mg/12 weeks; T 1000 mg/12 weeks
Study quality	**1+**
Reference	23: Gu YQ, Tong JS, Ma DZ, Wang XH, Yuan D, Tang WH, Bremner WJ. Male hormonal contraception: effects of injections of testosterone undecanoate and depot medroxyprogesterone acetate at eight-week intervals in Chinese men. J Clin Endocrinol Metab. 2004 May;89(5):2254–62.
Language	English

Compound	Medroxprogesterone acetate (G03AC06)
Disease treated	Contraception
Quantification of dysfunction	Semen
No. of patients treated	30
Age group	Young
Treatment period	Single dose
Treatment consequences	Azoospermia, induction
Efficacy	4 of 10 with T alone, 8 of 10 with T+MPA
Side effects compromising effectiveness	None
Randomization of patients	Yes
Dose arms 1–3	300 mg s.d. MPA+T 4×200 mg pellet; T 4×200 mg pellet; T 2×200 mg pellet
Study quality	**1–**
Reference	188: Handelsman DJ, Conway AJ, Howe CJ, Turner L, Mackey MA. Establishing the minimum effective dose and additive effects of depot progestin in suppression of human spermatogenesis by a testosterone depot. J Clin Endocrinol Metab. 1996 Nov;81(11):4113–21.
Language	English

Compound	Medroxprogesterone acetate (G03AC06)
Disease treated	Cancer, testicular
Quantification of adverse effects	Hormones
No. of patients treated	24
Age group	Young
Treatment period	During chemotherapy
Dose	500 mg/day
Treatment consequences	Spermatogenesis, impairment
Efficacy	No protection against cytotoxic therapy
Side effects compromising effectiveness	"Medical castration" (loss of libido and erections)
Randomization of patients	No
Study quality	**3**

Reference	346: Fossa SD, Klepp O, Norman N. Lack of gonadal protection by medroxyprogesterone acetate-induced transient medical castration during chemotherapy for testicular cancer. Br J Urol. 1988 Nov;62(5):449–53.
Language	English

Compound	Medroxprogesterone acetate (G03AC06)
Disease treated	Contraception
Quantification of dysfunction	Semen
No. of patients treated	23
Age group	Young
Treatment period	15 months
Dose	300 mg/day
Treatment consequences	Spermatogenesis, impairment
Efficacy	Most
Side effects compromising effectiveness	Acne, gynaecomastia
Randomization of patients	No
Dose arms 1–3	Various doses of MPA
Study quality	**2–**
Reference	592: Bain J, Rachlis V, Robert E, Khait Z. The combined use of oral medroxyprogesterone acetate and methyltestosterone in a male contraceptive trial programme. Contraception. 1980 Apr;21(4):365–79.
Language	English

Compound	Medroxprogesterone acetate (G03AC06)
Disease treated	Contraception
Quantification of dysfunction	Semen
No. of patients treated	10
Age group	Young
Treatment period	12 months
Dose	300 mg/day
Treatment consequences	Spermatogenesis, impairment
Efficacy	Hamster oocyte penetration, abolished

Side effects compromising effectiveness	Not mentioned
Randomization of patients	No
Study quality	**3**
Reference	332: Wu FC, Aitken RJ. Suppression of sperm function by depot medroxyprogesterone acetate and testosterone enanthate in steroid male contraception. Fertil Steril. 1989 Apr;51(4):691–8.
Language	English

Compound	Medroxprogesterone acetate (G03AC06)
Disease treated	Contraception
Quantification of dysfunction	Semen
No. of patients treated	9
Age group	Young
Treatment period	8 months
Treatment consequences	Spermatogenesis, impairment
Efficacy	All
Randomization of patients	No
Dose arms 1–3	MPA 150 mg/month+T 250/month; MPA 75 mg/month+T 250 mg/month
Study quality	**2–**
Reference	530: Frick J, Danner C, Kunit G, Joos H, Kohle R. Spermatogenesis in men treated with injections of medroxyprogesterone acetate combined with testosterone enanthate. Int J Androl. 1982 Jun;5(3):246–52.
Language	English

Compound	Medroxprogesterone acetate (G03AC06)
Disease treated	Contraception
Quantification of dysfunction	Pregnancy in the female partners
No. of patients treated	9
Age group	Young
Treatment period	12 months
Dose	n.g.

2

Treatment consequences	Spermatogenesis, impairment
Efficacy	Nine pregnancies in partners of men with sperm count <10 million, 5 of them in partners of men with <1 million/ml
Randomization of patients	No
Dose arms 1–3	MPA+T implant; MPA+T i.m.
Study quality	**2–**
Reference	616: Barfield A, Melo J, Coutinho E, Alvarez-Sanchez F, Faundes A, Brache V, Leon P, Frick J, Bartsch G, Weiske WH, Brenner P, Mishell D Jr, Bernstein G, Ortiz A. Pregnancies associated with sperm concentrations below 10 million/ml in clinical studies of a potential male contraceptive method, monthly depot medroxyprogesterone acetate and testosterone esters. Contraception. 1979 Aug;20(2):121–7.
Language	English

Compound	Medroxprogesterone acetate (G03AC06)
Disease treated	Contraception
Quantification of dysfunction	Semen
No. of patients treated	6
Age group	Young
Treatment period	12 months
Dose	MPA 20 mg/day+T 100 mg/day percutaneous
Treatment consequences	Spermatogenesis, impairment
Efficacy	95% reduction in respect to pretreatment values
Side effects compromising effectiveness	Hyperglycaemia
Randomization of patients	No
Study quality	**2–**
Reference	510: Soufir JC, Jouannet P, Marson J, Soumah A. Reversible inhibition of sperm production and gonadotrophin secretion in men following combined oral medroxyprogesterone acetate and percutaneous testosterone treatment. Acta Endocrinol (Copenh). 1983 Apr;102(4):625–32.
Language	English

Compound	Etonogestrel implant (G03AC08)
Disease treated	Contraception
Quantification of dysfunction	Semen
No. of patients treated	28
Age group	Young
Treatment period	24 weeks
Treatment consequences	Azoospermia, induction
Efficacy	64% (group 1); 73% (group 2)
Side effects compromising effectiveness	None
Randomization of patients	Yes
Dose arms 1–3	1× implant+T 400 mg/week; 2× implant+T 400 mg/week
Study quality	**1–**
Reference	66: Anderson RA, Kinniburgh D, Baird DT. Suppression of spermatogenesis by etonogestrel implants with depot testosterone: potential for long-acting male contraception. J Clin Endocrinol Metab. 2002 Aug;87(8):3640–9.
Language	English

Compound	Etonogestrel (G03AC08)
Disease treated	Contraception
Quantification of dysfunction	Semen
No. of patients treated	20
Age group	Young
Treatment period	12 months
Treatment consequences	Azoospermia, induction
Efficacy	In 16 of 20 men
Side effects compromising effectiveness	Body weight increase
Randomization of patients	No
Dose arms 1–3	One implant etonogrestrel+T implant; two implants etonogrestrel+T implant
Study quality	**2–**

Reference	57: Anderson RA, Zhu H, Cheng L, Baird DT. Investigation of a novel preparation of testosterone decanoate in men: pharmacokinetics and spermatogenic suppression with etonogestrel implants. Contraception. 2002 Nov;66(5):357–64.
Language	English

Compound	Etonogestrel (G03AC08)
Disease treated	Contraception
Quantification of dysfunction	Semen, hormones
No. of patients treated	15
Age group	Young
Treatment period	48 weeks
Dose	T 400 mg/12 weeks+3×68 mg etonogestrel implants
Treatment consequences	Azoospermia, induction
Efficacy	15 of 15 men
Side effects compromising effectiveness	No hypercholesterinaemia
Randomization of patients	No
Study quality	**3**
Reference	17: Brady BM, Walton M, Hollow N, Kicman AT, Baird DT, Anderson RA. Depot testosterone with etonogestrel implants result in induction of azoospermia in all men for long-term contraception. Hum Reprod. 2004 Nov;19(11):2658–67.
Language	English

Compound	Desogestrel (G03AC09)
Disease treated	Contraception
Quantification of dysfunction	Semen
No. of patients treated	66
Age group	Young
Treatment period	24 weeks
Treatment consequences	Azoospermia, induction
Efficacy	22 of 31 (group 1); 28 of 28 (group 2)
Side effects compromising effectiveness	Body weight increase

Randomization of patients	Yes
Dose arms 1–3	150 µg/day DSG+T 40 mg/day; 300 µg DSG+T 400 mg/12 weeks
Study quality	**1+**
Reference	72: Kinniburgh D, Zhu H, Cheng L, Kicman AT, Baird DT, Anderson RA. Oral desogestrel with testosterone pellets induces consistent suppression of spermatogenesis to azoospermia in both Caucasian and Chinese men. Hum Reprod. 2002 Jun;17(6):1490–501.
Language	English

Compound	Desogestrel (G03AC09)
Disease treated	Contraception
Quantification of dysfunction	Semen
No. of patients treated	52
Age group	Young
Treatment period	20 weeks
Treatment consequences	Azoospermia, induction
Efficacy	33 of 39 men
Side effects compromising effectiveness	None
Randomization of patients	Yes
Dose arms 1–3	150 µg/DSG+T 400 mg/12 weeks; 300 µg/day DSG+T 400 mg/12 weeks;
Study quality	**1+**
Reference	59: Anderson RA, Van Der Spuy ZM, Dada OA, Tregoning SK, Zinn PM, Adeniji OA, Fakoya TA, Smith KB, Baird DT. Investigation of hormonal male contraception in African men: suppression of spermatogenesis by oral desogestrel with depot testosterone. Hum Reprod. 2002 Nov;17(11):2869–77.
Language	English

Compound	Desogestrel (G03AC09)
Disease treated	Contraception
Quantification of dysfunction	Azoospermia
No. of patients treated	24
Age group	20–49 years

Treatment period	6 months
Treatment consequences	Azoospermia, induction
Efficacy	7 of 8 men (group 2); 8 of 8 men (group 3)
Side effects compromising effectiveness	Body weight increase, decrease of high-density lipoprotein (HDL) levels
Randomization of patients	Yes
Dose arms 1–3	DSG 150 µg/day+T 50 mg/week; DSG 150 µg/day+T 100 mg/week; DSG 300 µg/day+T 100 mg/week
Study quality	**1–**
Reference	108: Anawalt BD, Herbst KL, Matsumoto AM, Mulders TM, Coelingh-Bennink HJ, Bremner WJ. Desogestrel plus testosterone effectively suppresses spermatogenesis but also causes modest weight gain and high-density lipoprotein suppression. Fertil Steril. 2000 Oct;74(4):707–14.
Language	English

Compound	Desogestrel (G03AC09)
Disease treated	Contraception
Quantification of dysfunction	Semen
No. of patients treated	24
Age group	Young
Treatment period	24 weeks
Treatment consequences	Azoospermia, induction
Efficacy	78%
Randomization of patients	No
Dose arms 1–3	300 µg/day DSG+T 100 mg/week; 300 µg/day DSG+T 50 mg/week; 150 µg/day DSG+T 100 mg/week
Study quality	**2–**
Reference	141: Wu FC, Balasubramanian R, Mulders TM, Coelingh-Bennink HJ. Oral progestogen combined with testosterone as a potential male contraceptive: additive effects between desogestrel and testosterone enanthate in suppression of spermatogenesis, pituitary–testicular axis, and lipid metabolism. J Clin Endocrinol Metab. 1999 Jan;84(1):112–22.
Language	English

Compound	Desogestrel (G03AC09)
Disease treated	Contraception
Quantification of dysfunction	Semen, hormones
No. of patients treated	23
Age group	Young
Treatment period	32 weeks
Treatment consequences	Azoospermia, induction
Efficacy	57% in 300 μg/day DSG
Side effects compromising effectiveness	None
Randomization of patients	Yes
Dose arms 1–3	75 μg/day DSG+T patch; 150 μg/day DSG+T patch; 300 μg/day DSG+T patch
Study quality	**1–**
Reference	90: Hair WM, Kitteridge K, O'Connor DB, Wu FC. A novel male contraceptive pill-patch combination: oral desogestrel and transdermal testosterone in the suppression of spermatogenesis in normal men. J Clin Endocrinol Metab. 2001 Nov;86(11):5201–9.
Language	English

Compound	Desogestrel (G03AC09), finasteride
Disease treated	Contraception
Quantification of dysfunction	Semen
No. of patients treated	16
Age group	Young
Treatment period	24 weeks
Treatment consequences	Azoospermia, induction
Efficacy	5 of 7 men (group 1); 6 of 8 men (group 2)
Randomization of patients	Yes
Dose arms 1–3	150 μg DSG+T 400 mg/12 weeks+5 mg finasteride; 150 μg DSG+T 400 mg/12 weeks
Study quality	**1–**

Reference	102: Kinniburgh D, Anderson RA, Baird DT. Suppression of spermatogenesis with desogestrel and testosterone pellets is not enhanced by addition of finasteride. J Androl. 2001 Jan–Feb;22(1):88–95.
Language	English

G03 Sex Hormones and Modulators of the Genital System

G03B Androgens

Exogenously applied testosterone suppresses spermatogenesis via the inhibition of LH and FSH secretion from the pituitary gland, and as a consequence Leydig cell stimulation ceases. This effect has been used for different purposes:

1. The "rebound therapy" of spermatogenic dysfunction used the rebound phase after suppression by testosterone injections. A recovery in 29% of patients with oligozoospermia and in 8% with azoospermia and an increase of pregnancy rate has been quoted; however, no RCT are available.

Overall level of evidence of positive effects: D
Overall level of evidence of adverse effects compromising effectiveness: D

2. For contraceptive purposes, different modalities of testosterone were applied in healthy volunteers. In RCT, a significant depression of spermatogenesis (as observed histologically) or a decline of sperm count in conjunction with a decline of inhibin-B serum levels were observed; however, the azoospermia necessary for complete transient infertility was not observed in all cases. The reason for the individual difference in testosterone effects is not clear; one possibility is a polychromasy of androgen receptor. Pregnancies were observed in the partners of the treated men at a rate of about 1%.

   As generally mild side effects, reversible weight gain, acne, decrease of HDL levels were observed, it is questionable as to whether these side effects would inhibit the use of testosterone application in male contraception. The recovery after cessation of therapy was complete in all cases.

Overall level of evidence of positive effects: B
Overall level of evidence of adverse effects compromising effectiveness: B

3. In principle, the effect of testosterone on spermatogenesis is present also in prepubertal stages; thus, it is noticeable that testosterone therapy in hypogonadism does not deteriorate the success of subsequent stimulation of spermatogenesis by gonadotropins.

Overall level of evidence of positive effects: D
Overall level of evidence of adverse effects compromising effectiveness: D

Compound	Fluoxymesterone (G03BA01)
Disease treated	Contraception
Quantification of dysfunction	Semen
No. of patients treated	9
Age group	Young
Treatment period	12 weeks
Treatment consequences	Spermatogenesis, impairment
Efficacy	Insignificantly lower sperm count
Randomization of patients	No
Dose arms 1–3	10 mg/day; 20 mg/day; 30 mg/day
Study quality	**2–**
Reference	680: Jones TM, Fang VS, Landau RL, Rosenfield RL. The effects of fluoxymesterone administration on testicular function. J Clin Endocrinol Metab. 1977 Jan;44(1):121–9.
Language	English

Compound	Testosterone (G03BA03), rebound therapy
Disease treated	Infertility
Quantification of dysfunction	Semen
No. of patients treated	225
Age group	Young
Treatment period	6 months
Dose	3×50 mg/week until induction of azoospermia
Treatment consequences	Pregnancy induced
Efficacy	60% of oligozoospermic patients improvement, 25% pregnancy rate

Side effects compromising effectiveness	Body weight gain in 1 patient
Randomization of patients	No
Remarks	In 4% of patients no recovery from azoospermia
Study quality	**3**
Reference	655: Charny CW, Gordon JA. Testosterone rebound therapy: a neglected modality. Fertil Steril. 1978 Jan;29(1):64–8.
Language	English

Compound	Testosterone (G03BA03), rebound therapy
Disease treated	Infertility
Quantification of dysfunction	Semen
No. of patients treated	131
Age group	Young
Treatment period	Up to 20 weeks or until azoospermia
Dose	10 mg/week
Treatment consequences	Pregnancy rate induced, increase in rebound phase
Efficacy	29% in partners of patients with oligozoospermia, 8% with azoospermia
Side effects compromising effectiveness	Not mentioned
Randomization of patients	No
Study quality	**2–**
Reference	722: Lamensdorf H, Compere D, Begley G. Testosterone rebound therapy in the treatment of male infertility. Fertil Steril. 1975 May;26(5):469–72.
Language	English

Compound	Testosterone (G03BA03), rebound therapy
Disease treated	Infertility
Quantification of dysfunction	Semen
No. of patients treated	5
Age group	Young
Treatment period	12 weeks
Dose	3×80 mg/day

Treatment consequences	Spermatogenesis, impairment
Efficacy	In few men
Randomization of patients	No
Study quality	**3**
Reference	589: Kloer H, Hoogen H, Nieschlag E. Trial of high-dose testosterone undecanoate in treatment of male infertility. Int J Androl. 1980 Apr;3(2):121–9.
Language	English

Compound	Testosterone (G03BA03)
Disease treated	Contraception
Quantification of dysfunction	Semen
No. of patients treated	399
Age group	Young
Treatment period	12 months
Dose	200 mg/week
Treatment consequences	Pregnancies induced
Efficacy	4 of 349 in oligozoospermic men, none in azoospermic men
Side effects compromising effectiveness	Minimal
Randomization of patients	No
Study quality	**2–**
Reference	202: World Health Organization [No authors listed]. Contraceptive efficacy of testosterone-induced azoospermia and oligozoospermia in normal men. Fertil Steril. 1996 Apr;65(4):821–9.
Language	English

Compound	Testosterone (G03BA03)
Disease treated	Contraception
Quantification of dysfunction	Semen
No. of patients treated	308
Age group	Young
Treatment period	12 months
Dose	500 mg/month

Treatment consequences	Azoospermia, induction
Efficacy	95%
Side effects compromising effectiveness	No significant changes in serum chemistry
Randomization of patients	No
Study quality	**3**
Reference	53: Gu YQ, Wang XH, Xu D, Peng L, Cheng LF, Huang MK, Huang ZJ, Zhang GY. A multicenter contraceptive efficacy study of injectable testosterone undecanoate in healthy Chinese men. J Clin Endocrinol Metab. 2003 Feb;88(2):562–8.
Language	English

Compound	Testosterone (G03BA03)
Disease treated	Healthy
Quantification of dysfunction	Inhibin B
No. of patients treated	56
Age group	Young
Treatment period	65 weeks
Dose	200 mg/week
Treatment consequences	Inhibin-B recovery after suppression
Efficacy	Parallel to sperm count
Randomization of patients	No
Study quality	**3**
Reference	184: Anderson RA, Wallace EM, Groome NP, Bellis AJ, Wu FC. Physiological relationships between inhibin B, follicle stimulating hormone secretion and spermatogenesis in normal men and response to gonadotrophin suppression by exogenous testosterone. Hum Reprod. 1997 Apr;12(4):746–51.
Language	English

Compound	Testosterone (G03BA03)
Disease treated	Contraception
Quantification of dysfunction	Semen
No. of patients treated	51

Age group	Young
Treatment period	6 months
Treatment consequences	Spermatogenesis, impairment
Efficacy	Not 100% azoospermia
Side effects compromising effectiveness	Acne
Randomization of patients	Yes
Dose arms 1–3	300 mg/week; 100 mg/week; placebo
Study quality	**1–**
Reference	321: Matsumoto AM. Effects of chronic testosterone administration in normal men: safety and efficacy of high dosage testosterone and parallel dose-dependent suppression of luteinizing hormone, follicle-stimulating hormone, and sperm production. J Clin Endocrinol Metab. 1990 Jan;70(1):282–7.
Language	English

Compound	Testosterone (G03BA03)
Disease treated	Contraception
Quantification of dysfunction	Semen
No. of patients treated	47
Age group	Young
Treatment period	6 months
Treatment consequences	Spermatogenesis, impairment
Efficacy	38% sperm decrease in T implants, 77% in T enanthate
Randomization of patients	No
Dose arms 1–3	T implant 1200 mg; T enanthate 200 mg/week
Study quality	**2–**
Reference	273: Handelsman DJ, Conway AJ, Boylan LM. Suppression of human spermatogenesis by testosterone implants. J Clin Endocrinol Metab. 1992 Nov;75(5):1326–32.
Language	English

Compound	Testosterone (G03BA03)
Disease treated	Androgen receptor, type
Quantification of dysfunction	Semen

2

No. of patients treated	33
Age group	Young
Treatment period	16 weeks
Dose	200 mg/week
Treatment consequences	Azoospermia, induction
Efficacy	18 of 33 men; activity of type-2 5α–reductase in OAT increased
Randomization of patients	No
Study quality	**2–**
Reference	178: Anderson RA, Kelly RW, Wu FC. Comparison between testosterone enanthate-induced azoospermia and oligozoospermia in a male contraceptive study. V. Localization of higher 5 alpha-reductase activity to the reproductive tract in oligozoospermic men administered supraphysiological doses of testosterone. J Androl. 1997 Jul–Aug;18(4):366–71.
Language	English

Compound	Testosterone (G03BA03)
Disease treated	Contraception
Quantification of dysfunction	Semen
No. of patients treated	19
Age group	Young
Treatment period	20 weeks
Dose	200 mg/week
Treatment consequences	Spermatogenesis, impairment
Efficacy	Most
Side effects compromising effectiveness	Body weight increase, decrease of HDL levels, increase of parathormone levels
Randomization of patients	No
Study quality	**3**
Reference	235: Bagatell CJ, Heiman JR, Matsumoto AM, Rivier JE, Bremner WJ. Metabolic and behavioral effects of high-dose, exogenous testosterone in healthy men. J Clin Endocrinol Metab. 1994 Aug;79(2):561–7.
Language	English

Compound	Testosterone (G03BA03)
Disease treated	Contraception
Quantification of dysfunction	Semen
No. of patients treated	17
Age group	Young
Treatment period	6 months
Dose	200 mg/week
Treatment consequences	Spermatogenesis, recovery
Efficacy	To sperm count >20×10^6/ml) at a median time of 3.9 months, recovery to their own baseline in 13 of 17 (76.5%) at a median time of 4.9 months
Randomization of patients	No
Study quality	**3**
Reference	190: Aribarg A, Sukcharoen N, Chanprasit Y, Ngeamvijawat J, Kriangsinyos R. Suppression of spermatogenesis by testosterone enanthate in Thai men. J Med Assoc Thai. 1996 Oct;79(10):624–9.
Language	English

Compound	Testosterone (G03BA03)
Disease treated	Contraception
Quantification of dysfunction	Sperm function test
No. of patients treated	12
Age group	Young
Treatment period	15 months
Dose	200 mg/week
Treatment consequences	Spermatogenesis, impairment
Efficacy	In 12 men sperm function unchanged
Randomization of patients	No
Study quality	**3**
Reference	179: Wang C, Leung A, Superlano L, Steiner B, Swerdloff RS. Oligozoospermia induced by exogenous testosterone is associated with normal functioning residual spermatozoa. Fertil Steril. 1997 Jul;68(1):149–53.
Language	English

Compound	Testosterone (G03BA03)
Disease treated	Contraception
Quantification of dysfunction	Semen
No. of patients treated	12
Age group	Young
Treatment period	32 weeks
Treatment consequences	Azoospermia, induction
Efficacy	In 3 of 8 men with 1200 mg T, in 0 of 4 men with 600 mg T
Randomization of patients	No
Dose arms 1–3	1200 mg/12 weeks; 600 mg/12 weeks
Study quality	**2–**
Reference	213: Behre HM, Baus S, Kliesch S, Keck C, Simoni M, Nieschlag E. Potential of testosterone buciclate for male contraception: endocrine differences between responders and nonresponders. J Clin Endocrinol Metab. 1995 Aug;80(8):2394–403.
Language	English

Compound	Testosterone (G03BA03)
Disease treated	Contraception
Quantification of dysfunction	Testicular histology
No. of patients treated	10
Age group	31–46
Treatment period	24 weeks
Treatment consequences	Spermatogenesis, impairment
Efficacy	In 5 of 5 men
Randomization of patients	Yes
Dose arms 1–3	200 mg/week; placebo
Study quality	**1–**
Reference	159: Zhengwei Y, Wreford NG, Royce P, de Kretser DM, McLachlan RI. Stereological evaluation of human spermatogenesis After suppression by testosterone treatment: heterogeneous pattern of spermatogenic impairment. J Clin Endocrinol Metab. 1998 Apr;83(4):1284–91.
Language	English

Compound	Testosterone (G03BA03)
Disease treated	Contraception
Quantification of dysfunction	Semen
No. of patients treated	8
Age group	Young
Treatment period	12 weeks
Dose	3×80 mg/day
Treatment consequences	Azoospermia, induction
Efficacy	In 1 of 8 men
Randomization of patients	No
Study quality	**3**
Reference	637: Nieschlag E, Hoogen H, Bolk M, Schuster H, Wickings EJ. Clinical trial with testosterone undecanoate for male fertility control. Contraception. 1978 Dec;18(6):607–14.
Language	English

Compound	Testosterone (G03BA03)
Disease treated	Contraception
Quantification of dysfunction	Semen
No. of patients treated	7
Age group	Young
Treatment period	Long term
Dose	250 mg/week
Treatment consequences	Spermatogenesis, impairment
Efficacy	All men, recovery after withdrawal
Randomization of patients	No
Study quality	**3**
Reference	649: Mauss J, Borsch G, Richter E, Bormacher K. Demonstration of the reversibility of spermatozoa suppression by testosterone oenanthate. Andrologia. 1978 Mar–Apr;10(2):149–53.
Language	English

Compound	Testosterone (G03BA03)
Disease treated	Contraception
Quantification of dysfunction	Semen
No. of patients treated	7
Age group	20–27 years
Treatment period	21
Dose	250 mg/week
Treatment consequences	Spermatogenesis, impairment
Efficacy	To mean 3 millions/ml
Side effects compromising effectiveness	Weight gain, reversible
Randomization of patients	No
Study quality	**3**
Reference	733: Mauss J, Borsch G, Bormacher K, Richter E, Leyendecker G, Nocke W. Effect of long-term testosterone oenanthate administration on male reproductive function: clinical evaluation, serum FSH, LH, testosterone, and seminal fluid analyses in normal men. Acta Endocrinol (Copenh). 1975 Feb;78(2):373–84.
Language	English

Compound	Testosterone (G03BA03)
Disease treated	Contraception
Quantification of dysfunction	Semen
No. of patients treated	4
Age group	Young
Treatment period	4 months
Dose	200 mg/week
Treatment consequences	Spermatogenesis, impairment
Efficacy	All, severe
Randomization of patients	No
Study quality	**3**
Reference	445: Matsumoto AM, Bremner WJ. Stimulation of sperm production by human chorionic gonadotropin after prolonged gonadotropin suppression in normal men. J Androl. 1985 May–Jun;6(3):137–43.

Language	English

Compound	Testosterone (G03BA03)+letrozole
Disease treated	Delayed puberty
Quantification of dysfunction	Erythropoiesis
No. of patients treated	23
Age group	Pubertal
Treatment period	12 months
Treatment consequences	Erythropoiesis, increase
Efficacy	Better increase in T+letrozole than in T+placebo
Randomization of patients	Yes
Dose arms 1–3	T+letrozole; T+placebo
Study quality	**1–**
Reference	829: Hero M, Wickman S, Hanhijarvi R, Siimes MA, Dunkel L. Pubertal upregulation of erythropoiesis in boys is determined primarily by androgen. J Pediatr. 2005 Feb;146(2):245–52.
Language	English

Compound	Testosterone (G03BA03)+letrozole
Disease treated	Delayed puberty
Quantification of dysfunction	Pubertal growth
No. of patients treated	23
Age group	Pubertal
Treatment period	12 months
Treatment consequences	Growth acceleration increase
Efficacy	In the T+letrozole group, not in T+placebo group
Randomization of patients	Yes
Dose arms 1–3	T+letrozole; T+placebo
Study quality	**1–**
Reference	830: Dunkel L, Wickman S. Novel treatment of short stature with aromatase inhibitors. J Steroid Biochem Mol Biol. 2003 Sep;86(3–5):345–56.
Language	English

2

Compound	Testosterone (G03BA03)
Disease treated	Hypogonadism, secondary
Quantification of dysfunction	Semen
No. of patients treated	16
Age group	Young
Treatment period	>12 months
Dose	200 mg/week
Treatment consequences	spermatogenesis, recovery
Efficacy	4 of 12
Randomization of patients	No
Remarks	Men with acquired hypogonadism treated with testosterone are not necessarily sterile, in contrast to patients with IHH
Study quality	**3**
Reference	35: Drincic A, Arseven OK, Sosa E, Mercado M, Kopp P, Molitch ME. Men with acquired hypogonadotropic hypogonadism treated with testosterone may be fertile. Pituitary. 2003;6(1):5–10.
Language	English

Compound	Testosterone (G03BA03)
Disease treated	Idiopathic hypogonadotropic hypogonadism (IHH)
Quantification of dysfunction	Semen
No. of patients treated	3
Age group	Young
Treatment period	n.g.
Treatment consequences	Spermatogenesis, maturation
Efficacy	No inhibition if T is given prior to gonadotropins
Randomization of patients	No
Study quality	**3**
Reference	572: Burger HG, de Kretser DM, Hudson B, Wilson JD. Effects of preceding androgen therapy on testicular response to human pituitary gonadotropin in hypogonadotropic hypogonadism: a study of three patients. Fertil Steril. 1981 Jan;35(1):64–8.
Language	English

Compound	Mesterolone (G03BB01)+tamoxifen
Disease treated	Infertility
Quantification of dysfunction	Semen
No. of patients treated	79
Age group	Young
Treatment period	6 months
Dose	Mesterolone 100 mg/day+20 mg/day tamoxifen
Treatment consequences	Sperm morphology, improvement
Efficacy	Significant
Randomization of patients	No
Study quality	**3**
Reference	54: Caroppo E, Niederberger C, Iacovazzi PA, Correale M, Palagiano A, D'Amato G. Human chorionic gonadotropin free beta-subunit in the human seminal plasma: a new marker for spermatogenesis? Eur J Obstet Gynecol Reprod Biol. 2003 Feb 10;106(2):165–9.
Language	English

G03	Sex Hormones and Modulators of the Genital System
G03C	*Oestrogens*

Oestrogens show dose-dependent antiandrogenic effects in male reproductive development and severely impair spermatogenesis of the adult male. They are not suitable for inducing azoospermia. In trials used for contraception, the side effects were inacceptable. In addition, oestrogen treatment may enhance the risk of induction of testicular tumours.

Overall level of evidence of adverse effects: C

Compound	Oestrogens (G03CA03)
Disease treated	Contraception
Quantification of dysfunction	Semen
No. of patients treated	26
Age group	Young
Treatment period	6 months

Treatment consequences	Azoospermia, induction
Efficacy	In 6 of 26 men
Side effects compromising effectiveness	Gynaecomastia, loss of libido
Randomization of patients	Yes
Dose arms 1–3	Implant of T 600 mg+10 mg oestradiol; implant of 600 mg T+20 mg oestradiol; implant of T 600 mg alone
Study quality	**1–**
Reference	124: Handelsman DJ, Wishart S, Conway AJ. Oestradiol enhances testosterone-induced suppression of human spermatogenesis. Hum Reprod. 2000 Mar;15(3):672–9.
Language	English

Compound	Oestrogens (G03CA03)
Disease treated	Transsexualism
Quantification of dysfunction	DNA flow cytometry of spermatozoa
No. of patients treated	8
Age group	24–32
Treatment period	Continuous
Dose	n.g.
Treatment consequences	Spermatogenesis, impairment
Efficacy	Maturation arrest
Randomization of patients	No
Study quality	**3**
Reference	252: Chiu AW, Chen MT, Chiang H, Wu LH, Fang RH, Chang LS. Deoxyribonucleic acid histogram of testes in primary transsexualism. Br J Urol. 1993 Oct;72(4):495–7.
Language	English

Compound	Oestrogens (G03CA03)
Disease treated	Healthy, testicular physiology
Quantification of dysfunction	Oestrogen effects
Age group	Embryo
Treatment consequences	Antiandrogen effects in male reproductive development

Efficacy	Dose dependent
Remarks	Disorders of male reproductive health in phenotypically normal males, such as cancer, oligozoospermia and failure of testicular descent have a common origin.
Study quality	**4 (review)**
Reference	99: Sharpe RM. Hormones and testis development and the possible adverse effects of environmental chemicals. Toxicol Lett. 2001 Mar 31;120(1–3):221–32.
Language	English

G03	**Sex Hormones and Modulators of the Genital system**
G03F	*Other Progestins*

19-nortestosterone is also able to depress spermatogenesis. It has been applied in trials with male contraception with moderate success. The compound has not been investigated further.

Overall level of evidence of adverse effects: B

Compound	19-nortestosterone hexyloxyphenylpropionate (19NT-HPP) (G03FA05)+buserelin
Disease treated	Contraception
Quantification of dysfunction	Semen
No. of patients treated	24
Age group	Young
Treatment period	30 weeks
Treatment consequences	Azoospermia, induction
Efficacy	4 of 8 men with nortestosterone alone, 4 of 16 men with buserelin added
Side effects compromising effectiveness	Haematocrit, increase
Randomization of patients	Yes
Dose arms 1–3	19NT-HPP 200 mg/3 weeks+buserelin implant 3.3 mg; 19NT-HPP 200 mg/3 weeks+buserelin implant 6.6 mg; 19NT-HPP 200 mg/3 weeks alone
Study quality	**1–**

Reference	284: Behre HM, Nashan D, Hubert W, Nieschlag E. Depot gonadotropin-releasing hormone agonist blunts the androgen-induced suppression of spermatogenesis in a clinical trial of male contraception. J Clin Endocrinol Metab. 1992 Jan;74(1):84–90.
Language	English

Compound	19-nortestosterone (G03FA05)+cetrorelix (H01CC02)
Disease treated	Contraception
Quantification of dysfunction	Semen
No. of patients treated	6
Age group	Young
Treatment period	26 weeks
Dose	2 mg/day
Treatment consequences	Azoospermia, induction
Efficacy	1 of 6
Randomization of patients	No
Study quality	**2–**
Reference	88: Behre HM, Kliesch S, Lemcke B, von Eckardstein S, Nieschlag E. Suppression of spermatogenesis to azoospermia by combined administration of GnRH antagonist and 19-nortestosterone cannot be maintained by this non-aromatizable androgen alone. Hum Reprod. 2001 Dec;16(12):2570–7.
Language	English

Compound	19-nortestosterone (G03FA05)
Disease treated	Contraception
Quantification of dysfunction	Semen
No. of patients treated	5
Age group	Young
Treatment period	13 weeks
Dose	200 mg/week
Treatment consequences	Azoospermia, induction
Efficacy	Achieved at 7–13 weeks of treatment
Randomization of patients	No

Study quality	2–
Reference	473: Schurmeyer T, Knuth UA, Belkien L, Nieschlag E. Reversible azoospermia induced by the anabolic steroid 19-nortestosterone. Lancet. 1984 Feb 25;1(8374):417–20.
Language	English

G03 **Sex Hormones and Modulators of the Genital System**

G03G *Gonadotropins*

Insufficient gonadotropin secretion from the pituitary gland results in hypogonadism. In these cases, exogenously applied gonadotropins stimulate testicular testosterone secretion. In addition, maturation of spermatogenesis is successfully achieved, when LH (substituted by hCG) and FSH (substituted by hMG) are applied together, in up to 90% of the patients. They also become fertile: pregnancies were reported in about half of the treated patients. The treatment is virtually free of side effects. Reports on the occurrence of gynaecomastia has to consider that gynaecomastia is common also in normal pubertal development.

The FSH was applied also in spermatogenic dysfunction resulting from different causes. In these cases, the success rate was lower and amounted to 50% of treated patients. The FSH in earlier years was substituted by human menopausal gonadotropin (hMG), but today the recombinant hormone (rFSH) is used.

The LH in studies was generally substituted by human chorionic gonadotropin (hCG), which is produced presently as a recombinant protein.

Overall level of evidence of positive effects: C
Overall level of evidence of adverse effects compromising effectiveness: C

Compound	hCG (G03GA01), FSH
Disease treated	Idiopathic hypogonadotropic hypogonadism (IHH)
Quantification of dysfunction	Semen
No. of patients treated	60
Age group	Young
Treatment period	6 months

Dose	5000 IU/week hCG+FSH 450 IU/week
Treatment consequences	Spermatogenesis, maturation
Efficacy	48 of 60 patients positive for spermatozoa in semen
Side effects compromising effectiveness	Gynaecomastia
Randomization of patients	No
Study quality	**2–**
Reference	182: Burgues S, Calderon MD. Subcutaneous self-administration of highly purified follicle stimulating hormone and human chorionic gonadotrophin for the treatment of male hypogonadotrophic hypogonadism. Spanish Collaborative Group on Male Hypogonadotropic Hypogonadism. Hum Reprod. 1997 May;12(5):980–6.
Language	English

Compound	hCG (G03GA01)
Disease treated	Idiopathic hypogonadotropic hypogonadism (IHH)
Quantification of dysfunction	Clinically, semen
No. of patients treated	36
Age group	11–42
Treatment period	n.g.
Dose	n.g.
Treatment consequences	Spermatogenesis, maturation
Efficacy	36% (group 1); 71% (group 2)
Side effects compromising effectiveness	Not mentioned
Randomization of patients	No
Dose arms 1–3	Small testis volume; normal testis volume
Study quality	**2–**
Reference	2: Miyagawa Y, Tsujimura A, Matsumiya K, Takao T, Tohda A, Koga M, Takeyama M. Outcome of gonadotropin therapy for male hypogonadotropic hypogonadism at university affiliated male infertility centers: a 30-year retrospective study. J Urol. 2005 Jun;173(6):2072–5.
Language	English

Compound	hCG (G03GA01), hMG
Disease treated	Idiopathic hypogonadotropic hypogonadism (IHH)
Quantification of dysfunction	Semen
No. of patients treated	35
Age group	Young
Treatment consequences	Spermatogenesis, maturation
Efficacy	One of 16 patients with hCG alone, 5 of 7 with hCG+hMG
Randomization of patients	No
Dose arms 1–3	hCG alone; hCG+hMG;
Study quality	**2–**
Reference	429: Finkel DM, Phillips JL, Snyder PJ. Stimulation of spermatogenesis by gonadotropins in men with hypogonadotropic hypogonadism. N Engl J Med. 1985 Sep 12;313(11):651–5.
Language	English

Compound	hCG (G03GA01), rFSH
Disease treated	Idiopathic hypogonadotropic hypogonadism (IHH)
Quantification of dysfunction	Semen, hormones
No. of patients treated	30
Age group	16–48
Treatment period	48 weeks
Treatment consequences	Spermatogenesis, maturation
Efficacy	In 14 of 30 subjects
Randomization of patients	Yes, in part
Dose arms 1–3	hCG 3000 IU/week+FSH 2×225 IU/week; hCG 3000 IU/week+FSH 3×150 IU/week
Study quality	**1–**
Reference	42: Bouloux PM, Nieschlag E, Burger HG, Skakkebaek NE, Wu FC, Handelsman DJ, Baker GH, Ochsenkuehn R, Syska A, McLachlan RI, Giwercman A, Conway AJ, Turner L, van Kuijk JH, Voortman G. Induction of spermatogenesis by recombinant follicle-stimulating hormone (puregon) in hypogonadotropic azoospermic men who failed to respond to human chorionic gonadotropin alone. J Androl. 2003 Jul–Aug;24(4):604–11.
Language	English

2

Compound	hCG (G03GA01), hMG
Disease treated	Delayed puberty after orchidopexy
Quantification of dysfunction	Semen
No. of patients treated	23
Age group	Young
Treatment period	Long term
Dose	n.g.
Treatment consequences	Spermatogenesis, maturation
Efficacy	5 of 12 vs 9 of 11
Randomization of patients	No
Study quality	**3**
Reference	491: Okuyama A, Namiki M, Aono T, Matsumoto K, Utsunomiya M, Itoh H, Yoshioka T, Itatani H, Sonoda T. Improvement of spermatogenesis by hCG and hMG treatment in pubertal boys with history of orchiopexy at early childhood. Arch Androl. 1984;12 Suppl:29–33.
Language	English

Compound	hCG (G03GA01)
Disease treated	Idiopathic hypogonadotropic hypogonadism (IHH)
Quantification of dysfunction	Semen, testicular volume
No. of patients treated	22
Age group	Young
Treatment period	>12 months
Dose	n.g.
Treatment consequences	Spermatogenesis, maturation
Efficacy	6 of 11 with complete, 9 of 11 with partial gonadotropin deficiency
Randomization of patients	No
Study quality	**3**
Reference	349: Burris AS, Rodbard HW, Winters SJ, Sherins RJ. Gonadotropin therapy in men with isolated hypogonadotropic hypogonadism: the response to human chorionic gonadotropin is predicted by initial testicular size. J Clin Endocrinol Metab. 1988 Jun;66(6):1144–51.
Language	English

Compound	hCG (G03GA01), hMG
Disease treated	Idiopathic hypogonadotropic hypogonadism (IHH)
Quantification of dysfunction	Semen
No. of patients treated	20
Age group	23.8 (mean)
Treatment period	5 years
Treatment consequences	Spermatogenesis, maturation
Efficacy	19 of 20 patients at 2.19 years (mean)
Randomization of patients	No
Study quality	**3**
Reference	282: Okada Y, Kondo T, Okamoto S, Ogawa M. Induction of ovulation and spermatogenesis by hMG/hCG in hypogonadotropic GH-deficient patients. Endocrinol Jpn. 1992 Feb;39(1):31–43.
Language	English

Compound	hCG (G03GA01), hMG
Disease treated	Idiopathic hypogonadotropic hypogonadism (IHH)
Quantification of dysfunction	T, semen, testicular volume
No. of patients treated	17
Age group	Young
Treatment period	14–120 months
Dose	n.g.
Treatment consequences	Spermatogenesis, maturation
Efficacy	13 of 17 patients
Side effects compromising effectiveness	Not mentioned
Randomization of patients	No
Study quality	**3**
Reference	277: Vicari E, Mongioi A, Calogero AE, Moncada ML, Sidoti G, Polosa P, D'Agata R. Therapy with human chorionic gonadotrophin alone induces spermatogenesis in men with isolated hypogonadotrophic hypogonadism: long-term follow-up. Int J Androl. 1992 Aug;15(4):320–9.
Language	English

Compound	hCG (G03GA01), hMG
Disease treated	Idiopathic hypogonadotropic hypogonadism (IHH)
Quantification of dysfunction	Semen
No. of patients treated	17
Age group	Young
Treatment period	52 months
Treatment consequences	Spermatogenesis, maturation
Efficacy	12 pregnancies
Randomization of patients	No
Dose arms 1–3	hCG 4000 IU/week+FSH 225 IU/week
Study quality	**3**
Reference	232: Kung AW, Zhong YY, Lam KS, Wang C. Induction of spermatogenesis with gonadotrophins in Chinese men with hypogonadotrophic hypogonadism. Int J Androl. 1994 Oct;17(5):241–7.
Language	English

Compound	hCG (G03GA01), hMG
Disease treated	Idiopathic hypogonadotropic hypogonadism (IHH)
Quantification of dysfunction	Hormones
No. of patients treated	16
Age group	Young
Treatment period	2 years
Dose	Various
Treatment consequences	Spermatogenesis, maturation
Efficacy	None in both groups After 12 months, 2 in GnRH and 8 in gonadotropin group after 24 months
Randomization of patients	Yes
Dose arms 1–3	GnRH pulsatile; gonadotropins
Study quality	**1–**
Reference	345: Liu L, Banks SM, Barnes KM, Sherins RJ. Two-year comparison of testicular responses to pulsatile gonadotropin-releasing hormone and exogenous gonadotropins from the inception of therapy in men with isolated hypogonadotropic hypogonadism. J Clin Endocrinol Metab. 1988 Dec;67(6):1140–5.
Language	English

Compound	hCG (G03GA01), FSH
Disease treated	Idiopathic hypogonadotropic hypogonadism (IHH)
Quantification of dysfunction	Hormones, semen
No. of patients treated	14
Age group	14–17 years
Treatment period	>12 months
Dose	Various
Treatment consequences	Pubertal development
Efficacy	Good effect
Randomization of patients	No
Study quality	**3**
Reference	140: Barrio R, de Luis D, Alonso M, Lamas A, Moreno JC. Induction of puberty with human chorionic gonadotropin and follicle-stimulating hormone in adolescent males with hypogonadotropic hypogonadism. Fertil Steril. 1999 Feb;71(2):244–8.
Language	English

Compound	hCG (G03GA01)
Disease treated	Idiopathic hypogonadotropic hypogonadism (IHH)
Quantification of dysfunction	Semen, hormones
No. of patients treated	13
Age group	Young
Treatment period	12 months
Dose	Various
Treatment consequences	Spermatogenesis, maturation
Efficacy	12 of 13 patients
Randomization of patients	No
Study quality	**3**
Reference	56: Depenbusch M, von Eckardstein S, Simoni M, Nieschlag E. Maintenance of spermatogenesis in hypogonadotropic hypogonadal men with human chorionic gonadotropin alone. Eur J Endocrinol. 2002 Nov;147(5):617–24.
Language	English

Compound	hCG (G03GA01), FSH
Disease treated	Idiopathic hypogonadotropic hypogonadism (IHH)
Quantification of dysfunction	Semen, hormones
No. of patients treated	10
Age group	Young
Treatment period	24 months
Treatment consequences	Spermatogenesis, maturation
Efficacy	In all men after 24 months
Randomization of patients	No
Dose arms 1–3	hCG 4500 IU/week+hMG 450 IU/week; hMG450 IU/week+T 250 mg/week
Study quality	**2–**
Reference	247: Schaison G, Young J, Pholsena M, Nahoul K, Couzinet B. Failure of combined follicle-stimulating hormone-testosterone administration to initiate and/or maintain spermatogenesis in men with hypogonadotropic hypogonadism. J Clin Endocrinol Metab. 1993 Dec;77(6):1545–9.
Language	English

Compound	hCG (G03GA01)
Disease treated	Spermatogenic dysfunction
Quantification of dysfunction	Semen
No. of patients treated	10
Age group	Young
Treatment period	Short-term
Dose	n.g.
Treatment consequences	Spermatogenesis, improvement
Efficacy	In 5 of 10 patients
Randomization of patients	No
Study quality	**3**
Reference	234: Radicioni A, Paris E, Dondero F, Bonifacio V, Isidori A. Recombinant-growth hormone (rec-hGH) therapy in infertile men with idiopathic oligozoospermia. Acta Eur Fertil. 1994 Sep–Oct;25(5):311–7.
Language	English

Compound	hCG (G03GA01), hMG
Disease treated	Thalassaemia
Quantification of dysfunction	Semen
No. of patients treated	10
Age group	15–23 years
Treatment period	2.1 years
Dose	Various
Treatment consequences	Spermatogenesis, maturation
Efficacy	In 7 of 10 patients occurrence of sperm with hCG alone
Randomization of patients	No
Study quality	**3**
Reference	344: De Sanctis V, Vullo C, Katz M, Wonke B, Nannetti C, Bagni B. Induction of spermatogenesis in thalassaemia. Fertil Steril. 1988 Dec;50(6):969–75.
Language	English

Compound	hCG (G03GA01)
Disease treated	Hypogonadism, secondary
Quantification of dysfunction	Hormones
No. of patients treated	3
Age group	Young
Dose	5000 IU/week
Treatment consequences	Spermatogenesis, recovery
Efficacy	Only with hCG+T
Randomization of patients	No
Study quality	**3**
Reference	467: Levalle O, Bokser L, Pacenza N, Aszenmil G, Fiszlejder L, Chervin A, Guitelman A. Restoration and maintenance of spermatogenesis by HCG therapy in patients with hypothalamo-hypophyseal damage. Andrologia. 1984 Jul–Aug;16(4):303–9.
Language	English

Compound	hCG (G03GA01)
Disease treated	Idiopathic hypogonadotropic hypogonadism (IHH)
Quantification of dysfunction	Semen

No. of patients treated	3
Age group	Young
Treatment period	Long term
Dose	n.g.
Treatment consequences	Spermatogenesis, maturation
Efficacy	In 2 of 3
Randomization of patients	No
Study quality	**3**
Reference	485: D'Agata R, Heindel JJ, Vicari E, Aliffi A, Gulizia S, Polosa P. hCG-induced maturation of the seminiferous epithelium in hypogonadotropic men. Horm Res. 1984;19(1):23–32.
Language	English

Compound	hCG (G03GA01), hMG
Disease treated	Hypogonadism, secondary
Quantification of dysfunction	Semen
No. of patients treated	1
Age group	Young
Treatment period	5 weeks
Dose	n.g.
Treatment consequences	Spermatogenesis, maturation
Efficacy	Also after testosterone pretreatment
Randomization of patients	No
Study quality	**3**
Reference	320: Hammar M, Berg AA. Long-term androgen replacement therapy does not preclude gonadotrophin-induced improvement on spermatogenesis. Scand J Urol Nephrol. 1990;24(1):17–9.
Language	English

Compound	hCG (G03GA01)
Disease treated	Idiopathic hypogonadotropic hypogonadism (IHH)
Quantification of dysfunction	Hormones
No. of patients treated	1
Age group	21
Treatment period	20 months

Dose	n.g.
Treatment consequences	Spermatogenesis, maturation
Efficacy	Complete
Study quality	**3**
Reference	564: Luboshitzky R, Dickstein G, Barzilai D. Induction of spermatogenesis in isolated hypogonadotropic hypogonadism with exogenous human chorionic gonadotropin. J Endocrinol Invest. 1981 Apr–Jun;4(2):217–9.
Language	English

Compound	hCG (G03GA01), FSH
Disease treated	Idiopathic hypogonadotropic hypogonadism (IHH)
Quantification of dysfunction	Semen
No. of patients treated	1
Age group	37
Treatment period	19 months
Dose	3×150 IU/week FSH, 5000 IU/week hCG
Treatment consequences	Pregnancy induction
Efficacy	28.3×10^6/ml spermatozoa after 16 months, natural conception
Randomization of patients	No
Study quality	**3**
Reference	181: Yong EL, Lee KO, Ng SC, Ratnam SS. Induction of spermatogenesis in isolated hypogonadotrophic hypogonadism with gonadotrophins and early intervention with intracytoplasmic sperm injection. Hum Reprod. 1997 Jun;12(6):1230–2.
Language	English

Compound	hCG (G03GA01), hMG
Disease treated	Idiopathic hypogonadotropic hypogonadism (IHH)
Quantification of dysfunction	Semen
No. of patients treated	1
Age group	Young
Treatment period	7 years
Dose	n.g.

2

Treatment consequences	Spermatogenesis, maturation
Efficacy	After induction with hCG/hMG maintenance with hCG alone
Study quality	**3**
Reference	636: Johnsen SG. Maintenance of spermatogenesis induced by HMG treatment by means of continuous HCG treatment in hypogonadotrophic men. Acta Endocrinol (Copenh). 1978 Dec;89(4):763–9.
Language	English

Compound	hCG (G03GA01), hMG
Disease treated	Idiopathic hypogonadotropic hypogonadism (IHH)
Quantification of dysfunction	Semen
No. of patients treated	1
Age group	Young
Treatment period	n.g.
Dose	n.g.
Treatment consequences	Spermatogenesis, maturation
Efficacy	Pregnancy induced
Study quality	**3**
Reference	638: Spitz IM, Schumert Z, Steiner J, Rosen E, Segal S, Slonim A, Rabinowitz D. Induction of spermatogenesis in hypogonadotrophic hypogonadism. Postgrad Med J. 1978 Oct;54(636):694–7.
Language	English

Compound	hCG (G03GA01)
Disease treated	Spermatogenic dysfunction
Quantification of dysfunction	Semen
No. of patients treated	1
Age group	Young
Treatment period	n.g.
Dose	n.g.
Treatment consequences	Spermatogenesis, maturation
Efficacy	Only with combination of hMG
Randomization of patients	No

Dose arms 1–3	hCG alone; hCG+hMG
Study quality	**3**
Reference	342: Hammar M, Berg AA, Kjessler B. hCG-treatment alone is insufficient for restitution of spermatogenesis in a state with arrest at the spermatogonial level. Scand J Urol Nephrol. 1989;23(4):247–9.
Language	English

Compound	FSH (G03GA04)
Disease treated	Varicocele
Quantification of dysfunction	Semen
No. of patients treated	183
Age group	18–45 years
Treatment period	3 months
Treatment consequences	Spermatogenesis, improvement
Efficacy	Clear-cut improvement
Randomization of patients	No
Dose arms 1–3	High ligation+FSH 75 IU/2 days; high ligation alone
Study quality	**2–**
Reference	117: Zarrilli S, Paesano L, Colao A, Mirone V, Lombardi G, Rosa M de. FSH treatment improves sperm function in patients after varicocelectomy. J Endocrinol Invest. 2000 Feb;23(2):68–73.
Language	English

Compound	FSH (G03GA04)
Disease treated	Poor sperm parameters
Quantification of dysfunction	Semen
No. of patients treated	135
Age group	Young
Treatment period	3 months
Dose	75 IU/2 days
Treatment consequences	Spermatogenesis, improvement
Efficacy	Significant increase only in oligozoospermic subjects with normal basal FSH and inhibin-B plasma levels
Randomization of patients	No

Dose arms 1–3	Group A: normal FSH and inhibin B; group B: high FSH and normal inhibin B; group C: high FSH and low inhibin B
Study quality	**2–**
Reference	118: Foresta C, Bettella A, Merico M, Garolla A, Plebani M, Ferlin A, Rossato M. FSH in the treatment of oligozoospermia. Mol Cell Endocrinol. 2000 Mar 30;161(1–2):89–97.
Language	English

Compound	FSH (G03GA04)
Disease treated	Infertility
Quantification of dysfunction	Semen
No. of patients treated	108
Age group	Young
Treatment period	3 months
Dose	3×75 IU/week
Treatment consequences	Sperm retrieval by TESE
Efficacy	In 40 of 63 patients treated with pFSH and 15/45 patients not treated
Randomization of patients	No
Dose arms 1–3	FSH; no FSH
Study quality	**2–**
Reference	998: Aydos K, Unlu C, Demirel LC, Evirgen O, Tolunay O. The effect of pure FSH administration in non-obstructive azoospermic men on testicular sperm retrieval. Eur J Obstet Gynecol Reprod Biol. 2003 May 1;108(1):54–8.
Language	English

Compound	FSH (G03GA04)
Disease treated	Infertility
Quantification of dysfunction	Semen
No. of patients treated	90
Age group	Young
Treatment period	3 months
Dose	3×75 IU/week
Treatment consequences	Spermatogenesis, improvement
Efficacy	In 20 of 60 patients

Randomization of patients	Yes
Dose arms 1–3	FSH; placebo
Study quality	**1–**
Reference	160: Foresta C, Bettella A, Ferlin A, Garolla A, Rossato M. Evidence for a stimulatory role of follicle-stimulating hormone on the spermatogonial population in adult males. Fertil Steril. 1998 Apr;69(4):636–42.
Language	English

Compound	FSH (G03GA04)
Disease treated	Infertilility
Quantification of dysfunction	Semen
No. of patients treated	44
Age group	28–45 years
Treatment period	12 weeks
Dose	3×150 IU/week
Treatment consequences	Pregnancy rate induced, increase
Efficacy	33% in the treated group and 20% in the control group
Randomization of patients	Yes
Dose arms 1–3	FSH; placebo
Study quality	**1–**
Reference	30. Baccetti B, Piomboni P, Bruni E, Capitani S, Gambera L, Moretti E, Sterzik K, Strehler E. Effect of follicle-stimulating hormone on sperm quality and pregnancy rate. Asian J Androl. 2004 Jun;6(2):133–7.
Language	English

Compound	FSH (G03GA04)
Disease treated	Idiopathic hypogonadotropic hypogonadism (IHH)
Quantification of dysfunction	Hormones, semen
No. of patients treated	42
Age group	Young
Treatment period	12 months
Dose	Various
Treatment consequences	Spermatogenesis, maturation
Efficacy	Pregnancy in the partners of 36 of 42 patients

Randomization of patients	No
Dose arms 1–3	hCG+hMG; GnRH pulsatile
Study quality	**2–**
Reference	150: Buchter D, Behre HM, Kliesch S, Nieschlag E. Pulsatile GnRH or human chorionic gonadotropin/human menopausal gonadotropin as effective treatment for men with hypogonadotropic hypogonadism: a review of 42 cases. Eur J Endocrinol. 1998 Sep;139(3):298–303.
Language	English

Compound	FSH (G03GA04)
Disease treated	Infertility
Quantification of dysfunction	Semen
No. of patients treated	30
Age group	Young
Treatment period	4 months
Dose	300 IU/2 days
Treatment consequences	Sperm count, increase
Efficacy	Significant
Randomization of patients	Yes
Dose arms 1–3	FSH; placebo
Study quality	**1+**
Reference	8. Paradisi R, Busacchi P, Seracchioli R, Porcu E, Venturoli S. Effects of high doses of recombinant human follicle-stimulating hormone in the treatment of male factor infertility: results of a pilot study. Fertil Steril. 2006 Sep;86(3):728–31.
Language	English

Compound	hMG (G03GA04)
Disease treated	Idiopathic hypogonadotropic hypogonadism (IHH)
Quantification of dysfunction	Semen
No. of patients treated	9
Age group	Young
Treatment period	12 months
Dose	525 IU/week

Treatment consequences	Spermatogenesis, maturation
Efficacy	Pregnancy in the partners of 3 of 9 patients
Randomization of patients	No
Study quality	**3**
Reference	261: Jones TH, Darne JF. Self-administered subcutaneous human menopausal gonadotrophin for the stimulation of testicular growth and the initiation of spermatogenesis in hypogonadotrophic hypogonadism. Clin Endocrinol (Oxf). 1993 Feb;38(2):203–8.
Language	English

Compound	Gonadotropins (G03GA04)
Disease treated	Anabolic steroid abuse
Quantification of dysfunction	Semen
No. of patients treated	1
Age group	Young
Treatment period	5 years
Dose	n.g.
Treatment consequences	Azoospermia induced by anabolic steroids, reversal
Efficacy	Conception after 3 months
Randomization of patients	No
Study quality	**3**
Reference	217: Turek PJ, Williams RH, Gilbaugh JH III, Lipshultz LI. The reversibility of anabolic steroid-induced azoospermia. J Urol. 1995 May;153(5):1628–30.
Language	English

Compound	FSH (G03GA04)
Disease treated	Y-Deletion with azoospermia
Quantification of dysfunction	Semen
No. of patients treated	1
Age group	32
Treatment period	6 months
Dose	n.g.
Treatment consequences	Spermatogenesis, improvement

Efficacy	Small number of spermatozoa in semen
Study quality	**3**
Reference	20: Selman HA, Cipollone G, Stuppia L, Santo M de, Sterzik K, El-Danasouri I. Gonadotropin treatment of an azoospermic patient with a Y-chromosome microdeletion. Fertil Steril. 2004 Jul;82(1):218–9.
Language	English

G03	**Sex Hormones and Modulators of the Genital System**
G03H	*Antiandrogens*

Cyproterone acetate (CPA) depresses spermatogenic activity. This effect appears to be a consequence of the suppression of gonadotropin secretion, not of the antiandrogenic activity. As a consequence, testosterone levels decrease; together with the antiandrogenic activity in the other target organs, a depression of libido and erectile function occurs; thus, the compound is not suitable for male contraception.

Overall level of evidence of positive effects: B
Overall level of evidence of adverse effects compromising effectiveness: B

Compound	Cyproterone acetate (G03HA01)
Disease treated	Contraception
Quantification of dysfunction	Hormones, semen
No. of patients treated	25
Age group	Young
Treatment period	21 days
Treatment consequences	Gonadotropin levels, decline
Efficacy	Profound suppression
Side effects compromising effectiveness	None
Randomization of patients	Yes
Dose arms 1–3	10 mg/day CPA+10 mg/day dienogestrel; 10 mg/day CPA+5 mg/day dienogestrel; 10 mg/day CPA+placebo
Study quality	**1–**

Reference	77: Meriggiola MC, Bremner WJ, Costantino A, Bertaccini A, Morselli-Labate AM, Huebler D, Kaufmann G, Oettel M, Flamigni C. Twenty-one day administration of dienogest reversibly suppresses gonadotropins and testosterone in normal men. J Clin Endocrinol Metab. 2002 May;87(5):2107–13.
Language	English

Compound	Cyproterone acetate (G03HA01)
Disease treated	Contraception
Quantification of dysfunction	Semen, hormones
No. of patients treated	24
Age group	Young
Treatment period	32 weeks
Treatment consequences	Azoospermia, induction
Efficacy	In all men
Randomization of patients	Yes
Dose arms 1–3	2 mg/day CPA+T 1000 mg/6 weeks; 20 mg/day CPA+T 1000 mg/6 weeks; placebo+T 1000 mg/6 weeks
Study quality	**1–**
Reference	36: Meriggiola MC, Costantino A, Cerpolini S, Bremner WJ, Huebler D, Morselli-Labate AM, Kirsch B, Bertaccini A, Pelusi C, Pelusi G. Testosterone undecanoate maintains spermatogenic suppression induced by cyproterone acetate plus testosterone undecanoate in normal men. J Clin Endocrinol Metab. 2003 Dec;88(12):5818–26.
Language	English

Compound	Cyproterone acetate (G03HA01)
Disease treated	Contraception
Quantification of dysfunction	Semen
No. of patients treated	23
Age group	Young
Treatment period	16 weeks
Treatment consequences	Azoospermia, induction
Efficacy	In only 1 of 12, but lower sperm count in all men
Randomization of patients	No

Dose arms 1–3	10 mg/day CPA; 5 mg/day CPA; placebo
Study quality	**2–**
Reference	595: Wang C, Yeung KK. Use of low-dosage oral cyproterone acetate as a male contraceptive. Contraception. 1980 Mar;21(3):245–72.
Language	English

Compound	Cyproterone acetate (G03HA01)
Disease treated	Contraception
Quantification of dysfunction	Semen
No. of patients treated	18
Age group	21–45 years
Treatment period	16 weeks
Treatment consequences	Azoospermia, induction
Efficacy	Lower T dose leads to stronger suppression of sperm
Randomization of patients	No
Dose arms 1–3	5 mg/day CPA+T100 mg/day; 5 mg/day CPA+T200 mg/day
Study quality	**2–**
Reference	64: Meriggiola MC, Costantino A, Bremner WJ, Morselli-Labate AM. Higher testosterone dose impairs sperm suppression induced by a combined androgen–progestin regimen. J Androl. 2002 Sep–Oct;23(5):684–90.
Language	English

Compound	Cyproterone acetate (G03HA01)
Disease treated	Contraception
Quantification of dysfunction	Semen
No. of patients treated	10
Age group	Young
Treatment period	16 weeks
Treatment consequences	Azoospermia, induction
Efficacy	In 10 of 10 men
Side effects compromising effectiveness	Haemoglobin, depression
Randomization of patients	Yes

Dose arms 1–3	25 mg/day CPA+T; 12.5 mg/day CPA+T
Study quality	**1–**
Reference	154: Meriggiola MC, Bremner WJ, Costantino A, Cintio G di, Flamigni C. Low dose of cyproterone acetate and testosterone enanthate for contraception in men. Hum Reprod. 1998 May;13(5):1225–9.
Language	English

Compound	Cyproterone acetate (G03HA01)
Disease treated	Contraception
Quantification of dysfunction	Hormones
No. of patients treated	10
Age group	Young
Treatment period	12 weeks
Dose	10 mg/day
Treatment consequences	Gonadotropin levels, decline; sperm motility, impairment
Efficacy	Suppression by 30–40%; inhibition
Side effects compromising effectiveness	No serious
Randomization of patients	No
Study quality	**3**
Reference	590: Moltz L, Rommler A, Post K, Schwartz U, Hammerstein J. Medium dose cyproterone acetate (CPA): effects on hormone secretion and on spermatogenesis in men. Contraception. 1980 Apr;21(4):393–413.
Language	English

Compound	Cyproterone acetate (G03HA01)
Disease treated	Contraception
Quantification of dysfunction	Semen
No. of patients treated	n.g.
Age group	Young
Treatment period	28 weeks
Treatment consequences	Spermatogenesis, impairment
Efficacy	All

2

Side effects compromising effectiveness	Testosterone levels decreased, libido and potency were not altered
Randomization of patients	Yes
Dose arms 1–3	5 mg/day CPA; 10 mg/day CPA
Study quality	**2–**
Reference	618: Roy S, Chatterjee S. Studies with cyproterone acetate for male contraception. J Steroid Biochem. 1979 Jul;11(1B):675–80.
Language	English

Compound	Cyproterone acetate (G03HA01)
Disease treated	Infertility
Quantification of dysfunction	Semen
No. of patients treated	n.g.
Age group	Young
Treatment consequences	Spermatogenesis, impairment
Efficacy	Morphological anomalies of midpiece and tail after 2 weeks, and of heads after 4 weeks
Randomization of patients	No
Study quality	**4 (review)**
Reference	654: Fredricsson B. On the development of different morphologic abnormalities of human spermatozoa. Andrologia. 1978 Jan–Feb;10(1):43–8.
Language	English

G03	**Sex Hormones and Modulators of the Genital System**
G03X	*Other Sex Hormones and Modulators of the Genital System*

This group of drugs summarizes chemically and biologically extremely different compounds. Some drugs were used with the aim to improve spermatogenesis and fertility, such as *chlomiphene* and *kallikrein*. The efficacy of the two compounds remains questionable: they are no longer available as prescription drugs. Severe adverse effects, on the other hand, have not been reported.

Overall level of evidence of positive effects: C

Overall level of evidence of adverse effects compromising effectiveness: C

Other compounds have been designed for contraceptive purposes. None of them have been launched for clinical use, particularly because of severe adverse effects. The progestin gestrinone decreased severely sexual libido; the androgen 7-α-methyl-nortestosterone (MENT) is only weakly effective. Alpha-chlorhydrine, similarly to other halogenated sugars, inhibited epididymal maturation of spermatozoa effectively, but unfortunately it is not harmful to animals (rat, hamster, guinea pig, ram, rhesus monkey). It has never been tested in humans. Gossypol (extract from cotton seed) effectively inhibits spermatogenesis and has been described as an ideal male contraceptive; however, the recovery after cessation of application is insufficient, and up to 40% of men remained infertile. Nonoxinol inhibited sperm motility in vitro effectively. It is used as a vaginal contraceptive.

Overall level of evidence of positive effects: B
Overall level of evidence of adverse effects compromising effectiveness: C

Compound	Clomiphene (not listed)
Disease treated	Spermatogenic dysfunction
Quantification of dysfunction	Semen
No. of patients treated	35
Age group	Young
Treatment period	n.g.
Dose	n.g.
Treatment consequences	LH response to GnRH
Efficacy	Increase during treatment
Side effects compromising effectiveness	Not mentioned
Randomization of patients	No
Dose arms 1–3	Clomiphen in hypozoospermia; clomiphen in normozoospermia
Study quality	**2–**
Reference	565: Johnsen SG. Clomiphene stimulation test in men with idiopathic hypospermatogenesis. Acta Endocrinol (Copenh). 1981 Apr;96(4):557–63.
Language	English

Compound	Clomiphene (not listed)
Disease treated	Infertility
Quantification of dysfunction	Semen
No. of patients treated	35
Age group	Young
Treatment period	9 months
Dose	50 mg/day
Treatment consequences	Spermatogenesis, improvement
Efficacy	31 of 35 men, 8 pregnancies
Randomization of patients	No
Study quality	**3**
Reference	696: Paulson DF, Wacksman J. Clomiphene citrate in the management of male infertility. J Urol. 1976 Jan;115(1):73–6.
Language	English

Compound	Clomiphene (not listed)
Disease treated	Spermatogenic dysfunction
Quantification of dysfunction	Semen
No. of patients treated	30
Age group	Young
Treatment period	3 months
Dose	50 mg/day
Treatment consequences	Spermatogenesis, improvement
Efficacy	13.3 to 28.7–10^6 sperm in the verum group, no change in placebo group
Side effects compromising effectiveness	None
Randomization of patients	Yes
Dose arms 1–3	Clomiphene; placebo
Study quality	**1–**
Reference	578: Ronnberg L. The effect of clomiphene citrate on different sperm parameters and serum hormone levels in preselected infertile men: a controlled double-blind cross-over study. Int J Androl. 1980 Oct;3(5):479–86.
Language	English

Compound	Kallikrein (not listed)
Disease treated	Infertility
Quantification of dysfunction	Semen
No. of patients treated	90
Age group	Young
Treatment period	7 weeks
Dose	600 U/day
Treatment consequences	Pregnancy induction
Efficacy	38% in kallikrein group, 16% in placebo group
Side effects compromising effectiveness	None
Randomization of patients	Yes
Dose arms 1–3	Kallikrein 600 U/day; placebo
Study quality	**1+**
Reference	625: Schill WB. Treatment of idiopathic oligozoospermia by kallikrein: results of a double-blind study. Arch Androl. 1979 Mar;2(2):163–70.
Language	English

Compound	Kallikrein (not listed)
Disease treated	Infertility
Quantification of dysfunction	Semen
No. of patients treated	51
Age group	Young
Treatment period	7 weeks
Dose	600 U/day
Treatment consequences	Pregnancy induction
Efficacy	In partners of 31% of patients
Side effects compromising effectiveness	None
Randomization of patients	No
Study quality	**3**
Reference	666: Kienitz T, Schill WB. Oral kallikrein-therapy of asthenozoospermia. Fortschr Med. 1977 Sep 15;95(34):2102–5.

Language	German

Compound	Kallikrein (not listed)
Disease treated	Spermatogenic dysfunction
Quantification of dysfunction	Semen
No. of patients treated	16
Age group	Young
Treatment period	120 days
Dose	600 U/day
Treatment consequences	Spermatogenesis, improvement
Efficacy	Significant
Side effects compromising effectiveness	None
Randomization of patients	Yes
Dose arms 1–3	Kallikrein 200 mg/day; vitamin E 200 mg/day
Study quality	**1–**
Reference	388: Giovenco P, Amodei M, Barbieri C, Fasani R, Carosi M, Dondero F. Effects of kallikrein on the male reproductive system and its use in the treatment of idiopathic oligozoospermia with impaired motility. Andrologia. 1987 Jun;19 Spec No:238–41.
Language	English

Compound	Gestrinone (G03XA02)
Disease treated	Contraception
Quantification of dysfunction	Semen
No. of patients treated	20
Age group	25–35 years
Treatment period	Long term
Treatment consequences	Spermatogenesis, impairment
Efficacy	8 azoospermic with T+gestrinone, 7 with gestrinone alone
Side effects compromising effectiveness	Decrease of libido and other sexual functions
Randomization of patients	Yes

Dose arms 1–3	50 µg/week gestrinone+T; 100 µg/day gestrinone+T; 100 µg/day gestrinone+placebo
Study quality	**1–**
Reference	685: Salat-Baroux J, Le Lorier G, Sakiz E, Rotman J, Piquet JM. Preliminary trials of an oral chemical contraceptive for men. J Gynecol Obstet Biol Reprod (Paris). 1976 Sep;5(6):831–42.
Language	French

Compound	7-α-methyl-nortestosterone (MENT) (not listed)
Disease treated	Contraception
Quantification of dysfunction	Semen, hormone
No. of patients treated	35
Age group	Young
Treatment period	6 months
Dose	MENT implants, releasing 400 µg/day
Treatment consequences	Spermatogenesis, impairment
Efficacy	Dose-related depression of spermatogenesis
Side effects compromising effectiveness	Not mentioned
Randomization of patients	Yes
Dose arms 1–3	MENT 1 implant; MENT 2 implants; MENT implants
Study quality	**1+**
Reference	37: Eckardstein S von, Noe G, Brache V, Nieschlag E, Croxatto H, Alvarez F, Moo-Young A, Sivin I, Kumar N, Small M, Sundaram K. International Committee for Contraception Research, The Population Council. A clinical trial of 7 alpha-methyl-19-nortestosterone implants for possible use as a long-acting contraceptive for men. J Clin Endocrinol Metab. 2003 Nov;88(11):5232–9.
Language	English

Compound	α chlorhydrine (not listed)
Disease treated	Contraception
Quantification of dysfunction	Sperm motility
Age group	Rat
Treatment consequences	Spermatogenesis, impairment

Efficacy	S-enantiomer is more effective.
Side effects compromising effectiveness	Kidney toxicity by R-enantiomer
Randomization of patients	No
Remarks	α-chlorohydrins are not harmful to animals (rat, hamster, guinea pig, ram, rhesus monkey), not tested in humans
Study quality	**4 (review)**
Reference	138: Jones AR, Cooper TG. A re-appraisal of the post-testicular action and toxicity of chlorinated antifertility compounds. Intern J Androl 1999;22;130–138.
Language	English

Compound	α chlorhydrine (not listed)
Disease treated	Contraception
Quantification of dysfunction	Semen
Age group	Men and animals
Treatment consequences	Spermatogenesis, impairment
Efficacy	Recovery after withdrawal
Side effects compromising effectiveness	Neurotoxic
Randomization of patients	No
Remarks	Toxicity of α-chlorohydrin in humans is unknown
Study quality	**4 (review)**
Reference	518: Jones AR. Antifertility actions of alpha-chlorohydrin in the male. Aust J Biol Sci. 1983;36(4):333–50.
Language	English

Compound	Gossypol (not listed)
Disease treated	Contraception
Quantification of dysfunction	Semen
No. of patients treated	151
Age group	Young
Treatment period	56 weeks
Treatment consequences	Spermatogenesis, impairment

Efficacy	81 of 81
Side effects compromising effectiveness	None
Randomization of patients	Yes
Dose arms 1–3	gossypol 7.5 mg/day; gossypol 10 mg/day
Study quality	**1+**
Reference	119: Coutinho EM, Athayde C, Atta G, Gu ZP, Chen ZW, Sang GW, Emuveyan E, Adekunle AO, Mati J, Otubu J, Reidenberg MM, Segal SJ. Gossypol blood levels and inhibition of spermatogenesis in men taking gossypol as a contraceptive. A multicenter, international, dose-finding study. Contraception. 2000 Jan;61(1):61–7.
Language	English

Compound	Gossypol (not listed)
Disease treated	Contraception
Quantification of dysfunction	Semen
No. of patients treated	46
Age group	Young
Treatment period	12 months
Dose	Total mean dose 8.5 g (range 2.5–27.5 g)
Treatment consequences	Spermatogenesis, recovery after cessation
Efficacy	61% in 1.1 years
Randomization of patients	No
Study quality	**3**
Reference	360: Meng GD, Zhu JC, Chen ZW, Wong LT, Zhang GY, Hu YZ, Ding JH, Wang XH, Qian SZ, Wang C et al. Recovery of sperm production following the cessation of gossypol treatment: a two-centre study in China. Int J Androl. 1988 Feb;11(1):1–11.
Language	English

Compound	Gossypol (not listed)
Disease treated	Contraception
Quantification of dysfunction	Semen
No. of patients treated	35

Age group	Young
Treatment period	70 days
Dose	20 mg
Treatment consequences	Azoospermia, induction
Efficacy	100%, after recovery 8 men azoospermic
Randomization of patients	No
Study quality	**3**
Reference	314: Gu ZP, Wang YX, Sang GW, Wang WC, Chen ZX, Zhao XJ, Shao QX, Jiang Y. Relationship between hormone profiles and the restoration of spermatogenesis in men treated with gossypol. Int J Androl. 1990 Aug;13(4):253–7.
Language	English

Compound	Gossypol (not listed)
Disease treated	Contraception
Quantification of dysfunction	Semen, hormones
No. of patients treated	26
Age group	27–51 years
Treatment period	52 weeks
Dose	20 mg/day
Treatment consequences	Spermatogenesis, impairment; FSH levels, increase
Efficacy	Low sperm count after 3 months; FSH continuously elevated
Randomization of patients	No
Study quality	**3**
Reference	439: Zhang GY, Xiao B, Chen ZW, Zhu JC, Meng GD. Dynamic study of serum gonadotrophin and testosterone levels in gossypol-treated men. Long-term follow-up study of 60 cases. Int J Androl. 1985 Jun;8(3):177–85.
Language	English

Compound	Nonoxinol (not listed)
Disease treated	Healthy
Quantification of dysfunction	Sperm motility in vitro
No. of patients treated	50
Treatment period	In vitro

Treatment consequences	Sperm motility, decrease
Efficacy	Complete, not based on Ca2+ influx
Randomization of patients	No
Study quality	**2–**
Reference	885: White DR, Clarkson JS, Ratnasooriya WD, Aitken RJ. Complementary effects of propranolol and nonoxynol-9 upon human sperm motility. Contraception. 1995 Oct;52(4):241–7.
Language	English

G04 Urologicals

Because of the widespread use of 5-phosphodiesterase inhibitors in men with erectile dysfunction, it is essential to test these substances for adverse effects on spermatogenesis, even if the majority of patients treated is beyond the fertile age. Some randomized prospective trials did not reveal arguments for this concern.

Finasteride, which is used for androgenic alopecia also in young men, did not exert unfavourable effects on spermatogenesis.

The inhibition of testosterone effects by casodex in prostatic carcinoma was not associated with severe impairment of spermatogenesis.

Overall level of evidence of adverse effects: A

Compound	Sildenafil (G04BE03)
Disease treated	Healthy
Quantification of adverse effects	Semen
No. of patients treated	20
Age group	32 years (mean)
Treatment period	Single dose
Dose	100 mg
Treatment consequences	Sperm parameters, alteration
Efficacy	No changes in seminal parameters when compared with placebo
Randomization of patients	Yes

Dose arms 1–3	Sildenafil; placebo
Study quality	**1–**
Reference	130: Aversa A, Mazzilli F, Rossi T, Delfino M, Isidori AM, Fabbri A. Effects of sildenafil (Viagra) administration on seminal parameters and post-ejaculatory refractory time in normal males. Hum Reprod. 2000 Jan; 15(1): 131–4.
Language	English

Compound	Sildenafil (G04BE03)
Disease treated	Healthy
Quantification of adverse effects	Semen
No. of patients treated	17
Age group	19–34 years
Treatment period	Single dose
Dose	100 mg
Treatment consequences	Sperm parameters, alteration
Efficacy	No statistically significant effect
Randomization of patients	Yes
Dose arms 1–3	Sildenafil; placebo
Study quality	**1–**
Reference	129: Purvis K, Muirhead GJ, Harness JA. The effects of sildenafil on human sperm function in healthy volunteers. Br J Clin Pharmacol. 2002;53 Suppl 1:53S–60S.
Language	English

Compound	Tadalafil (G04BE08)
Disease treated	Erectile dysfunction
Quantification of adverse effects	Semen, hormones
No. of patients treated	421
Age group	>45 years
Treatment period	6 months
Dose	20 mg
Treatment consequences	Spermatogenesis, impairment
Efficacy	No effect
Randomization of patients	Yes
Dose arms 1–3	Tadalafil; placebo

Study quality	**1++**
Reference	40: Hellstrom WJ, Overstreet JW, Yu A, Saikali K, Shen W, Beasley CM Jr, Watkins VS. Tadalafil has no detrimental effect on human spermatogenesis or reproductive hormones. J Urol. 2003 Sep;170(3):887–91.
Language	English

Compound	Finasteride (G04CB01)
Disease treated	Healthy
Quantification of adverse effects	Semen
No. of patients treated	181
Age group	19–41 years
Treatment period	48 weeks
Dose	1 mg/day
Treatment consequences	Spermatogenesis, impairment
Efficacy	No effect
Randomization of patients	Yes
Dose arms 1–3	Finasteride 5 mg/day; placebo
Study quality	**1++**
Reference	131: Overstreet JW, Fuh VL, Gould J, Howards SS, Lieber MM, Hellstrom W, Shapiro S, Carroll P, Corfman RS, Petrou S, Lewis R, Toth P, Shown T, Roy J, Jarow JP, Bonilla J, Jacobsen CA, Wang DZ, Kaufman KD. Chronic treatment with finasteride daily does not affect spermatogenesis or semen production in young men. J Urol. 1999 Oct;162(4):1295–300.
Language	English

Compound	Casodex (not listed)
Disease treated	Cancer, prostate
Quantification of adverse effects	Testicular histology
No. of patients treated	34
Age group	Old
Treatment period	n.g.
Dose	50 mg/day
Treatment consequences	Leydig cells, hyperplasia
Efficacy	Not increased in comparison with controls

Randomization of patients	No
Dose arms 1–3	Casodex; orchidectomy
Study quality	**2–**
Reference	43: Jones HB, Betton GR, Bowdler AL, McFarquhar RL, Middleton BJ, Lunglmayr G. Pathological and morphometric assessment of testicular parameters in patients with metastatic prostate cancer following treatment with either the antiandrogen Casodex (ZM176,334) or bilateral orchidectomy. Urol Res. 1994;22(3):191–5.
Language	English

Compound	Casodex (not listed)
Disease treated	Cancer, prostate
Quantification of adverse effects	Testicular histology
No. of patients treated	5
Age group	55–78 years
Treatment period	12 months
Dose	50 mg/day
Treatment consequences	Spermatogenesis, impairment
Efficacy	Not significantly
Randomization of patients	No
Study quality	**3**
Reference	242: Bjerklund Johansen TE, Majak M, Nesland JM. Testicular histology after treatment with the new antiandrogen Casodex for carcinoma of the prostate. A preliminary report. Scand J Urol Nephrol. 1994 Mar;28(1):67–70.
Language	English

H01 Pituitary and Hypothalamic Hormones and Analogues

It has been suggested that somatotropin might have a positive effect on spermatogenesis owing to its general effect as a growth hormone. This was, however, demonstrated neither in hypogonadal boys nor in infertile men. The addition of somatotropin did not improve the effect of gonadotropins, but a higher rate of side effects was observed.

Since oxytocin plays a role in epididymal motility, the application of oxytocin was expected to improve sperm parameters. No significant effects could be proven.

Overall level of evidence of positive effects: B
Overall level of evidence of adverse effects compromising effectiveness: C

Compound	Somatotropin (H01AC01)
Disease treated	Spermatogenic dysfunction
Quantification of dysfunction	Semen, fertility
No. of patients treated	18
Age group	Young
Treatment period	12 weeks
Dose	6 U/day
Treatment consequences	Pregnancy induced
Efficacy	Three pregnancies in the nine couples from the asthenozoospermic group, 0 pregnancies in the oligozoospermic group
Side effects compromising effectiveness	Not mentioned
Randomization of patients	No
Dose arms 1–3	Oligo-astheno-teratozoospermia; asthenozoospermia
Study quality	**3**
Reference	194: Ovesen P, Jorgensen JO, Ingerslev J, Ho KK, Orskov H, Christiansen JS. Growth hormone treatment of subfertile males. Fertil Steril. 1996 Aug;66(2):292–8.
Language	English

Compound	Somatotropin (H01AC01)
Disease treated	Infertility
Quantification of dysfunction	Semen
No. of patients treated	15
Age group	Young
Treatment period	n.g.
Dose	n.g.
Treatment consequences	Spermatogenesis, improvement

Efficacy	Not statistically significant
Study quality	**3**
Reference	193: Ng SC, Lee KO. Treatment of male infertility with growth hormone. Clin Sci (Lond). 1996 Sep;91(3):254–5.
Language	English

Compound	Somatotropin (H01AC01)
Disease treated	Somatotropin deficiency
Quantification of dysfunction	Semen
No. of patients treated	15
Age group	Children
Treatment period	5.3 months (mean)
Dose	0.7 IU/kg week^{-1}
Treatment consequences	Spermatogenesis, maturation
Efficacy	In all patients
Side effects compromising effectiveness	Not mentioned
Randomization of patients	No
Dose arms 1–3	Somatotropin deficiency; panhypopituitarism
Study quality	**2–**
Reference	201: Tato L, Zamboni G, Antoniazzi F, Piubello G. Gonadal function and response to growth hormone (GH) in boys with isolated GH deficiency and to GH and gonadotropins in boys with multiple pituitary hormone deficiencies. Fertil Steril. 1996 Apr;65(4):830–4.
Language	English

Compound	Somatotropin (H01AC01)
Disease treated	Hypogonadism, secondary
Quantification of dysfunction	Hormone
No. of patients treated	11
Age group	33–54 years
Treatment period	12 months
Dose	0.25 IU/kg week^{-1}
Treatment consequences	Spermatogenesis, improvement

Efficacy	No effect
Randomization of patients	No
Study quality	**3**
Reference	139: Carani C, Granata AR, De Rosa M, Garau C, Zarrilli S, Paesano L, Colao A, Marrama P, Lombardi G. The effect of chronic treatment with GH on gonadal function in men with isolated GH deficiency. Eur J Endocrinol. 1999 Mar;140(3):224–30.
Language	English

Compound	Somatotropin (H01AC01)+hCG (G03GA01)
Disease treated	Idiopathic hypogonadotropic hypogonadism (IHH)
Quantification of dysfunction	Semen
No. of patients treated	7
Age group	Young
Treatment period	24 weeks
Dose	5000 IU/week, somatotropin 8 IU/week
Treatment consequences	Spermatogenesis, maturation
Efficacy	In 2 of 4 patients increase of sperm count, 1 pregnancy
Randomization of patients	No
Dose arms 1–3	Somatotropin after unsuccessful stimulation
Study quality	**3**
Reference	279: Shoham Z, Conway GS, Ostergaard H, Lahlou N, Bouchard P, Jacobs HS. Cotreatment with growth hormone for induction of spermatogenesis in patients with hypogonadotropic hypogonadism. Fertil Steril. 1992 May;57(5):1044–51.
Language	English

Compound	Somatotropin (H01AC01)+gonadotropins (G03GA04)
Disease treated	Idiopathic hypogonadotropic hypogonadism (IHH)
Quantification of dysfunction	Hormones
No. of patients treated	4
Age group	Young
Treatment period	12 months
Dose	n.g.

2

Treatment consequences	Spermatogenesis, maturation
Efficacy	All patients remained azoospermic after 6 months of gonadotropin treatment alone as well as after 6 months subsequent addition of somatotropin.
Randomization of patients	No
Study quality	**3**
Reference	135: Giagulli VA. Absence of effect of recombinant growth hormone to classic gonadotropin treatment on spermatogenesis of patients with severe hypogonadotropic hypogonadism. Arch Androl. 1999 Jul–Aug;43(1):47–53.
Language	English

Compound	Somatotropin (H01AC01)+gonadotropins (G03GA04)
Disease treated	Idiopathic hypogonadotropic hypogonadism (IHH)
Quantification of dysfunction	Semen
No. of patients treated	4
Age group	Young
Treatment period	>12 months
Dose	n.g.
Treatment consequences	Spermatogenesis, maturation
Efficacy	2× production of sperm, 1 pregnancy
Randomization of patients	No
Remarks	Addition of GH is suitable in induction of puberty, not in improving spermatogenesis in the adult.
Study quality	**3**
Reference	302: Jacobs HS, Bouchard P, Conway GS, Homburg R, Lahlou N, Mason B, Ostergaard H, Owen EJ, Shoham Z. Role of growth hormone in infertility. Horm Res. 1991;36 Suppl 1:61–5.
Language	English

Compound	Somatotropin (H01AC01)+gonadotropins (G03GA04)
Disease treated	Spermatogenic dysfunction
Quantification of dysfunction	Semen
No. of patients treated	4
Age group	Young

Treatment period	24 weeks
Dose	n.g.
Treatment consequences	Spermatogenesis, improvement
Efficacy	In 0 of 4
Randomization of patients	No
Study quality	**3**
Reference	204: Zalel Y, Draysen E, Goldschmit R, Zadik Z, Shoham Z. A prospective pilot study of co-treatment with growth hormone and gonadotropins for improving spermatogenesis in normogonadotropic patients with severe oligoteratoasthenospermia. Gynecol Endocrinol. 1996 Feb;10(1):23–8.
Language	English

Compound	Oxytocin (H01BB02)
Disease treated	Infertility
Quantification of dysfunction	Semen
No. of patients treated	49
Age group	Young
Treatment period	Single dose
Dose	n.g.
Treatment consequences	Sperm parameters, improvement
Efficacy	No effect
Side effects compromising effectiveness	None
Randomization of patients	Yes
Dose arms 1–3	Oxytocin; placebo
Study quality	**1–**
Reference	38: Byrne MM, Rolf C, Depenbusch M, Cooper TG, Nieschlag E. Lack of effect of a single i.v. dose of oxytocin on sperm output in severely oligozoospermic men. Hum Reprod. 2003 Oct;18(10):2098–102.
Language	English

2

H02	Corticosteroids for Systemic Use
	A number of randomized studies which treated immune infertility and the associated deterioration of sperm parameters with corticosteroids have been published, but only one of them describes a significant positive effect. In spite of the disappointing results, the treatment is still in use. **Overall level of evidence of positive effects: C** **Overall level of evidence of adverse effects compromising effectiveness: D**

Compound	Glucocorticoids (H02AB)
Disease treated	Infertility, immune
Quantification of dysfunction	Semen
No. of patients treated	36
Age group	Young
Treatment period	10 days
Dose	40 mg/day
Treatment consequences	Sperm parameters, improvement
Efficacy	None
Side effects compromising effectiveness	Thirteen patients (42%) reported mild side effects; dyspepsia (10), acne (6), mood changes (5), weight gain (4) flushes (4).
Randomization of patients	No
Study quality	**2–**
Reference	145: Grigoriou O, Konidaris S, Antonaki V, Papadias C, Antoniou G, Gargaropoulos A. Corticosteroid treatment does not improve the results of intrauterine insemination in male subfertility caused by antisperm antibodies. Eur. J. Obstet. Gynecol Reprod Biol. 1996;65:227–30.
Language	English

Compound	Methylprednisolon (H02AB04)
Disease treated	Infertility, immune
Quantification of dysfunction	Semen
No. of patients treated	43
Age group	Young
Treatment period	7 days

Dose	96 mg
Treatment consequences	Sperm parameters, improvement
Efficacy	None
Randomization of patients	Yes
Dose arms 1–3	Methylprednisolone; placebo
Study quality	**1–**
Reference	147: Haas GG Jr, Manganiello P. A double-blind, placebo-controlled study of the use of methylprednisolone in infertile men with sperm-associated immunoglobulins. Fertil Steril. 1987;47:295–301.
Language	English

Compound	Prednisolone (H02AB06)
Disease treated	Infertility, immune
Quantification of dysfunction	Semen, flow cytometry
No. of patients treated	n.g.
Age group	Young
Treatment period	7 days
Dose	20 mg
Treatment consequences	Sperm parameters, improvement
Efficacy	None
Randomization of patients	Yes
Dose arms 1–3	Prednisolone; placebo
Study quality	**1–**
Reference	164: Rasanen M, Lahteenmaki A, Agrawal YP, Saarikoski S, Hovatta O. A placebo-controlled flow cytometric study of the effect of low-dose prednisolone treatment on sperm-bound antibody levels. Int J Androl. 1996;19:150–4.
Language	English

Compound	Prednisolone (H02AB06)
Disease treated	Infertility, immune
Quantification of dysfunction	Semen
No. of patients treated	77
Age group	Young
Treatment period	7 days

Dose	20 mg
Treatment consequences	Sperm parameters, improvement
Efficacy	None
Randomization of patients	No
Study quality	**3**
Reference	161: Omu AE, al-Qattan F, Abdul Hamada B. Effect of low dose continuous corticosteroid therapy in men with antisperm antibodies on spermatozoal quality and conception rate. Eur J Obstet Gynecol Reprod Biol. 1996;69:129–34.
Language	English

Compound	Prednisolone (H02AB06)
Disease treated	Infertility, immune
Quantification of dysfunction	In vitro fertilization
No. of patients treated	53
Age group	Young
Treatment period	7 days
Dose	20 mg
Treatment consequences	Sperm parameters, improvement
Efficacy	None
Randomization of patients	No
Study quality	**3**
Reference	156: Lahteenmaki A, Rasanen M, Hovatta O. Low-dose prednisolone does not improve the outcome of in-vitro fertilization in male immunological infertility. Hum Reprod. 1995;10:3124–9.
Language	English

Compound	Prednisolone (H02AB06)
Disease treated	Infertility, immune
Quantification of dysfunction	Semen
No. of patients treated	43
Age group	Young
Treatment period	7 days

Dose	20 mg
Treatment consequences	Sperm parameters, improvement
Efficacy	Pregnancy rate, increase
Side effects compromising effectiveness	Mild
Randomization of patients	Yes
Dose arms 1–3	Prednisolone; placebo
Study quality	**1–**
Reference	152: Hendry WF, Hughes L, Scammell G, Pryor JP, Hargreave TB. Comparison of prednisolone and placebo in subfertile men with antibodies to spermatozoa. Lancet 1990;335(8681):85–8.
Language	English

Compound	Prednisolone (H02AB06)
Disease treated	Infertility, immune
Quantification of dysfunction	Semen
No. of patients treated	20
Age group	Young
Treatment period	7 days
Dose	40 mg/day
Treatment consequences	Sperm parameters, improvement
Efficacy	None
Side effects compromising effectiveness	Mild
Randomization of patients	Yes
Dose arms 1–3	Prednisolone; placebo
Study quality	**1–**
Reference	132: Bals-Pratsch M, Doren M, Karbowski B, Schneider HP, Nieschlag E. Cyclic corticosteroid immunosuppression is unsuccessful in the treatment of sperm antibody-related male infertility: a controlled study. Hum Reprod. 1992;7:99–104.
Language	English

Compound	Prednisolone (H02AB06)
Disease treated	Infertility, immune
Quantification of dysfunction	Semen
No. of patients treated	10
Age group	Young
Treatment period	9 days
Dose	1 mg/kg day^{-1}
Treatment consequences	Sperm parameters, improvement
Efficacy	None
Randomization of patients	Yes
Dose arms 1–3	Prednisolone; placebo
Study quality	**1–**
Reference	133: Almeida M de, Feneux D, Rigaud C, Jouannet P. Steroid therapy for male infertility associated with antisperm antibodies. Results of a small randomized clinical trial. Int J Androl. 1985;8:111–7.
Language	English

Compound	Prednisone (H02AB07)
Disease treated	Infertility, immune
Quantification of dysfunction	Semen
No. of patients treated	47
Age group	Young
Treatment period	12 months
Dose	5 mg/day
Treatment consequences	Male accessory gland inflammation, improvement
Efficacy	Decline of antibody titres, three pregnancies induced
Randomization of patients	No
Study quality	**3**
Reference	610: Hendry WF, Stedronska J, Hughes L, Cameron KM, Pugh RC. Steroid treatment of male subfertility caused by antisperm antibodies. Lancet. 1979 Sep 8;2(8141):498–501.
Language	English

Compound	Cortisone (H02AB10)
Disease treated	Sarcoidosis, testicular
Quantification of adverse effects	Semen
No. of patients treated	1
Age group	27 years
Treatment period	5 months
Dose	60 down to 15 mg/day
Treatment consequences	Spermatogenesis, improvement
Efficacy	Good effect
Study quality	**3**
Reference	11: Rees DA, Dodds AL, Rathbone N, Davies JS, Scanlon MF. Azoospermia in testicular sarcoidosis is an indication for corticosteroid therapy. Fertil Steril. 2004 Dec;82(6):1672–4.
Language	English

Compound	Cortisone (H02AB10)
Disease treated	Hydroxylase deficiency
Quantification of adverse effects	Semen
No. of patients treated	1
Age group	45 years
Treatment period	6 months
Treatment consequences	Spermatogenesis, improvement
Efficacy	Good effect
Side effects compromising effectiveness	Not mentioned
Study quality	**3**
Reference	71: Tiitinen A, Valimaki M. Primary infertility in 45-year-old man with untreated 21-hydroxylase deficiency: successful outcome with glucocorticoid therapy. J Clin Endocrinol Metab. 2002 Jun;87(6):2442–5.
Language	English

2

J01 Antibacterials for Systemic Use

Infections of the genito-urinary system, as well as systemic infections, enhances the risk of altered sperm parameters as demonstrated in case-control studies. It remains unclear as to whether the alteration is a consequence of the infection or the antibiotic treatment used.

In experimental studies, no impairment of sperm parameters in vivo and in vitro has been observed. No unfavourable effects have been described in the literature.

Overall level of evidence of adverse effects: C

Compound	Antibacterial for systemic use (J01)
Disease treated	Infertility
Quantification of adverse effects	Semen
No. of patients treated	3698
Age group	20–55 years
Treatment period	Various
Dose	Various
Treatment consequences	History of infection
Efficacy	Incidence increasing with age
Randomization of patients	No
Study quality	**3**
Reference	2179: Rolf C, Kenkel S, Nieschlag E. Age-related disease pattern in infertile men: increasing incidence of infections in older patients. Andrologia. 2002 Sep;34(4):209–17.
Language	English

Compound	Antibacterial for systemic use (J01)
Disease treated	Infertility
Quantification of adverse effects	History, semen
No. of patients treated	430
Age group	31.2 years (mean)
Treatment period	Various
Dose	Various
Treatment consequences	History urinary infection

Efficacy	79 cases of men with abnormal semen parameters, 63 in men with normal semen parameters; $p<0.01$
Randomization of patients	No
Study quality	**2–**
Reference	2175: Bayasgalan G, Naranbat D, Radnaabazar J, Lhagvasuren T, Rowe PJ. Male infertility: risk factors in Mongolian men. Asian J Androl. 2004 Dec;6(4):305–11.
Language	English

Compound	Antibacterial for systemic use (J01)
Disease treated	Infertility
Quantification of adverse effects	History, semen
No. of patients treated	150; 150
Age group	30–50 years
Treatment period	Various
Dose	Various
Treatment consequences	Sexually transmitted diseases as risk factors
Efficacy	Significantly more urethritis, genital ulcer and testicular swelling in infertile men than in fertile men
Randomization of patients	No
Study quality	**2–**
Reference	2173: Okonofua F, Menakaya U, Onemu SO, Omo-Aghoja LO, Bergstrom S. A case-control study of risk factors for male infertility in Nigeria. Asian J Androl. 2005 Dec;7(4):351–61.
Language	English

Compound	Antibacterial for systemic use (J01)
Disease treated	Infertility
Quantification of adverse effects	Semen
No. of patients treated	92; 73
Age group	34.4 years (mean)
Treatment period	Various
Dose	Various
Treatment consequences	Oligozoospermia

Efficacy	OR 8.0 (95% CI 1.7–37.3), p=0.002
Randomization of patients	No
Study quality	**2–**
Reference	2177: Wong WY, Zielhuis GA, Thomas CM, Merkus HM, Steegers-Theunissen RP. New evidence of the influence of exogenous and endogenous factors on sperm count in man. Eur J Obstet Gynecol Reprod Biol. 2003 Sep 10;110(1):49–54.
Language	English

Compound	Tetracycline (J01AA07)
Disease treated	Male accessory gland infection
Quantification of adverse effects	Sperm motility
No. of patients treated	243
Age group	Young
Treatment period	2 weeks
Dose	Various
Treatment consequences	Sperm motility, increase
Efficacy	By 80%
Randomization of patients	No
Study quality	**3**
Reference	753: Toth A, Lesser ML. Urea plasma, urea lyticum and infertility: the effect of various antibiotic regimens on semen quality. J Urol. 1982 Oct;128(4):705–7.
Language	English

Compound	Tetracycline (J01AA07)
Disease treated	Male accessory gland infection
Quantification of adverse effects	Sperm functions in vitro
Age group	Young
Treatment period	In vitro
Dose	50 mg/ml
Treatment consequences	Sperm motility, decrease
Efficacy	Dose dependent
Randomization of patients	No
Study quality	**2–**

Reference	745: Hargreaves CA, Rogers S, Hills F, Rahman F, Howell RJ, Homa ST. Effects of co-trimoxazole, erythromycin, amoxycillin, tetracycline and chloroquine on sperm function in vitro. Hum Reprod. 1998 Jul;13(7):1878–86.
Language	English

Compound	Amoxycillin (J01CA04)
Disease treated	Male accessory gland infection
Quantification of adverse effects	Sperm functions in vitro
No. of patients treated	n.g.
Age group	Young
Dose	500 mg/ml
Treatment period	24 h
Treatment consequences	Sperm motility, alteration
Efficacy	No effect
Randomization of patients	No
Study quality	**2–**
Reference	745: Hargreaves CA, Rogers S, Hills F, Rahman F, Howell RJ, Homa ST. Effects of co-trimoxazole, erythromycin, amoxycillin, tetracycline and chloroquine on sperm function in vitro. Hum Reprod. 1998 Jul;13(7):1878–86.
Language	English

Compound	Co-trimoxazole (J01EE01)
Disease treated	Male accessory gland infection
Quantification of adverse effects	Sperm functions in vitro
Age group	Young
Treatment period	24 h
Dose	96 mg/ml
Treatment consequences	Sperm motility, alteration
Efficacy	No effect
Randomization of patients	No
Study quality	**2–**
Reference	745: Hargreaves CA, Rogers S, Hills F, Rahman F, Howell RJ, Homa ST. Effects of co-trimoxazole, erythromycin, amoxycillin, tetracycline and chloroquine on sperm function in vitro. Hum Reprod. 1998 Jul;13(7):1878–86.

Language	English

Compound	**Erythromycin (J01FA01)**
Disease treated	Male accessory gland infection
Quantification of adverse effects	Sperm functions in vitro
Age group	Young
Dose	50 mg/ml
Treatment period	24 h
Treatment consequences	Sperm motility, decrease
Efficacy	Significant effect
Randomization of patients	No
Study quality	**2-**
Reference	745: Hargreaves CA, Rogers S, Hills F, Rahman F, Howell RJ, Homa ST. Effects of co-trimoxazole, erythromycin, amoxycilin, tetracycline and chloroquine on sperm function in vitro. Hum Reprod. 1998 Jul;13(7):1878–86.
Language	English

Compound	**Ofloxacin (J01MA01)**
Disease treated	Male accessory gland infection
Quantification of adverse effects	Leucocyte count, sperm parameter
No. of patients treated	122
Age group	Young
Treatment period	3 months
Dose	n.g.
Treatment consequences	Leucocytes in semen decrease; sperm parameters, increase
Efficacy	Positive effects
Randomization of patients	No
Study quality	**2–**
Reference	751: Vicari E. Effectiveness and limits of antimicrobial treatment on seminal leukocyte concentration and related reactive oxygen species production in patients with male accessory gland infection. Hum Reprod. 2000 Dec;15(12):2536–44.
Language	English

Compound	Ciprofloxacine (J01MA02)
Disease treated	Healthy
Quantification of adverse effects	Hormones
No. of patients treated	8
Age group	Young
Treatment period	4 days
Dose	500 mg/day
Treatment consequences	Testosterone level, alteration
Efficacy	No effect
Randomization of patients	No
Study quality	**3**
Reference	926: Waite NM, Edwards DJ, Arnott WS, Warbasse LH. Effects of ciprofloxacin on testosterone and cortisol concentrations in healthy males. Antimicrob Agents Chemother. 1989 Nov;33(11):1875–7.
Language	English

Compound	Enoxacin (J01MA04)
Disease treated	Male accessory gland infection
Quantification of adverse effects	Semen
No. of patients treated	30
Age group	32 years (mean)
Treatment period	10 weeks
Dose	600 mg/day
Treatment consequences	Sperm parameters, impairment
Efficacy	50% hyperviscosity of semen
Randomization of patients	No
Study quality	**3**
Reference	323: Giorgi PM, Giorgi P, Canale D, Turchi P, Poggi MS, Coscio M di, Bartelloni M, Meschini P, Andreini F, Campa M et al. Treatment of male genital infections with enoxacin. Arch Ital Urol Nefrol Androl. 1989 Sep;61(3):235–41.
Language	Italian

Compound	Enoxacin (J01MA04)
Disease treated	Spermatogenic dysfunction
Quantification of adverse effects	Semen
No. of patients treated	20
Age group	Young
Treatment period	7 days
Dose	600 mg/day
Treatment consequences	Spermatogenesis, impairment
Efficacy	No effect
Randomization of patients	No
Study quality	**3**
Reference	214: Barletta D, Monzani F, Gasperi M, Caraccio N, Maccanti O, Bellitti P, Bonadio M, Pucci E. Efficacy of enoxacin in the treatment of prostatitis–vesiculitis: its absence of toxicity on spermatogenesis. Presse Med. 1995 Jun 17;24(22):1025–7.
Language	English

Compound	Metronidazol (J01XD01)
Disease treated	Healthy
Quantification of dysfunction	Sperm motility in vitro
Treatment period	In vitro
Dose	10 mg/ml
Treatment consequences	Sperm motility, depression; hamster oocyte test, alteration
Efficacy	Significant
Study quality	**3**
Reference	855: Foote RH. Effects of metronidazole, ipronidazole, and dibromochloropropane on rabbit and human sperm motility and fertility. Reprod Toxicol. 2002 Nov–Dec;16(6):749–55.
Language	English

J02	Antimycotics for Systemic Use
	Ketoconazole inhibits testosterone synthesis (see also Chap. 2.4) and sperm production. Other antimycotics, however, do not show this effect.
	Overall level of evidence of adverse effects: B

Compound	Ketoconazole (J02AB02), terbinafine
Disease treated	Healthy
Quantification of adverse effects	Hormones
No. of patients treated	n.g. (low)
Age group	Young
Treatment period	Three times
Dose	n.g.
Treatment consequences	Testosterone level decreased, LH pulse alteration
Efficacy	Marginal
Randomization of patients	Cross-over
Dose arms 1–3	Ketoconazole 200 mg/3 times; terbinafine 500 g/3 times; placebo
Study quality	**1–**
Reference	949: Nashan D, Knuth UA, Weidinger G, Nieschlag E. The antimycotic drug terbinafine in contrast to ketoconazole lacks acute effects on the pituitary–testicular function of healthy men: a placebo-controlled double-blind trial. Acta Endocrinol (Copenh). 1989 May;120(5):677–81.
Language	English

Compound	Fluconazole (J02AC01), ketoconazole
Disease treated	Healthy
Quantification of adverse effects	Hormones
No. of patients treated	9
Age group	Young
Treatment period	5 days
Dose	400 mg/200 mg
Treatment consequences	Testosterone level
Efficacy	Increase after fluconazol, decrease after ketoconazole

2

Randomization of patients	Cross-over
Dose arms 1–3	Fluconazole 400 mg/day; ketoconazole 200 mg/day
Study quality	**1–**
Reference	940: Touchette MA, Chandrasekar PH, Milad MA, Edwards DJ. Contrasting effects of fluconazole and ketoconazole on phenytoin and testosterone disposition in man. Br J Clin Pharmacol. 1992 Jul;34(1):75–8.
Language	English

Compound	Fluconazole (J02AC01)
Disease treated	Healthy
Quantification of adverse effects	Hormones
No. of patients treated	n.g.
Age group	Young
Treatment period	Continuous
Dose	n.g.
Treatment consequences	Cytochrome-P-450-dependent enzymes of steroid hormone synthesis
Efficacy	No influences in male
Study quality	**Phase–II study**
Reference	904: Rieth H, Sauerbrey N. Interaction studies with fluconazole, a new triazole antifungal drug. Wien Med Wochenschr. 1989 Aug 31;139(15–16):370–4.
Language	German

Compound	Itraconazole (J02AC02)
Disease treated	Mycosis
Quantification of adverse effects	Hormones
No. of patients treated	15
Age group	Young
Treatment period	12 months
Dose	200–400 mg/day
Treatment consequences	Testerone level, alteration
Efficacy	None
Randomization of patients	No
Study quality	**3**

Reference	826: Queiroz-Telles F, Purim KS, Boguszewski CL, Afonso FC, Graf H. Adrenal response to corticotrophin and testosterone during long-term therapy with itraconazole in patients with chromoblastomycosis. J Antimicrob Chemother. 1997 Dec;40(6):899–902.
Language	English

J04	**Antimycobacterials**
	There are some reports that spermatogenesis is not impaired by antimycobacterials.
	Overall level of evidence of adverse effects: D

Compound	Rifampicin (J04AB02)
Disease treated	Healthy
Quantification of adverse effects	Hormones
No. of patients treated	18
Age group	Young
Treatment period	7 days
Dose	600 mg/day
Treatment consequences	Testosterone level and response to hCG, alteration
Efficacy	Significant
Randomization of patients	No
Study quality	**3**
Reference	877: Bammel A, van der Mee K, Ohnhaus EE, Kirch W. Divergent effects of different enzyme-inducing agents on endogenous and exogenous testosterone. Eur J Clin Pharmacol. 1992;42(6):641–4.
Language	English

Compound	Isoniazide (J04AC01)
Disease treated	Spermatogenic dysfunction
Quantification of adverse effects	Semen
No. of patients treated	n.g.
Age group	n.g.
Treatment period	n.g.

Dose	n.g.
Treatment consequences	Spermatogenesis, impairment
Efficacy	No effect of combined antituberculous therapy
Randomization of patients	No
Study quality	**3**
Reference	65: Kul'chavenia EV, Brizhitiuk EV, Medvedev SA. Toxic effect of antituberculous drugs on spermatogenesis. Probl Tuberk. 2002;(5):29–32. (text in Russian, abstract in English)
Language	Russian

J05	**Antivirals for Systemic Use**
	No impairment of sperm parameters was shown in a randomized controlled study with aciclovir. **Overall level of evidence of adverse effects: B**

Compound	Aciclovir (J05AB01)
Disease treated	Herpes simplex, recurrent
Quantification of adverse effects	Semen
No. of patients treated	33
Age group	19–35 years
Treatment period	6 months
Treatment consequences	Sperm parameters, impairment
Efficacy	No difference between treated and control men
Randomization of patients	Yes
Dose arms 1–3	Aciclovir 1000 mg/day; placebo
Study quality	**1–**
Reference	916: Douglas JM Jr, Davis LG, Remington ML, Paulsen CA, Perrin EB, Goodman P, Conner JD, King D, Corey L. A double-blind, placebo-controlled trial of the effect of chronically administered oral acyclovir on sperm production in men with frequently recurrent genital herpes. J Infect Dis. 1988 Mar;157(3):588–93.
Language	English

L01 Antineoplastic Agents and Radiation

Antineoplastic agents used for the treatment of cancers and lymphomas cause spermatogenic dysfunction in the majority of cases. At a cellular level, they also induce chromosomal abnormalities. The aneuploidy rates of sperm chromosomes was found to be enhanced after antineoplastic chemotherapy. The toxic effect was clearly dose related. Radiation aggravated the effect. Malformations in the children fathered, on the other hand, were not more frequent than in controls, but conception should be avoided for at least 90 days after the end of antineoplastic therapy, and an interval of 1 year is favourable.

Cyclophosphamide is the antineoplastic agent best studied. If the cumulative dose exceeds 640 mg/kg, azoospermia occurs and persists regularly, whereas in lower doses a recovery was possible in up to 31 months, but was also observed even after 19 years. This held true also for prepubertal antineoplastic treatment, after which the majority of adolescents demonstrate small testis volume. For chlorambucil, a cumulative dose <8.2 mg/kg is safe.

Cisplatin caused irreversible azoospermia at a dose of >400 mg/cm^2; in other doses the rate of azoospermia was 80–87%. A recovery was observed in 78% of patients after 2 years if the dose of cisplatin was >600 mg/month. Frequently, Leydig cell dysfunction persisted.

The application of the ABVD protocol is clearly less hazardous to the spermatogenesis than that of the COPP protocol. The relative risk of azoospermia induction was increased fivefold (95% CI 1.3–18.8) after vincristine, 3.4-fold (95% CI 0.95–12.3) after cyclophosphamide and 8.2-fold after testicular irradiation.

Some of the combined drug regimens were of lesser toxicity, e.g. after treatment with the BEC protocol (bleomycin, ectoposide, carboplatine), 93% remained normozoosperm. Methotrexate is far less toxic to spermatogenesis.

An increase of FSH levels was associated with lower sperm count. The recovery of spermatogenesis was poorer in patients with elevated FSH levels in serum. A decrease of FSH levels preceded recovery.

There is no pharmacological prohibition against cytotoxic damage of spermatogenesis, and the sparse studies failed to demonstrate a protective effect of testosterone or GnRH agonists.

The studies cited below are usually based on observation after treatment; RCTs are not available. Only in a few studies were patients randomized to various regimens.

Overall level of evidence of adverse effects: C

2

Compound	Antineoplastic agents in general
Disease treated	Spermatogenic dysfunction
Quantification of adverse effects	Sperm chromosomes
Age group	Young
Treatment consequences	Germ cells, chromosomal abnormalities, induction
Efficacy	Highest in the first weeks after treatment
Randomization of patients	No
Study quality	**4 (review)**
Reference	4: Wyrobek AJ, Schmid TE, Marchetti F. Relative susceptibilities of male germ cells to genetic defects induced by cancer chemotherapies. J Natl Cancer Inst Monogr. 2005;(34):31–5.
Language	English

Compound	Antineoplastic agents in general
Disease treated	Cancers
Quantification of adverse effects	Progeny outcome
Age group	Young
Treatment consequences	Alteration of number and quality of progeny
Efficacy	Within the first cycle of spermatogenesis
Randomization of patients	No
Study quality	**4 (review)**
Reference	2044: Hales BF, Robaire B. Paternal exposure to drugs and environmental chemicals: effects on progeny outcome. J Androl. 2001 Nov–Dec;22(6):927–36.
Language	English

Compound	Antineoplastic agents in general
Disease treated	Infertility
Quantification of adverse effects	History, semen
No. of patients treated	430
Age group	31.2 years (mean)
Treatment period	Various
Dose	Various

Treatment consequences	History of other infection
Efficacy	84 cases in men with abnormal semen parameters, 91 cases in men with normal semen parameters; $p>0.05$
Randomization of patients	No
Study quality	**2–**
Reference	2175: Bayasgalan G, Naranbat D, Radnaabazar J, Lhagvasuren T, Rowe PJ. Male infertility: risk factors in Mongolian men. Asian J Androl. 2004 Dec;6(4):305–11.
Language	English

Compound	Antineoplastic agents in general
Disease treated	Leukemia
Quantification of adverse effects	Testicular histology
No. of patients treated	29
Age group	Young
Treatment period	Post mortem
Treatment consequences	Spermatogenesis, impairment
Efficacy	In longer treatment
Randomization of patients	No
Dose arms 1–3	Various treatment periods
Study quality	**2–**
Reference	550: Maguire LC, Dick FR, Sherman BM. The effects of anti-leukemic therapy on gonadal histology in adult males. Cancer. 1981 Nov 1;48(9):1967–71.
Language	English

Compound	Cyclophosphamide (L01AA01)
Disease treated	Cancer, in childhood
Quantification of adverse effects	Semen
No. of patients treated	43
Age group	Young
Treatment period	Various
Dose	Various
Treatment consequences	Sperm parameters after puberty, impairment

2

Efficacy	8 of 43 patients azoospermia, 16 of 43 patients normospermia
Study quality	**3**
Reference	122: Lopez Andreu JA, Fernandez PJ, Ferris i Tortajada J, Navarro I, Rodriguez-Ineba A, Antonio P, Muro MD, Romeu A. Persistent altered spermatogenesis in long-term childhood cancer survivors. Pediatr Hematol Oncol. 2000 Jan–Feb;17(1):21–30.
Language	English

Compound	Cyclophosphamide (L01AA01)
Disease treated	Cancer
Quantification of adverse effects	Semen
No. of patients treated	26
Age group	Young
Treatment period	31 months
Treatment consequences	Spermatogenesis, recovery after treatment
Efficacy	31 months after cessation of therapy despite >100 mg/day
Study quality	**3**
Reference	716: Buchanan JD, Fairley KF, Barrie JU. Return of spermatogenesis after stopping cyclophosphamide therapy. Lancet. 1975 Jul 26;2(7926):156–7.
Language	English

Compound	Cyclophosphamide (L01AA01)
Disease treated	Nephrotic syndrome in childhood
Quantification of adverse effects	Semen
No. of patients treated	19
Age group	Young
Treatment period	8 weeks
Dose	Various
Treatment consequences	Spermatogenesis, impairment
Efficacy	Most
Study quality	**3**
Reference	562: Trompeter RS, Evans PR, Barratt TM. Gonadal function in boys with steroid-responsive nephrotic syndrome treated with cyclophosphamide for short periods. Lancet. 1981 May 30;1(8231):1177–9.
Language	English

Compound	Cyclophosphamide (L01AA01)
Disease treated	Nephrotic syndrome
Quantification of adverse effects	Hormones
No. of patients treated	19
Age group	Children
Treatment period	Various
Dose	Various
Treatment consequences	Spermatogenesis, impairment
Efficacy	In all boys
Study quality	**3**
Reference	668: Lentz RD, Bergstein J, Steffes MW, Brown DR, Prem K, Michael AF, Vernier RL. Postpubertal evaluation of gonadal function following cyclophosphamide therapy before and during puberty. J Pediatr. 1977 Sep;91(3):385–94.
Language	English

Compound	Cyclophosphamide (L01AA01)
Disease treated	Nephrotic syndrome
Quantification of adverse effects	Semen
No. of patients treated	17
Age group	Children
Treatment period	Various
Dose	Up to 640 mg/kg
Treatment consequences	Spermatogenesis, impairment
Efficacy	5α-, 1 oligo-, 11 normozoospermia
Study quality	**3**
Reference	310: Bogdanovic R, Banicevic M, Cvoric A. Testicular function following cyclophosphamide treatment for childhood nephritic syndrome: long-term follow-up study. Pediatr Nephrol. 1990 Sep;4(5):451–4.
Language	English

Compound	Cyclophosphamide (L01AA01)
Disease treated	Nephrotic syndrome
Quantification of adverse effects	Semen
No. of patients treated	16
Age group	Children

Treatment period	6 months
Dose	5 mg/kg
Treatment consequences	Spermatogenesis, impairment
Efficacy	No effect
Study quality	**3**
Reference	731: Pennisi AJ, Grushkin CM, Lieberman E. Gonadal function in children with nephrosis treated with cyclophosphamide. Am J Dis Child. 1975 Mar;129(3):315–8.
Language	English

Compound	Cyclophosphamide (L01AA01)
Disease treated	Cancer
Quantification of adverse effects	Semen
No. of patients treated	15
Age group	Young
Treatment period	Various
Dose	Various
Treatment consequences	Spermatogenesis, recovery after treatment
Efficacy	One of 10 without T suppression during treatment, 5 of 5 with T suppression during treatment
Randomization of patients	Yes
Dose arms 1–3	Cyclophosphamide daily; cyclophosphamide bolus monthly Cyclophosphamide monthly+T
Study quality	**1–**
Reference	801: Masala A, Faedda R, Alagna S et al. Use of testosterone to prevent cyclophoshamide-induced azoospermia. Ann Int Med 1997;126:292–5.
Language	English

Compound	Cyclophosphamide (L01AA01)
Disease treated	Nephrotic syndrome
Quantification of adverse effects	Testicular histology
No. of patients treated	8
Age group	Children
Treatment period	Up to 489 days
Treatment consequences	Azoospermia, induction

Efficacy	In all after puberty
Randomization of patients	No
Dose arms 1–3	2–4 mg/day; 2–5 mg/day
Study quality	**2–**
Reference	694: Etteldorf JN, West CD, Pitcock JA, Williams DL. Gonadal function, testicular histology, and meiosis following cyclophosphamide therapy in patients with nephrotic syndrome. J Pediatr. 1976 Feb;88(2):206–12.
Language	English

Compound	Chlorambucil (L01AA02)
Disease treated	Nephrotic syndrome
Quantification of adverse effects	Semen
No. of patients treated	21
Age group	Children
Treatment period	Long term
Dose	Various
Treatment consequences	Azoospermia, induction
Efficacy	In 17 of 21 patients
Study quality	**3**
Reference	652: Guesry P, Lenoir G, Broyer M. Gonadal effects of chlorambucil given to prepubertal and pubertal boys for nephrotic syndrome. J Pediatr. 1978 Feb;92(2):299–303.
Language	English

Compound	Chlorambucil (L01AA02)
Disease treated	Nephrotic syndrome
Quantification of adverse effects	Semen
No. of patients treated	16
Age group	Prepubertal
Treatment period	Various
Dose	Various
Treatment consequences	Spermatogenesis, impairment
Efficacy	Total safe dose <8.2 mg/kg
Study quality	**3**

2

Reference	577: Callis L, Nieto J, Vila A, Rende J. Chlorambucil treatment in minimal lesion nephrotic syndrome: a reappraisal of its gonadal toxicity. J Pediatr. 1980 Oct;97(4):653–6.
Language	English

Compound	Chlorambucil (L01AA02)
Disease treated	Lymphoma
Quantification of adverse effects	Semen
No. of patients treated	6
Age group	Young
Treatment period	Various
Dose	Various
Treatment consequences	Spermatogenesis, impairment
Efficacy	In all men, treatment with T improved only fructose concentration
Study quality	**3**
Reference	634: Calamera JC, Morgenfeld MC, Mancini RE, Vilar O. Biochemical changes of the human semen produced by chlorambucil, testosterone propionate and human chorionic gonadotropin administration. Andrologia. 1979 Jan;11(1):43–50.
Language	English

Compound	Chlorambucil (L01AA02)
Disease treated	Nephrotic syndrome
Quantification of adverse effects	Semen
No. of patients treated	2
Age group	Young
Treatment period	14 years
Dose	3000–6500 mg cumulative
Treatment consequences	Spermatogenesis, recovery after treatment
Efficacy	After 19 years
Study quality	**3**
Reference	275: Marmor D, Grob-Menendez F, Duyck F, Delafontaine D. Very late return of spermatogenesis after chlorambucil therapy: case reports. Fertil Steril. 1992 Oct;58(4):845–6.
Language	English

Compound	Dacarbazine (L01AX04)
Disease treated	Cancer, in childhood
Quantification of adverse effects	Semen
No. of patients treated	7
Age group	Young
Treatment period	24 weeks
Dose	Various
Treatment consequences	Spermatogenesis, impairment
Efficacy	Azoospermia in all men
Study quality	**3**
Reference	69: Thomson AB, Anderson RA, Irvine DS, Kelnar CJ, Sharpe RM, Wallace WH. Investigation of suppression of the hypoth alamic–pituitary–gonadal axis to restore spermatogenesis in azoospermic men treated for childhood cancer. Hum Reprod. 2002 Jul;17(7):1715–23.
Language	English

Compound	Methotrexate (L01BA01)
Disease treated	Psoriasis
Quantification of adverse effects	Semen
No. of patients treated	26
Age group	Young
Treatment period	Various
Dose	Various
Treatment consequences	Spermatogenesis, impairment
Efficacy	None
Study quality	**3**
Reference	633: El-Beheiry A, El-Mansy E, Kamel N, Salama N. Methotrexate and fertility in men. Arch Androl. 1979;3(2):177–9.
Language	English

Compound	Methotrexate (L01BA01)
Disease treated	Psoriasis arthritis
Quantification of adverse effects	Semen
No. of patients treated	1
Age group	26

Treatment period	10 years
Dose	728 mg cumulative
Treatment consequences	Spermatogenesis, impairment
Efficacy	Partial
Remarks	Avoid conception for at least 90 days
Study quality	**3**
Reference	250: Morris LF, Harrod MJ, Menter MA, Silverman AK. Methotrexate and reproduction in men: case report and recommendations. J Am Acad Dermatol. 1993 Nov;29(5 Pt 2):913–6.
Language	English

Compound	6-mercaptopurine (L01BB02)
Disease treated	Chronic hepatitis
Quantification of adverse effects	Semen, sperm chromosomes
No. of patients treated	1
Age group	36
Treatment period	4 years
Dose	50–70 mg/day
Treatment consequences	Sperm parameters, impairment
Efficacy	No difference against controls
Study quality	**3**
Reference	981: Jenderny J, Jacobi ML, Ruger A, Rohrborn G. Chromosome aberrations in 450 sperm complements from eight controls and lack of increase after chemotherapy in two patients. Hum Genet. 1992 Sep–Oct;90(1–2):151–4.
Language	English

Compound	6-mercaptopurine (L01BB02)
Disease treated	Inflammatory bowel disease
Quantification of adverse effects	Offspring
No. of patients treated	54
Age group	Young
Treatment period	Various
Dose	Various
Treatment consequences	Malformations in the children fathered
Efficacy	No more frequent than in controls

Remarks	The risk/benefit ratio still weighs heavily in favour of continuing therapy in men attempting conception in their female partners.
Study quality	**3**
Reference	980: Cohen RD. sperm, sex, and 6-MP: the perception on conception. Gastroenterology. 2004 Oct;127(4):1263–4.
Language	English

Compound	Doxorubicine (L01DB01)
Disease treated	Cancer
Quantification of adverse effects	Semen
No. of patients treated	14
Age group	Young
Treatment period	Various
Dose	Various
Treatment consequences	Spermatogenesis, impairment
Efficacy	In contrast to protocols with mechlorethamine, vincristine, procarbazine and prednisone sperm production after short-time recovery is possible after treatment with protocols that include doxorubicin.
Study quality	**3**
Reference	493: Da Cunha MF, Meistrich ML, Ried HL, Gordon LA, Watchmaker G, Wyrobek AJ. Active sperm production after cancer chemotherapy with doxorubicin. J Urol. 1983 Nov;130(5):927–30.
Language	English

Compound	Cisplatin (L01XA01)
Disease treated	Cancer, testicular
Quantification of adverse effects	Hormones
No. of patients treated	63
Age group	19–53 years
Treatment period	Various
Dose	Various
Treatment consequences	Hormone levels, impairment
Efficacy	Elevated FSH levels in 63% of patients, elevated LH levels in 24%, subnormal T levels in 10%. Gonadotropin elevation was highly significantly correlated with the cumulative platinum dose.

Randomization of patients	No
Study quality	**3**
Reference	2113: Berger CC, Bokemeyer C, Schuppert F, Schmoll HJ. Endocrinological late effects after chemotherapy for testicular cancer. Br J Cancer. 1996 May;73(9):1108–14.
Language	English

Compound	Cisplatin (L01XA01)
Disease treated	Cancer, testicular
Quantification of adverse effects	Semen
No. of patients treated	27
Age group	Young
Treatment period	Various
Dose	1250 mg/cm^2
Treatment consequences	Spermatogenesis, impairment
Efficacy	In all 27 men
Study quality	**3**
Reference	32: Ishikawa T, Kamidono S, Fujisawa M. Fertility after high-dose chemotherapy for testicular cancer. Urology. 2004 Jan;63(1):137–40.
Language	English

Compound	Cisplatin (L01XA01)
Disease treated	Cancer, testicular
Quantification of adverse effects	Semen
No. of patients treated	n.g
Age group	Young
Treatment period	Various
Dose	Various
Treatment consequences	Spermatogenesis, recovery after treatment
Efficacy	2–3 years after chemotherapy
Study quality	**3**
Reference	262: Fossa SD, Aabyholm T, Vespestad S, Norman N, Ous S. Semen quality after treatment for testicular cancer. Eur Urol. 1993;23(1):172–6.
Language	English

Compound	Cisplatin (L01XA01)
Disease treated	Cancer
Quantification of adverse effects	Semen
Age group	Young
Treatment consequences	Azoospermia, induction
Efficacy	>400 mg/cm^2 cisplatin irreversible
Study quality	**4 (review)**
Reference	180: Pont J, Albrecht W. Fertility after chemotherapy for testicular germ cell cancer. Fertil Steril. 1997 Jul;68(1):1–5.
Language	English

Compound	Cisplatin (L01XA01)
Disease treated	Cancer, testicular
Quantification of adverse effects	Semen, histology
Age group	Young
Treatment consequences	Spermatogenesis, impairment
Efficacy	Increase of apoptosis
Remarks	Cisplatin induces leakage of blood–testis barrier and germ cell apoptosis
Study quality	**4 (review)**
Reference	5: Boekelheide K. Mechanisms of toxic damage to spermatogenesis. J Natl Cancer Inst Monogr. 2005;(34):6–8.
Language	English

Compound	Cisplatin (L01XA01)
Disease treated	Spermatogenic dysfunction
Quantification of adverse effects	Semen
Age group	Young
Treatment consequences	Azoospermia, induction
Efficacy	In 50% of patients
Remarks	Hormonal protection of spermatogenesis has thus far succeeded only in animals. The mechanism is unclear, since there are no changes in number of spermatogonia.
Study quality	**4 (review)**

Reference	87: Schrader M, Muller M, Straub B, Miller K. The impact of chemotherapy on male fertility: a survey of the biologic basis and clinical aspects. Reprod Toxicol. 2001 Nov–Dec;15(6):611–7.
Language	English

Compound	Cisplatin (L01XA01)
Disease treated	Cancer, testicular
Quantification of adverse effects	Semen
Age group	Young
Treatment consequences	Spermatogenesis, recovery after treatment
Efficacy	Most in the following years, but persistent Leydig cell dysfunction
Study quality	**4 (review)**
Reference	268: Hansen PV, Hansen SW. Gonadal function in men with testicular germ cell cancer: the influence of cisplatin-based chemotherapy. Eur Urol. 1993;23(1):153–6.
Language	English

Compound	Procarbazine (L01XB01)
Disease treated	Cancer
Quantification of adverse effects	Semen
Age group	Young
Treatment consequences	Spermatogenesis, recovery after treatment
Efficacy	80% by 5 years
Remarks	"Permanent azoospermia suggests that all spermatogonia may be eradicated, in these cases there is no possibility of recovery".
Study quality	**4 (review)**
Reference	94: Howell SJ, Shalet SM. Testicular function following chemotherapy. Hum Reprod Update. 2001 Jul–Aug;7(4):363–9.
Language	English

Compound	Asparaginase (L01XX02), prednisolone, vincristine
Disease treated	Lymphoma
Quantification of adverse effects	Semen, flow cytometry

No. of patients treated	6
Age group	Young
Treatment period	42 months
Dose	Various
Treatment consequences	Sperm chromosomes, impairment
Efficacy	None as determined by flow cytometry
Randomization of patients	No
Study quality	**3**
Reference	476: Evenson DP, Arlin Z, Welt S, Claps ML, Melamed MR. Male reproductive capacity may recover following drug treatment with the L-10 protocol for acute lymphocytic leukemia. Cancer. 1984 Jan 1;53(1):30–6.
Language	English

Compound	Imatinib (L01XX28)
Disease treated	Leukemia, chronic myeloid
Quantification of adverse effects	Hormones
No. of patients treated	38
Age group	Old
Treatment period	23 months
Dose	Various
Treatment consequences	Testosterone synthesis, inhibition
Efficacy	Observed in 7 men with gynaecomastia
Randomization of patients	No
Study quality	**3**
Reference	818: Gambacorti-Passerini C, Tornaghi L, Cavagnini F, Rossi P, Pecori-Giraldi F, Mariani L, Cambiaghi N, Pogliani E, Corneo G, Gnessi L. Gynaecomastia in men with chronic myeloid leukaemia after imatinib. Lancet. 2003 Jun 7;361(9373):1954–6.
Language	English

Compound	MOPP/ABVD (mechlorethamine, vincristine, procarbazine, prednisone)/(bleomycin, dacarbazine, doxorubicin, vinblastine) (L01XY)
Disease treated	Lymphoma, Hodgkin
Quantification of adverse effects	Semen

No. of patients treated	92
Age group	Young
Treatment period	Various
Dose	Various
Treatment consequences	Spermatogenesis, impairment
Efficacy	87% azoospermic, recovery in 27 of 42 patients
Randomization of patients	No
Study quality	**3**
Reference	301: Viviani S, Ragni G, Santoro A, Perotti L, Caccamo E, Negretti E, Valagussa P, Bonadonna G. Testicular dysfunction in Hodgkin's disease before and after treatment. Eur J Cancer. 1991;27(11):1389–92.
Language	English

Compound	Combinations (L01XY)
Disease treated	Lymphoma, Hodgkin
Quantification of adverse effects	Semen
No. of patients treated	79
Age group	Young
Treatment period	Various
Dose	Various
Treatment consequences	Spermatogenesis, impairment
Efficacy	In 80% azoospermia
Study quality	**3**
Reference	391: Redman JR, Bajorunas DR, Goldstein MC, Evenson DP, Gralla RJ, Lacher MJ, Koziner B, Lee BJ, Straus DJ, Clarkson BD et al. Semen cryopreservation and artificial insemination for Hodgkin's disease. J Clin Oncol. 1987 Feb;5(2):233–8.
Language	English

Compound	Combinations (L01XY)
Disease treated	Cancer, testicular
Quantification of adverse effects	Semen, flow cytometry
No. of patients treated	77
Age group	Young
Treatment period	Various

Dose	Various
Treatment consequences	Spermatogenesis, impairment
Efficacy	Useful information by flow cytometry
Study quality	**3**
Reference	298: Fossa SD, Melvik JE, Juul NO, Pettersen EO, Amellem O, Theodorsen L. DNA flow cytometry in sperm cells from testicular cancer patients. Impact of different treatment modalities on spermatogenesis. Eur Urol. 1991;19(2):125–31.
Language	English

Compound	OPPA and COPP (cyclophosphamide, prednisone, procarbacine, vincristine (L01XY)
Disease treated	Cancer, in childhood
Quantification of adverse effects	Semen
No. of patients treated	75
Age group	Young
Treatment period	Various
Dose	Various
Treatment consequences	Gonadotropin levels, increase
Efficacy	18 of 75 (24.0%) elevated basal and 65 of 74 (87.8%) elevated stimulated LH levels
Remarks	Procarbacine is the major gonadotoxic agent
Study quality	**3**
Reference	318: Bramswig JH, Heimes U, Heiermann E, Schlegel W, Nieschlag E, Schellong G. The effects of different cumulative doses of chemotherapy on testicular function. Results in 75 patients treated for Hodgkin's disease during childhood or adolescence. Cancer. 1990 Mar 15;65(6):1298–302.
Language	English

Compound	Combinations (L01XY)
Disease treated	Lymphoma, Hodgkin
Quantification of adverse effects	Semen
No. of patients treated	74
Age group	Young
Treatment period	Various

Dose	Various
Treatment consequences	Spermatogenesis, recovery after treatment
Efficacy	Four of 74 recovered after mean 27 months.
Study quality	**3**
Reference	630: Chapman RM, Sutcliffe SB, Rees LH, Edwards CR, Malpas JS. Cyclical combination chemotherapy and gonadal function. Retrospective study in males. Lancet. 1979 Feb 10;1(8111):285–9.
Language	English

Compound	BEC (bleomycin, ectoposide, carboplatine) (L01XY)
Disease treated	Cancer, testicular
Quantification of adverse effects	Semen
No. of patients treated	69
Age group	Young
Treatment period	Various
Dose	Various
Treatment consequences	Spermatogenesis, impairment
Efficacy	93% remained normozoosperm following chemotherapy
Study quality	**2–**
Reference	24: Pectasides D, Pectasides M, Farmakis D, Nikolaou M, Koumpou M, Kostopoulou V, Mylonakis N. Testicular function in patients with testicular cancer treated with bleomycin–etoposide–carboplatin (BEC(90)) combination chemotherapy. Eur Urol. 2004 Feb;45(2):187–93.
Language	English

Compound	Combinations (L01XY)
Disease treated	Cancer, in childhood
Quantification of adverse effects	Semen, testicular volume
No. of patients treated	66
Age group	Young
Treatment period	Various
Dose	Various
Treatment consequences	Spermatogenesis, impairment
Efficacy	51 of 66 patients had small testis volume; cyclophosphamide most toxic
Study quality	**3**

Reference	317: Siimes MA, Rautonen J. Small testicles with impaired production of sperm in adult male survivors of childhood malignancies. Cancer. 1990 Mar 15;65(6):1303-6.
Language	English

Compound	POMB-ACE (bleomycin, cisplatin, cyclophosphamide, dactinomycin, etoposide, methotrexate, vincristine) (L01XY)
Disease treated	Cancer, testicular
Quantification of adverse effects	Semen
No. of patients treated	59
Age group	Young
Treatment period	Various
Dose	Various
Treatment consequences	Spermatogenesis, recovery after treatment
Efficacy	In 81% without radiation, in 32% with radiation
Study quality	**3**
Reference	394: Rustin GJ, Pektasides D, Bagshawe KD, Newlands ES, Begent RH. Fertility after chemotherapy for male and female germ cell tumours. Int J Androl. 1987 Feb;10(1):389–92.
Language	English

Compound	NOVP (mitoxantrone, prednisone, vinblastine, vincristine) (L01XY)
Disease treated	Lymphoma, Hodgkin
Quantification of adverse effects	Semen
No. of patients treated	58
Age group	Young
Treatment period	Various
Dose	Various
Treatment consequences	Spermatogenesis, impairment
Efficacy	Azoospermia 100% in first month, 0% after 1 year
Study quality	**3**
Reference	172: Meistrich ML, Wilson G, Mathur K, Fuller LM, Rodriguez MA, McLaughlin P, Romaguera JE, Cabanillas FF, Ha CS, Lipshultz LI, Hagemeister FB. Rapid recovery of spermatogenesis after mitoxantrone, vincristine, vinblastine, and prednisone chemotherapy for Hodgkin's disease. J Clin Oncol. 1997 Dec;15(12):3488–95.

Language	English

Compound	Combination (L01XY)
Disease treated	Cancer, in childhood
Quantification of adverse effects	Semen
No. of patients treated	55
Age group	>18 years
Treatment period	Various
Dose	Various
Treatment consequences	Azoospermia, induction
Efficacy	In multivariate analysis, RR of azoospermia after vincristine 5 (95% CI 1.3–18.8), after cyclophosphamide 3.4-fold (0.95–12.3), after testicular irradiation it was 8.2-fold.
Randomization of patients	No
Dose arms 1–3	Radiation; protocol including vincristine; protocol including cyclophosphamide
Study quality	**2+**
Reference	2070: Rautonen J, Koskimies AI, Siimes MA. Vincristine is associated with the risk of azoospermia in adult male survivors of childhood malignancies. Eur J Cancer. 1992;28A(11):1837–41.
Language	English

Compound	MOPP (mechlorethamine, vincristine, procarbazine, prednisone) (L01XY)
Disease treated	Lymphoma, Hodgkin
Quantification of adverse effects	Semen
No. of patients treated	47
Age group	Young
Treatment period	Various
Dose	Various
Treatment consequences	Spermatogenesis, impairment
Efficacy	Azoospermia in 26 of47 patients after 89.4 months
Study quality	**3**
Reference	219: Marmor D, Duyck F. Male reproductive potential after MOPP therapy for Hodgkin's disease: a long-term survey. Andrologia. 1995 Mar–Apr;27(2):99–106.

Language	English

Compound	Combinations (L01XY)
Disease treated	Cancer, testicular
Quantification of adverse effects	Semen
No. of patients treated	44
Age group	Young
Treatment period	Various
Dose	Various
Treatment consequences	Spermatogenesis, recovery after treatment
Efficacy	In 77% of patients 25–60 months after treatment
Study quality	**3**
Reference	331: Kreuser ED, Kurrle E, Hetzel WD, Heymer B, Porzsolt F, Hautmann R, Gaus W, Schlipf U, Pfeiffer EF, Heimpel H. Reversible germ cell toxicity following aggressive chemotherapy in patients with testicular tumors: results of a prospective study. Klin Wochenschr. 1989 Apr 3;67(7):367–78.
Language	German

Compound	CIVPP (lomustine, prednisone, procarbazine, vinblastine) (L01XY)
Disease treated	Cancer
Quantification of adverse effects	Semen
No. of patients treated	40
Age group	Prepubertal
Treatment period	Various
Dose	Various
Treatment consequences	Spermatogenesis, recovery after treatment
Efficacy	None when FSH levels were elevated
Study quality	**3**
Reference	248: Shafford EA, Kingston JE, Malpas JS, Plowman PN, Pritchard J, Savage MO, Eden OB. Testicular function following the treatment of Hodgkin's disease in childhood. Br J Cancer. 1993 Dec;68(6):1199–204.
Language	English

Compound	Combination (L01XY)
Disease treated	Lymphoma, Hodgkin
Quantification of adverse effects	Semen
No. of patients treated	38
Age group	Young
Treatment period	Various
Dose	Various
Treatment consequences	Spermatogenesis, impairment
Efficacy	Azoospermia was seen in one patient from theABVD group and 10 patients from the COPP/ABVD group
Randomization of patients	No
Study quality	**3**
Reference	2064: Kulkarni SS, Sastry PS, Saikia TK, Parikh PM, Gopal R, Advani SH. Gonadal function following ABVD therapy for Hodgkin's disease. Am J Clin Oncol. 1997 Aug;20(4):354–7.
Language	English

Compound	NOVP (mitoxantrone, prednisone, vinblastine, vincristine) (L01XY)+radiation
Disease treated	Lymphoma, Hodgkin
Quantification of adverse effects	Semen
No. of patients treated	34
Age group	Young
Treatment period	8 weeks
Dose	Various
Treatment consequences	Spermatogenesis, impairment
Efficacy	At 4.5 months to nadir of sperm
Study quality	**2–**
Reference	121: Dubey P, Wilson G, Mathur KK, Hagemeister FB, Fuller LM, Ha CS, Cox JD, Meistrich ML. Recovery of sperm production following radiation therapy for Hodgkin's disease after induction chemotherapy with mitoxantrone, vincristine, vinblastine, and prednisone (NOVP). Int J Radiat Oncol Biol Phys. 2000 Feb 1;46(3):609–17.
Language	English

Compound	PADIC (cisplatin, dacarbazine, doxorubicin) (L01XY)
Disease treated	Osteosarcoma
Quantification of adverse effects	Semen
No. of patients treated	32
Age group	Young
Treatment period	Various
Dose	Various
Treatment consequences	Spermatogenesis, recovery after treatment
Efficacy	In 78% after 2 years, lower in cisplatin >600 mg/month
Study quality	**3**
Reference	236: Meistrich ML, Chawla SP, Da Cunha MF, Johnson SL, Plager C, Papadopoulos NE, Lipshultz LI, Benjamin RS. Recovery of sperm production after chemotherapy for osteosarcoma. Cancer. 1989 Jun 1;63(11):2115–23.
Language	English

Compound	Combinations (L01XY)
Disease treated	Lymphoma
Quantification of adverse effects	Semen
No. of patients treated	32
Age group	Young
Treatment period	Various
Dose	Various
Treatment consequences	Spermatogenesis, recovery after treatment
Efficacy	70% in group 1, 17% in group 2
Randomization of patients	No
Dose arms 1–3	Group 1: cyclophosphamide / vincristine / prednisone; group 2: mustine / procarbazine / vincristine / prednisone
Study quality	**2–**
Reference	647: Roeser HP, Stocks AE, Smith AJ. Testicular damage due to cytotoxic drugs and recovery after cessation of therapy. Aust N Z J Med. 1978 Jun;8(3):250–4.
Language	English

2

Compound	Combinations (L01XY)
Disease treated	Sarcoma
Quantification of adverse effects	Hormones
No. of patients treated	26
Age group	Young
Treatment period	Various
Dose	Various
Treatment consequences	Hormone levels, impairment
Efficacy	FSH and LH levels increased, T levels normal; 8 of 12 patients low sperm count
Randomization of patients	No
Dose arms 1–3	Chemotherapy; chemotherapy+radiation
Study quality	**3**
Reference	2135: Shamberger RC, Sherins RJ, Rosenberg SA. The effects of postoperative adjuvant chemotherapy and radiotherapy on testicular function in men undergoing treatment for soft tissue sarcoma. Cancer. 1981 May 15;47(10):2368–74.
Language	English

Compound	CVB (cisplatin, vindesine, bleomycin) (L01XY)
Disease treated	Cancer, testicular
Quantification of adverse effects	Semen
No. of patients treated	25
Age group	Young
Treatment period	Various
Dose	Various
Treatment consequences	Spermatogenesis, recovery after treatment
Efficacy	In 46% after 5 years
Study quality	**3**
Reference	324: Hansen PV, Trykker H, Helkjoer PE, Andersen J. Testicular function in patients with testicular cancer treated with orchiectomy alone or orchiectomy plus cisplatin-based chemotherapy. J Natl Cancer Inst. 1989 Aug 16;81(16):1246–50.
Language	English

Compound	MOPP (mechlorethamine, vincristine, procarbazine, prednisone) (L01XY)
Disease treated	Lymphoma, Hodgkin I
Quantification of adverse effects	Semen
No. of patients treated	25
Age group	Young
Treatment period	Various
Dose	Various
Treatment consequences	Spermatogenesis, recovery after treatment
Efficacy	Better after only two cycles than after five cycles
Randomization of patients	No
Dose arms 1–3	Two cycles MOPP; five cycles MOPP
Study quality	**2–**
Reference	468: da Cunha MF, Meistrich ML, Fuller LM, Cundiff JH, Hagemeister FB, Velasquez WS, McLaughlin P, Riggs SA, Cabanillas FF, Salvador PG. Recovery of spermatogenesis after treatment for Hodgkin's disease: limiting dose of MOPP chemotherapy. J Clin Oncol. 1984 Jun;2(6):571–7.
Language	English

Compound	Combinations (L01XY)
Disease treated	Lymphoma, Hodgkin
Quantification of adverse effects	Semen
No. of patients treated	24
Age group	30 mean
Treatment period	Various
Dose	Various
Treatment consequences	Sperm parameters, impairment
Efficacy	In 3 of 9 patients return to pretherapeutic status
Randomization of patients	No
Study quality	**3**
Reference	2065: Naccache P, Decaudin D, Koscielny S, Bendahmane B, Auger J, Munck JN. Semen preservation and gonadal toxicity in the treatment of non-Hodgkin lymphoma. Experience at the Gustave-Roussy Institute from 1980 to 1993. Bull Cancer. 1996 Apr;83(4):307–14.
Language	French

Compound	Combinations (L01XY)
Disease treated	Cancer, testicular
Quantification of adverse effects	FSH serum levels
No. of patients treated	20
Age group	Young
Treatment period	Various
Dose	Various
Treatment consequences	Spermatogenesis, recovery after treatment
Efficacy	Reduction of FSH precedes recovery
Study quality	**3**
Reference	300: Kader HA, Rostom AY. Follicle stimulating hormone levels as a predictor of recovery of spermatogenesis following cancer therapy. Clin Oncol (R Coll Radiol). 1991 Jan;3(1):37–40.
Language	English

Compound	VBP±A (bleomycin, vinblastine, cisplatin, adrimycin) (L01XY)
Disease treated	Cancer, testicular
Quantification of adverse effects	Semen
No. of patients treated	18
Age group	Young
Treatment period	Various
Dose	Various
Treatment consequences	Spermatogenesis, recovery after treatment
Efficacy	In 5 of 6 patients spermaozoa after 24 m
Study quality	**3**
Reference	490: Johnson DH, Hainsworth JD, Linde RB, Greco FA. Testicular function following combination chemotherapy with cis-platin, vinblastine, and bleomycin. Med Pediatr Oncol. 1984;12(4):233–8.
Language	English

Compound	MVPP (mustine, vinblastine, procarbazine, prednisolone) (L01XY)
Disease treated	Lymphoma, Hodgkin
Quantification of adverse effects	Hormones

No. of patients treated	18
Age group	18–30 years
Treatment period	Various
Dose	Various
Treatment consequences	Leydig cell function, alteration
Efficacy	Identical stimulability by hCG in comparison with controls
Randomization of patients	No
Dose arms 1–3	MVPP; healthy
Study quality	**2–**
Reference	374: Tsatsoulis A, Whitehead E, St. John J, Shalet SM, Robertson WR. The pituitary–Leydig cell axis in men with severe damage to the germinal epithelium. Clin Endocrinol (Oxf). 1987 Dec;27(6):683–9.
Language	English

Compound	Combinations (L01XY)
Disease treated	Cancer
Quantification of adverse effects	ICSI–TESE outcome
No. of patients treated	17
Age group	28–54 years
Treatment period	Various
Dose	Various
Treatment consequences	Interval chemotherapy to ICSI 16 years
Efficacy	9 of 20 patients positive for TESE, 3 pregnancies in 9 successful egg fertilizations
Study quality	**3**
Reference	790: Chan PTK, Palermo GD, Veeck LL, Rosenwaks Z, Schlegel PN. Testicular sperm extraction combined with intracytoplasmatic sperm injection in the treatment of men with persistent azoospermia porstchemotherapy. Cancer 2001, 166: 45–50.
Language	English

Compound	Combinations (L01XX02)
Disease treated	Lymphoma and leukemia
Quantification of adverse effects	Hormones
No. of patients treated	15

Age group	Young
Treatment period	Various
Dose	Various
Treatment consequences	Hormone levels, impairment
Efficacy	Elevated FSH in 14 of 15, elevated LH levels in 7 of 15, low T in 2 of 15 patients
Randomization of patients	No
Study quality	**3**
Reference	2136: Wang C, Ng RP, Chan TK, Todd D. Effect of combination chemotherapy on pituitary–gonadal function in patients with lymphoma and leukemia. Cancer. 1980 Apr 15;45(8):2030–7.
Language	English

Compound	NOVP (novanthrone, oncovin, vinblastine, prednisone) (L01XX02)
Disease treated	Lymphoma, Hodgkin
Quantification of adverse effects	FISH of sperm chromosomes
No. of patients treated	8
Age group	Young
Treatment period	Various
Dose	Various
Treatment consequences	Sperm aneuploidy rates of chromosomes X, Y, 8, increased
Efficacy	Fivefold increases in sperm with disomies, diploids and complex genotypes involving chromosome X, Y and 8
Randomization of patients	No
Study quality	**3**
Reference	2090: Robbins WA, Meistrich ML, Moore D, Hagemeister FB, Weier HU, Cassel MJ, Wilson G, Eskenazi B, Wyrobek AJ. Chemotherapy induces transient sex chromosomal and autosomal aneuploidy in human sperm. Nat Genet. 1997 May;16(1):74–8.
Language	English

Compound	Combinations (L01XY)
Disease treated	Lymphoma, Hodgkin
Quantification of adverse effects	Semen

No. of patients treated	8
Age group	Young
Treatment period	Various
Dose	Various
Treatment consequences	Spermatogenesis, impairment
Efficacy	In 7 of 8 patients azoospermia after 24 months
Study quality	**3**
Reference	695: Asbjornsen G, Molne K, Klepp O, Aakvaag A. Testicular function after combination chemotherapy for Hodgkin's disease. Scand J Haematol. 1976 Jan;16(1):66–9.
Language	English

Compound	Combinations (L01XY)
Disease treated	Cancer
Quantification of adverse effects	Semen
Age group	Young
Treatment consequences	Spermatogenesis, impairment
Efficacy	Various according to regimen
Remarks	"There is no pharmacologically prohibiton against cytotoxic damage of spermatogenesis".
Study quality	**4 (review)**
Reference	27: Puscheck E, Philip PA, Jeyendran RS. Male fertility preservation and cancer treatment. Cancer Treat Rev. 2004 Apr;30(2):173–80.
Language	English

Compound	Combinations (L01XY)
Disease treated	Cancer
Quantification of adverse effects	Semen
Age group	Young
Treatment consequences	Spermatogenesis, impairment
Efficacy	Most
Study quality	**4 (review)**
Reference	584: Schilsky RL, Lewis BJ, Sherins RJ, Young RC. Gonadal dysfunction in patients receiving chemotherapy for cancer. Ann Intern Med. 1980 Jul;93(1):109–14.
Language	English

2

Compound	Acridinyl anisidide (amsacrine) (not listed)
Disease treated	Melanoma
Quantification of adverse effects	Semen
No. of patients treated	1
Age group	Young
Treatment period	n.g.
Dose	n.g.
Treatment consequences	Spermatogenesis, impairment
Efficacy	After six courses of azoospermia
Randomization of patients	No
Remarks	No further references on this compound
Study quality	**3**
Reference	529: da Cunha MF, Meistrich ML, Haq MM, Gordon LA, Wyrobek AJ. Temporary effects of AMSA (4'-(9-acridinylamino) methanesulfon-m-anisidide) chemotherapy on spermatogenesis. Cancer. 1982 Jun 15;49(12):2459–62.
Language	English

Compound	Mustard gas (not listed)
Disease treated	Poisoning
Quantification of adverse effects	Hormones
No. of patients treated	42
Age group	Young
Treatment period	Various
Dose	Not available
Treatment consequences	Testosterone level, decrease
Efficacy	Three months after exposition
Randomization of patients	No
Study quality	**3**
Reference	223: Azizi F, Keshavarz A, Roshanzamir F, Nafarabadi M. Reproductive function in men following exposure to chemical warfare with sulphur mustard. Med War. 1995 Jan–Mar;11(1):34–44.
Language	English

Compound	Hydroxyurea (not listed)
Disease treated	Sickle cell anemia
Quantification of adverse effects	Semen
No. of patients treated	8
Age group	Young
Treatment period	Various
Dose	Not available
Treatment consequences	Spermatogenesis, impairment
Efficacy	All patients had OAT syndrome
Randomization of patients	No
Study quality	**3**
Reference	744: Friedman G, Freeman R, Bookchin R, Boyar R, Murthy G, Hellman L. Testicular function in sickle cell disease. Fertil Steril. 1974 Dec;25(12):1018–21.
Language	English

Radiation

Although radiation is not a drug, numerous reports on the effects on testicular function with effects similar to antineoplastic drugs have to be considered here. They occurred after radiation for testicular cancer as well as for other diseases.

Testicular cancer: The disease itself impairs spermatogenesis. Of 232 patients, 35% had sperm count below the normal limits.

Radiotherapy in testicular cancer had a much more deleterious effect on spermatogenesis and fertility in patients than chemotherapy alone. A direct radiation to the testis for testicular intraepithelial neoplasia (TIN) with a dose of 14–20 Gy deleted spermatogenic activity. Also after radiation of para-aortal lymph nodes, a testicular scatter dose of 0.22 Gy, a transient increase of FSH levels indicating depression of spermatogenesis was observed. In 10 of 14 patients, in which a gonadal dose of 0.65 Gy was calculated, azoospermia occurred. In higher doses, the effect was more pronounced, and azoospermia was observed in more than 50% of patients. In the spermatozoa in semen an increase of chromosome abnormalities after radiation with a testicular dose of 0.4–5.0 Gy, significantly correlated to testicular radiation dose, was demonstrated. Recovery of spermatogenesis was observed within 2 years; the period appeared to be dose dependent.

Not only spermatogenic activity, but also steroid hormone production was impaired. T levels in blood decreased, and gonadotropin levels increased as a regulatory response. T levels showed a stable decrease for more than 5 years after treatment by 3.6% per year without dose dependency.

Fertility was severely impaired. In a randomized prospective trial 67% of patients treated for testicular cancer achieved a pregnancy in their female partners, but 85% in the wait-and-see group. In another study, 91.2% of patients before diagnosis of testicular cancer, who had tried to induce a pregnancy in their partners, had succeeded, compared with 67.1% of patients after treatment. There was, however, no influence of radiation on gender ratio, weight, height and malformation of children in comparison with a control group.

Prostate cancer: After external beam radiation in prostate cancer, a dose-dependent decrease of testosterone levels in a study with 666 patients was observed, and only 60% had recovery to their individual pretreatment level. The FSH and LH levels were increased. This alteration was less severe than in GnRH treatment. Smaller studies had the same results. If the total dose to the testis was <18.88 cGy, sperm parameters were not impaired.

Rectum cancer: A testicular dose of up to 8.4 Gy in radiation for increased FSH levels in 100%, LH levels in 70% and testosterone in 25% of patients.

Thyroid cancer: Treatment of thyroid cancer with 3.7–5.5 GBq of 131I resulted in an increase of FSH levels in 31 of 52 patients. At a higher dose of 9.8±0.89 GBq mean FSH levels increased to 21 IU/ml and inhibin levels decreased to 29 pg/ml. The LH and testosterone were within the normal range during the whole study. Dose-dependent elevation of serum FSH, 350 mCi and 131I induced impairment of spermatogenesis resulting in azoospermia

Other cancers and lymphoma: If the testicular dose exceeded 20 Gy (200 rad) in radiation of soft tissue sarcoma or Hodgkin's lymphoma, an increase of gonadotropin levels was observed. A return to normal values occurred within 24 months. Up to 25 Gy no significant changes in total testosterone levels occurred. Following an estimated testicular dose of 0.4–5.0 Gy in radiation therapy for other cancers, 8 of 11 men were azoospermic at 3–12 months, but by 24 months they were producing sperm again.

Pituitary adenoma: Radiation resulted in deficiencies of adrenal, thyroidal and gonadal function in 67, 55 and 67% of the patients, respectively. The rate was significantly higher in patients who were only surgically treated with 13, 13 and 0%.

Bone marrow transplantation: Total body irradiation resulted in decreased gonadotropin and testosterone levels.

Acute lymphoblastic leukemia (ALL) in childhood per se did not cause reduction in fertility. Total body irradiation in the course of bone marrow transplantation resulted in hypogonadism in all patients treated, and the T levels were low for more than 4 years After radiotherapy. A testicular dose exceeding 24 Gy in childhood resulted in azoospermia after puberty in all boys. In these cases, also T levels were low and LH and FSH levels increased. The response of T levels to hCG was diminished if the dose exceeded 24 Gy. Pubertal growth was impaired: the final body height and the testis size were reduced. Fertility was severely reduced in cases with high dose (up to 24 cGy) of cranial radiotherapy, although no significant alteration of hormone levels in the course of radiotherapy was found.

Brain cancer in childhood, which did not include the hypothalamo-hypophyseal region, resulted in impaired gonadal function in adulthood. The FSH levels were significantly higher than in controls, inhibin-B levels were significantly lower and also the testicular volume was significantly lower.

Nephroblastoma in childhood: Radiotherapy with an estimated testicular dose of less than 10 Gy resulted in low sperm count and elevated FSH levels after puberty.

Other cancers in childhood: Pubertal maturation was found to be impaired. The mean adult standing height and mean adult leg length were not significantly different from the normal boys; however, the mean adult sitting height was found to be shorter. This was due mainly to radiation-induced skeletal dysplasia attenuating the growth of the spine.

Hypertrophic adenoid or otitis media serosa: In a large study of over 5000 cases and 5000 controls a slight, but insignificant, increase of fertility disorders after nasopharyngeal radium irradiation with a mean dose of 2.75 Gy in childhood was observed (OR: 1.4; 1.0–2.1).

In the following tables, the treatment period of radiation is not given, since it comprised usually only one cycle which consisted of fractionated doses. The influence of fractionation was not studied.

Overall level of evidence of adverse effects: B

Compound	Radiation
Disease treated	Cancer, testicular
Quantification of adverse effects	Fertility

2

No. of patients treated	446
Age group	Young
Dose	Various
Treatment consequences	Children fathered
Efficacy	Before diagnosis of testicular cancer, 91.2% of patients who had tried to get their partners pregnant had succeeded, compared with 67.1% of patients after treatment. Radiotherapy had much more deleterious effect on fertility than chemotherapy alone.
Randomization of patients	No
Dose arms 1–3	Radiation; no radiation
Study quality	**2–**
Reference	2055: Huyghe E, Matsuda T, Daudin M, Chevreau C, Bachaud JM, Plante P, Bujan L, Thonneau P. Fertility after testicular cancer treatments: results of a large multicenter study. Cancer. 2004 Feb 15;100(4):732–7.
Language	English

Compound	Radiation
Disease treated	Cancer, testicular
Quantification of adverse effects	Semen
No. of patients treated	232
Age group	Young
Dose	Before treatment
Treatment consequences	Sperm parameters, impairment
Efficacy	Normal mean of the semen parameters, but 35% below the lower limit of sperm count
Randomization of patients	No
Study quality	**3**
Reference	2085: Gandini L, Lombardo F, Salacone P, Paoli D, Anselmo AP, Culasso F, Dondero F, Lenzi A. Testicular cancer and Hodgkin's disease: evaluation of Semen quality. Hum Reprod. 2003 Apr;18(4):796–801.
Language	English

Compound	Radiation
Disease treated	Cancer, testicular
Quantification of adverse effects	Pregnancy in the female partner
No. of patients treated	172
Age group	29.7 years (mean)
Dose	50 Gy inguinal
Treatment consequences	Pregnancies induced
Efficacy	Gender ratio, weight, height and malformation of children not different from control group
Randomization of patients	No
Study quality	**2+**
Reference	2075: Fossa SD, Almaas B, Jetne V, Bjerkedal T. Paternity after irradiation for testicular cancer. Acta Radiol Oncol. 1986 Jan–Feb;25(1):33–6.
Language	English

Compound	Radiation
Disease treated	Cancer, testicular
Quantification of adverse effects	Semen, hormones
No. of patients treated	158
Age group	Young
Dose	Various
Treatment consequences	Hormone levels; fertility
Efficacy	Decrease of T, increase of gonadotropin levels, fertility in 67% of patients compared with wait-and-see (85%)
Randomization of patients	No
Dose arms 1–3	Chemotherapy; radiation; surveillance
Study quality	**2–**
Reference	2050: Huddart RA, Norman A, Moynihan C, Horwich A, Parker C, Nicholls E, Dearnaley DP. Fertility, gonadal and sexual function in survivors of testicular cancer. Br J Cancer. 2005 Jul 25;93(2):200–7.
Language	English

2

Compound	Radiation
Disease treated	Cancer, testicular
Quantification of adverse effects	Semen
No. of patients treated	62
Age group	18–54 years
Dose	Inverted Y field 6000 rad
Treatment consequences	Sperm parameters, impairment
Efficacy	17 normozoospermia, 28 azoospermia
Randomization of patients	No
Study quality	**3**
Reference	2079: Meyer A, Greiner R. Fertility of semi-castrated and irradiated patients with testicular tumors. Schweiz Med Wochenschr. 1977 Sep 3;107(35):1225–8.
Language	German

Compound	Radiation
Disease treated	Cancer, testicular+para-aortal lymph nodes
Quantification of adverse effects	FSH levels
No. of patients treated	58
Age group	Young
Dose	28.07 Gy, mean testicular scatter dose 0.22 Gy
Treatment consequences	FSH levels, increase
Efficacy	Transient in 27%
Randomization of patients	No
Study quality	**3**
Reference	2062: Sedlmayer F, Joos H, Deutschmann H, Rahim H, Merz F, Kogelnik HD. Long-term tumor control and fertility after para-aortic limited radiotherapy of stage I seminoma. Strahlenther Onkol. 1999 Jul;175(7):320–4.
Language	German

Compound	Radiation
Disease treated	Testicular intraepithelial neoplasia (TIN)
Quantification of adverse effects	Hormones
No. of patients treated	48

Age group	Young
Dose	14–20 Gy
Treatment consequences	Hormone levels, impairment
Efficacy	T level showed a stable decrease for more than 5 years after treatment (3.6% per year) without dose dependency. The levels of LH and FSH were increased after radiotherapy.
Randomization of patients	No
Study quality	**3**
Reference	2104: Petersen PM, Giwercman A, Daugaard G, Rorth M, Petersen JH, Skakkeaek NE, Hansen SW, Maase H von der. Effect of graded testicular doses of radiotherapy in patients treated for carcinoma-in-situ in the testis. J Clin Oncol. 2002 Mar 15;20(6):1537–43.
Language	English

Compound	Radiation
Disease treated	Cancer, testicular
Quantification of adverse effects	FISH of sperm chromosomes
No. of patients treated	38
Age group	Young
Dose	n.g.
Treatment consequences	Sperm aneuploidy rates of chromosomes X, Y, 13, 18 and 21, increased
Efficacy	No significant alterations
Randomization of patients	No
Study quality	**3**
Reference	2083: Thomas C, Cans C, Pelletier R, De Robertis C, Hazzouri M, Sele B, Rousseaux S, Hennebicq S. No long-term increase in sperm aneuploidy rates after anticancer therapy: sperm fluorescence in situ hybridization analysis in 26 patients treated for testicular cancer or lymphoma. Clin Cancer Res. 2004 Oct 1;10(19):6535–43.
Language	English

Compound	Radiation
Disease treated	Cancer, testicular
Quantification of adverse effects	Hormones
No. of patients treated	38

Age group	Young
Dose	Infradiaphragmatic
Treatment consequences	Pretreatment FSH level
Efficacy	Normal levels (12 patients) associated with lower increase after radiation more than high levels (8 patients)
Randomization of patients	No
Dose arms 1–3	Normal FSH levels; high FSH levels
Study quality	**2–**
Reference	2110: Brennemann W, Stoffel-Wagner B, Wichers M, Helmers A, Albers P, Mezger J, Klingmuller D. Pretreatment follicle-stimulating hormone: a prognostic serum marker of spermatogenesis status in patients treated for germ cell cancer. J Urol. 1998 Jun;159(6):1942–6.
Language	English

Compound	Radiation
Disease treated	Cancer, testicular
Quantification of adverse effects	Semen
No. of patients treated	29
Age group	Young
Dose	n.g.
Treatment consequences	Sperm parameters, impairment
Efficacy	Improvement up to 2 years, FSH levels increased 50% up to 3 years
Randomization of patients	No
Study quality	**3**
Reference	2073: Fossa SD, Abyholm T, Normann N, Jetne V. Post-treatment fertility in patients with testicular cancer. III. Influence of radiotherapy in seminoma patients. Br J Urol. 1986 Jun;58(3):315–9.
Language	English

Compound	Radiation
Disease treated	Cancer, testicular
Quantification of adverse effects	Semen
No. of patients treated	16

Age group	Young
Dose	Various
Treatment consequences	Sperm morphology, impairment
Efficacy	Morphological abnormalities of sperm head and neck identical to that of fertile men but in higher percentage
Randomization of patients	No
Study quality	**3**
Reference	2058: Panidis D, Rousso D, Matalliotakis I, Kourtis A, Mavromatidis G, Mamopoulos M, Koumantakis E. Do characteristic spermatozoal morphological abnormalities exist in patients whom have undergone unilateral orchiectomy and preventive radiotherapy? Int J Fertil Womens Med. 2003 Mar–Apr;48(2):83–7.
Language	English

Compound	Radiation
Disease treated	Cancer, testicular
Quantification of adverse effects	Fertility
No. of patients treated	16
Age group	Young
Dose	<2 Gy
Treatment consequences	Pregnancy in the female partner
Efficacy	11 of 16 pregnancies if the dose to the remaining testis was <2 Gy No genetic abnormalities in the offspring
Randomization of patients	No
Study quality	**3**
Reference	2068: Malas S, Levin V, Sur RK, Donde B, Krawitz HE, Pacella JA. Fertility in patients treated with radiotherapy following orchidectomy for testicular seminoma. Clin Oncol (R Coll Radiol). 1994;6(6):377–80.
Language	English

Compound	Radiation
Disease treated	Cancer, testicular
Quantification of adverse effects	Sperm morphology
No. of patients treated	16

Age group	Young
Dose	n.g.
Treatment consequences	Sperm deformity and the sperm multiple anomalies index, impairment
Efficacy	No alteration
Randomization of patients	No
Dose arms 1–3	Radiation; no tumor
Study quality	**2–**
Reference	2089: Panidis D, Matalliotakis I, Papathanasiou K, Roussos C, Koumantakis E. The sperm deformity and the sperm multiple anomalies indexes in patients who underwent unilateral orchectomy and preventive radiotherapy. Eur J Obstet Gynecol Reprod Biol. 1998 Oct;80(2):247–50.
Language	English

Compound	Radiation
Disease treated	Cancer, testicular
Quantification of adverse effects	Semen
No. of patients treated	14
Age group	Young
Treatment period	
Dose	Mean: 78.4±7.4 rad
Treatment consequences	Azoospermia, induction
Efficacy	10 of 14 patients, if >65 rad; recovery after 30–80 weeks
Randomization of patients	No
Study quality	**3**
Reference	2076: Hahn EW, Feingold SM, Simpson L, Batata M. Recovery from aspermia induced by low-dose radiation in seminoma patients. Cancer. 1982 Jul 15;50(2):337–40.
Language	English

Compound	Radiation
Disease treated	Cancer, testicular
Quantification of adverse effects	Sperm chromosomes
No. of patients treated	13
Age group	19–47 years
Dose	0.4–5.0 Gy

Treatment consequences	Sperm chromosome abnormalities, increase
Efficacy	From 0 to 13%, significantly correlated to testicular radiation dose
Randomization of patients	No
Study quality	**3**
Reference	2071: Martin RH, Hildebrand K, Yamamoto J, Rademaker A, Barnes M, Douglas G, Arthur K, Ringrose T, Brown IS. An increased frequency of human sperm chromosomal abnormalities after radiotherapy. Mutat Res. 1986 Jul;174(3):219–25.
Language	English

Compound	Radiation
Disease treated	Cancer, testicular
Quantification of adverse effects	Hormones
No. of patients treated	12
Age group	Young
Treatment period	20 years ago
Dose	Various
Treatment consequences	Hormone levels, impairment
Efficacy	In 9 of 12 patients levels of FSH and LH, in 1 of 12 patients T level outside the normal ranges
Randomization of patients	No
Study quality	**3**
Reference	2129: Nader S, Schultz PN, Cundiff JH, Hussey DH, Samaan NA. Endocrine profiles of patients with testicular tumors treated with radiotherapy. Int J Radiat Oncol Biol Phys. 1983 Nov;9(11):1723–6.
Language	English

Compound	Radiation
Disease treated	Testicular intraepithelial neoplasia (TIN)
Quantification of adverse effects	Hormones
No. of patients treated	9
Age group	Young
Dose	13 Gy

Treatment consequences	Hormone levels, impairment
Efficacy	FSH levels continued to increase 1 year after radiotherapy
Randomization of patients	No
Study quality	**3**
Reference	2087: Sedlmayer F, Holtl W, Kozak W, Hawliczek R, Gebhart F, Gerber E, Joos H, Albrecht W, Pummer K, Kogelnik HD. Australian Uro-Oncology Group (AUO). Radiotherapy of testicular intraepithelial neoplasia (TIN): a novel treatment regimen for a rare disease. Int J Radiat Oncol Biol Phys. 2001 Jul 15;50(4):909–13.
Language	English

Compound	Radiation
Disease treated	Cancer, testicular
Quantification of adverse effects	Semen
No. of patients treated	8
Age group	32.9 years (mean)
Dose	44 cGy
Treatment consequences	Sperm parameters, impairment
Efficacy	At 3 months sperm count decreased to $<10\times10^6$/ml (range $4.4–8.6\times10^6$ in all except one, who decreased from 189×10^6/ml to 58×10^6/ml.
Randomization of patients	No
Study quality	**3**
Reference	2067: Centola GM, Keller JW, Henzler M, Rubin P. Effect of low-dose testicular irradiation on sperm count and fertility in patients with testicular seminoma. J Androl. 1994 Nov–Dec;15(6):608–13.
Language	English

Compound	Radiation
Disease treated	Cancer, testicular
Quantification of adverse effects	Semen, hormones
No. of patients treated	8
Age group	Young
Dose	15–157.5 rad

Treatment consequences	Sperm parameters, impairment
Efficacy	Decrease of sperm count, hamster-oocyte-penetration test normal
Randomization of patients	No
Study quality	**3**
Reference	2093: Freund I, Zenzes MT, Muller RP, Potter R, Knuth UA, Nieschlag E. Testicular function in eight patients with seminoma after unilateral orchidectomy and radiotherapy. Int J Androl. 1987 Apr;10(2):447–55.
Language	English

Compound	Radiation
Disease treated	Cancer, prostate
Quantification of adverse effects	Hormones
No. of patients treated	666
Age group	Old
Dose	External beam radiation without neoadjuvant or adjuvant androgen ablation
Treatment consequences	Testosterone level, decline
Efficacy	At 6 months decreased to 83% of baseline. Only 60% had recovery to their individual pretreatment level. Nadir dependent on radiation volume.
Randomization of patients	No
Study quality	**2+**
Reference	2102: Pickles T, Graham P. Members of the British Columbia Cancer Agency Prostate Cohort Outcomes Initiative. What happens to testosterone after prostate radiation monotherapy and does it matter? J Urol. 2002 Jun;167(6):2448–52.
Language	English

Compound	Radiation
Disease treated	Cancer, prostate
Quantification of adverse effects	Hormones
No. of patients treated	85
Age group	Old

2

Dose	External beam radiation
Treatment consequences	Hormone levels, impairment
Efficacy	Pretreatment T levels 185–783 ng/day, postradiation 3-month T 163–796 ng/day (significant mean difference)
Randomization of patients	No
Study quality	**3**
Reference	2112: Zagars GK, Pollack A. Serum testosterone levels after external beam radiation for clinically localized prostate cancer. Int J Radiat Oncol Biol Phys. 1997 Aug 1;39(1):85–9.
Language	English

Compound	Radiation
Disease treated	Cancer, prostate
Quantification of adverse effects	Hormones
No. of patients treated	58
Age group	Old
Dose	n.g.
Treatment consequences	Hormone levels, impairment
Efficacy	Severe by GnRH, lesser by radiotherapy, none in healthy men
Randomization of patients	No
Dose arms 1–3	Radiation; GnRH agonist; healthy
Study quality	**2–**
Reference	2101: Basaria S, Lieb J 2nd, Tang AM, DeWeese T, Carducci M, Eisenberger M, Dobs AS. Long-term effects of androgen deprivation therapy in prostate cancer patients. Clin Endocrinol (Oxf). 2002 Jun;56(6):779–86.
Language	English

Compound	Radiation
Disease treated	Cancer, prostate
Quantification of adverse effects	Hormones
No. of patients treated	33
Age group	>70 years
Dose	n.g.
Treatment consequences	Hormone levels, impairment, 3–8 years post treatment

Efficacy	Decline of testosterone levels 27.3%, increase of LH levels 52.7% Greater, increase of FSH levels 100%
Randomization of patients	No
Study quality	**3**
Reference	2107: Daniell HW, Clark JC, Pereira SE, Niazi ZA, Ferguson DW, Dunn SR, Figueroa ML, Stratte PT. Hypogonadism following prostate-bed radiation therapy for prostate carcinoma. Cancer. 2001 May 15;91(10):1889–95.
Language	English

Compound	Radiation
Disease treated	Cancer, prostate
Quantification of adverse effects	Hormones
No. of patients treated	17
Age group	Old
Dose	Total tumor dose 63.5 Gy
Treatment consequences	Hormone levels, impairment
Efficacy	T levels lower, LH and FSH levels higher than in controls. T levels decreased 3 months after treatment, but pretreatment values again 6 and 12 months after treatment.
Randomization of patients	No
Study quality	**3**
Reference	2130: Tomic R, Bergman B, Damber JE, Littbrand B, Lofroth PO. Effects of external radiation therapy for cancer of the prostate on the serum concentrations of testosterone, follicle-stimulating hormone, luteinizing hormone and prolactin. J Urol. 1983 Aug;130(2):287–9.
Language	English

Compound	Radiation
Disease treated	Cancer, prostate
Quantification of adverse effects	Hormones
No. of patients treated	11
Age group	68–78 years
Dose	20 Gy
Treatment consequences	Hormone levels, impairment

Efficacy	Decrease of T levels to an average of 70.3% of the initial values
Randomization of patients	No
Study quality	**3**
Reference	2134: Fleck H, Stahl F, Mau S. Suppression of testicular testosterone production by irradiation of the testis in prostatic cancer. Z Urol Nephrol. 1981 Jun;74(6):443–6.
Language	German

Compound	Radiation
Disease treated	Cancer, prostate
Quantification of adverse effects	Semen
No. of patients treated	4
Age group	Young
Dose	Total dose to the testis 18.88 cGy ^{125}I
Treatment consequences	Sperm parameters, impairment
Efficacy	No significant alterations
Randomization of patients	No
Remarks	This value is considered too low to have any significant effect on testicular tissues.
Study quality	**3**
Reference	2084: Mydlo JH, Lebed B. Does brachytherapy of the prostate affect sperm quality and/or fertility in younger men? Scand J Urol Nephrol. 2004;38(3):221–4.
Language	English

Compound	Radiation
Disease treated	Cancer, prostate
Quantification of adverse effects	Hormones
No. of patients treated	n.g.
Age group	Old
Dose	n.g.
Treatment consequences	Hormone levels, impairment
Efficacy	Increase of FSH and LH levels, no alteration of T levels at 3 and 12 months

Study quality	**3**
Reference	2137: Seal US. FSH and LH elevation after radiation for treatment of cancer of the prostate. Invest Urol. 1979 Jan;16(4):278–80.
Language	English

Compound	Radiation
Disease treated	Cancer, rectum
Quantification of adverse effects	Hormones
No. of patients treated	25
Age group	65 years (mean)
Dose	Testicular dose 8.4 Gy
Treatment consequences	Hormone levels, impairment
Efficacy	100% increase in serum FSH, 70% increase in LH, 25% reduction in testosterone levels
Randomization of patients	No
Study quality	**3**
Reference	2099: Dueland S, Guren MG, Olsen DR, Poulsen JP, Magne Tveit K. Radiation therapy induced changes in male sex hormone levels in rectal cancer patients. Radiother Oncol. 2003 Sep;68(3):249–53.
Language	English

Compound	Radiation
Disease treated	Cancer, rectum
Quantification of adverse effects	Hormones
No. of patients treated	11
Age group	55.2 years (mean)
Dose	Testicular dose 3.56 Gy (0.7–8.4 Gy)
Treatment consequences	Hormone levels, impairment
Efficacy	Levels of LH increased to 350%, of FSH levels to 185%, of testosterone decreased to 78%.
Randomization of patients	No
Study quality	**3**

2

Reference	2097: Hermann RM, Henkel K, Christiansen H, Vorwerk H, Hille A, Hess CF, Schmidberger H. Testicular dose and hormonal changes after radiotherapy of rectal cancer. Radiother Oncol. 2005 Apr;75(1):83–8.
Language	English

Compound	Radiation
Disease treated	Cancer, thyroid
Quantification of adverse effects	Hormones
No. of patients treated	52
Age group	All ages
Dose	3.7–5.5 GBq ^{131}I
Treatment consequences	Hormone levels, impairment
Efficacy	FSH levels increased in 31 of 52 patients, testosterone levels unaltered
Randomization of patients	No
Study quality	**3**
Reference	2082: Rosario PW, Barroso AL, Rezende LL, Padrao EL, Borges MA, Guimaraes VC, Purisch S. Testicular function after radioiodine therapy in patients with thyroid cancer. Thyroid. 2006 Jul;16(7):667–70.
Language	English

Compound	Radiation
Disease treated	Cancer, thyroid
Quantification of adverse effects	Hormones
No. of patients treated	25
Age group	23–73 years
Dose	Radioiodine dose 9.8±0.89 GBq
Treatment consequences	Hormone levels, impairment
Efficacy	FSH increased significantly to 21.32.4 IU/l after 6 months, decreased to 7.41.3 IU/l after 18 months. Inhibin B significantly decreased to 29.4 pg/ml after 6 months, increased to 154 pg/ml after 18 months. LH and testosterone were within the normal range during the whole study.
Randomization of patients	No

Study quality	**3**
Reference	2088: Wichers M, Benz E, Palmedo H, Biersack HJ, Grunwald F, Klingmuller D. Testicular function after radioiodine therapy for thyroid carcinoma. Eur J Nucl Med. 2000 May;27(5):503–7.
Language	English

Compound	Radiation
Disease treated	Cancer, thyroid
Quantification of adverse effects	Hormones
No. of patients treated	12
Age group	Young
Dose	^{131}I
Treatment consequences	Hormone levels, impairment
Efficacy	Dose-dependent elevation of serum FSH
Randomization of patients	No
Study quality	**3**
Reference	2133: Handelsman DJ, Turtle JR. Testicular damage after radioactive iodine (I-131) therapy for thyroid cancer. Clin Endocrinol (Oxf). 1983 May;18(5):465–72.
Language	English

Compound	Radiation
Disease treated	Cancer, thyroid
Quantification of adverse effects	Semen
No. of patients treated	1
Age group	32 years
Treatment period	Single dose
Dose	350 mCi ^{131}I
Treatment consequences	Spermatogenesis, impairment
Efficacy	Azoospermia
Study quality	**3**
Reference	2077: Handelsman DJ, Conway AJ, Donnelly PE, Turtle JR. Azoospermia after iodine-131 treatment for thyroid carcinoma. Br Med J. 1980 Dec 6;281(6254):1527.
Language	English

Compound	Radiation
Disease treated	Lymphoma and leukemia
Quantification of adverse effects	Hormones
No. of patients treated	66
Age group	All ages
Dose	n.g.
Treatment consequences	Fatigue, mood and sexual function by questionnaire; decrease
Efficacy	No significant differences between men with normal and low T levels
Randomization of patients	No
Dose arms 1–3	Normal T levels; low T levels
Study quality	**2–**
Reference	2108: Howell SJ, Radford JA, Smets EM, Shalet SM. Fatigue, sexual function and mood following treatment for haematological malignancy: the impact of mild Leydig cell dysfunction. Br J Cancer. 2000 Feb;82(4):789–93.
Language	English

Compound	Radiation
Disease treated	Lymphoma, Hodgkin
Quantification of adverse effects	Hormones
No. of patients treated	17
Age group	Young
Dose	Testicular dose 6–70 cGy
Treatment consequences	Hormone levels, impairment
Efficacy	In patients receiving more than 20 cGy, increase in serum FSH values following up to 6 months, return to normal within 24 months. No significant changes in LH and T. Two patients with transient oligospermia with complete recovery by 18 months following treatment
Randomization of patients	No
Study quality	**3**
Reference	2118: Kinsella TJ, Trivette G, Rowland J, Sorace R, Miller R, Fraass B, Steinberg SM, Glatstein E, Sherins RJ. Long-term follow-up of testicular function following radiation therapy for early-stage Hodgkin's disease. J Clin Oncol. 1989 Jun;7(6):718–24.

Language	English

Compound	Radiation
Disease treated	Lymphoma and leukemia
Quantification of adverse effects	Hormones
No. of patients treated	16
Age group	Young
Dose	Total body irradiation and bone marrow transplantation
Treatment consequences	Hormone levels, impairment
Efficacy	T and LH low levels, in the posttransplant period, return to the normal range, but not the sexual steroids.
Randomization of patients	No
Study quality	**3**
Reference	2119: Feyer P, Titlbach O, Hoffmann FA, Kubel M, Helbig W. Endocrine dysfunction after total body irradiation and bone marrow transplantation. Folia Haematol Int Mag Klin Morphol Blutforsch. 1989;116(3–4):547–52.
Language	English

Compound	Radiation
Disease treated	Lymphoma, malignant
Quantification of adverse effects	Semen
No. of patients treated	9
Age group	Young
Dose	Inverted Y field, mantle field
Treatment consequences	Sperm count, decrease
Efficacy	Eight men with sperm count zero or low; FSH levels elevated, three pregnancies in the female partner
Randomization of patients	No
Study quality	**3**
Reference	2081: Asbjornsen G, Molne K, Klepp O, Aakvaag A. Testicular function after radiotherapy to inverted "Y" field for malignant lymphoma. Scand J Haematol. 1976 Aug;17(2):96–100.
Language	English

2

Compound	Radiation
Disease treated	Lymphoma, non-Hodgkin
Quantification of adverse effects	Semen
No. of patients treated	7
Age group	29 years (median)
Dose	2.46–5.3 Gy+cyclophosphamide, doxorubicine, vincristine, bleomycin
Treatment consequences	Sperm parameters, impairment
Efficacy	Sperm count between 0 and 44×10^6
Randomization of patients	No
Study quality	**3**
Reference	2069: Pryzant RM, Meistrich ML, Wilson G, Brown B, McLaughlin P. Long-term reduction in sperm count after chemotherapy with and without radiation therapy for non-Hodgkin's lymphomas. J Clin Oncol. 1993 Feb;11(2):239–47.
Language	English

Compound	Radiation
Disease treated	Lymphoma, Hodgkin
Quantification of adverse effects	FISH of sperm chromosomes
No. of patients treated	1
Age group	Young
Dose	n.g.
Treatment consequences	Sperm aneuploidy rates of chromosomes X, Y, 1, 6, 11, increased
Efficacy	Day 0 as well as at day 38
Remarks	Lymphoma itself affects spermatogenic cell divisions.
Study quality	**3**
Reference	2091: Monteil M, Rousseaux S, Chevret E, Pelletier R, Cozzi J, Sele B. Increased aneuploid frequency in spermatozoa from a Hodgkin's disease patient after chemotherapy and radiotherapy. Cytogenet Cell Genet. 1997;76(3–4):134–8.
Language	English

Compound	Radiation
Disease treated	Soft tissue sarcoma
Quantification of adverse effects	Hormones

No. of patients treated	27
Age group	14–67 years
Dose	Testicular dose 1–2500 rad
Treatment consequences	Hormone levels, impairment
Efficacy	Only patients receiving greater than 200 rad had significant LH changes; no significant changes in total testosterone levels.
Randomization of patients	No
Study quality	**3**
Reference	2124: Shapiro E, Kinsella TJ, Makuch RW, Fraass BA, Glatstein E, Rosenberg SA, Sherins RJ. Effects of fractionated irradiation of endocrine aspects of testicular function. J Clin Oncol. 1985 Sep;3(9):1232–9.
Language	English

Compound	Radiation
Disease treated	Cancer, others
Quantification of adverse effects	Semen
No. of patients treated	11
Age group	Young
Dose	0.4–5.0 Gy
Treatment consequences	Sperm parameters, impairment
Efficacy	At 3 and 12 months post-radiotherapy 8 of 11 men were azoospermic, by 24 months 8 of 11 were producing sperm. Hamster-oocyte-penetration test >15%
Randomization of patients	No
Study quality	**3**
Reference	2094: Martin RH, Rademaker A, Barnes M, Arthur K, Ringrose T, Douglas G. A prospective serial study of the effects of radiotherapy on semen parameters, and hamster egg penetration rates. Clin Invest Med. 1985;8(3):239–43.
Language	English

Compound	Radiation
Disease treated	Pituitary adenoma
Quantification of adverse effects	Hormones

No. of patients treated	35
Age group	Young
Dose	n.g.
Treatment consequences	Hormone levels, impairment
Efficacy	Deficiencies of adrenal, thyroid and gonadal function in 67, 55 and 67% of the patients; in patients only surgically treated deficiencies in 13, 13 and 0%
Randomization of patients	No
Dose arms 1–3	Pituitary radiation; surgical intervention
Study quality	**2–**
Reference	2121: Snyder PJ, Fowble BF, Schatz NJ, Savino PJ, Gennarelli TA. Hypopituitarism following radiation therapy of pituitary adenomas. Am J Med. 1986 Sep;81(3):457–62.
Language	English

Compound	Radiation
Disease treated	Acromegaly
Quantification of adverse effects	Hormones
No. of patients treated	8
Age group	Young
Dose	Pituitary dose 5500 rad
Treatment consequences	Hormone levels, impairment
Efficacy	Low T levels in 1 of 6 patients
Randomization of patients	No
Study quality	**3**
Reference	2139: Aloia JF, Archambeau JO. Hypopituitarism following pituitary irradiation for acromegaly. Horm Res. 1978;9(4):201–7.
Language	English

Compound	Radiation
Disease treated	Pineal gland germinoma
Quantification of adverse effects	IVF outcome
No. of patients treated	1
Age group	Young
Dose	n.g.

Treatment consequences	Pregnancy in the female partner
Efficacy	ICSI was successful
Study quality	**3**
Reference	2061: Ramsewak S, Naraynsingh A, Kuruvilla A, Duffy S. Successful pregnancy by intracytoplasmic sperm injection after radiotherapy-induced azoospermia. West Indian Med J. 1999 Dec;48(4):240–1.
Language	English

Compound	Radiation
Disease treated	Acute lymphoblastic leukemia (ALL) in childhood
Quantification of adverse effects	Fertility
No. of patients treated	213; 145
Age group	Young
Dose	Various
Treatment consequences	Fertility disorders, increased
Efficacy	Relative fertility (RF)=0.95, 95% (CI 0.63–1.43), with high dose (24 cGy) cranial radiotherapy reduced fertility RR=0.09, 95% (CI 0.01–0.82)
Randomization of patients	No
Dose arms 1–3	Radiation; no radiation
Study quality	**2++**
Reference	2054: Byrne J, Fears TR, Mills JL, Zeltzer LK, Sklar C, Meadows AT, Reaman GH, Robison LL. Fertility of long-term male survivors of acute lymphoblastic leukemia diagnosed during childhood. Pediatr Blood Cancer. 2004 Apr;42(4):364–72.
Language	English

Compound	Radiation
Disease treated	Acute lymphoblastic leukemia (ALL) in childhood
Quantification of adverse effects	Hormones
No. of patients treated	93
Age group	Prepubertal
Dose	2400 rad cranial+methotrexate intrathecal
Treatment consequences	Hormone levels, impairment

2

Efficacy	No significant alterations
Randomization of patients	No
Dose arms 1–3	Radiation+methotrexate; methotrexate
Study quality	**2–**
Reference	2122: Voorhess ML, Brecher ML, Glicksman AS, Jones B, Harris M, Krischer J, Boyett J, Forman E, Freeman AI. Hypothalamic-pituitary function of children with acute lymphocytic leukemia after three forms of central nervous system prophylaxis. A retrospective study. Cancer. 1986 Apr 1;57(7):1287–91.
Language	English

Compound	Radiation
Disease treated	Acute lymphoblastic leukemia (ALL) in childhood
Quantification of adverse effects	Hormones
No. of patients treated	28
Age group	Prepubertal
Dose	Testicular dose 2000 rad
Treatment consequences	Hormone levels, impairment
Efficacy	Basal and stimulated FSH and LH levels increased, T response to hCG low
Randomization of patients	No
Dose arms 1–3	Radiation; radiation+chemotherapy
Study quality	**2–**
Reference	2127: Carrascosa A, Audi L, Ortega JJ, Javier G, Toran N. Hypothalamo-hypophyseal-testicular function in prepubertal boys with acute lymphoblastic leukemia following chemotherapy and testicular radiotherapy. Acta Paediatr Scand. 1984 May;73(3):364–71.
Language	English

Compound	Radiation
Disease treated	Acute lymphoblastic leukemia (ALL) in childhood
Quantification of adverse effects	Hormones
No. of patients treated	21
Age group	Prepubertal
Treatment period	

Dose	Testicular irradiation 24 Gy
Treatment consequences	Hormone levels, impairment
Efficacy	Low T levels and response to hCG, increase in LH levels in 19 of 21 patients
Randomization of patients	No
Study quality	**3**
Reference	2120: Brauner R, Caltabiano P, Rappaport R, Leverger G, Schaison G. Leydig cell insufficiency after testicular irradiation for acute lymphoblastic leukemia. Horm Res. 1988;30(2–3):111–4.
Language	English

Compound	Radiation
Disease treated	Acute lymphoblastic leukemia (ALL) in childhood
Quantification of adverse effects	Pubertal maturation
No. of patients treated	17
Age group	Prepubertal
Dose	Total body irradiation+bone marrow transplantation
Treatment consequences	Pubertal stages, development
Efficacy	Hypogonadism in all boys
Randomization of patients	No
Study quality	**3**
Reference	2098: Frisk P, Arvidson J, Gustafsson J, Lonnerholm G. Pubertal development and final height after autologous bone marrow transplantation for acute lymphoblastic leukemia. Bone Marrow Transplant. 2004 Jan;33(2):205–10.
Language	English

Compound	Radiation
Disease treated	Acute lymphoblastic leukemia (ALL) in childhood
Quantification of adverse effects	Hormones, semen
No. of patients treated	15
Age group	Prepubertal
Dose	Testicular dose 12–24 Gy
Treatment consequences	Hormone levels, impairment

Efficacy	Normal in all boys; azoospermia in all boys
Randomization of patients	No
Study quality	**3**
Reference	2117: Castillo LA, Craft AW, Kernahan J, Evans RG, Aynsley-Green A. Gonadal function after 12-Gy testicular irradiation in childhood acute lymphoblastic leukaemia. Med Pediatr Oncol. 1990;18(3):185–9.
Language	English

Compound	Radiation
Disease treated	Acute lymphoblastic leukemia (ALL) in childhood
Quantification of adverse effects	Hormones
No. of patients treated	12
Age group	Prepubertal
Dose	Various
Treatment consequences	Hormone levels, impairment
Efficacy	T levels low more than 4 years after testicular irradiation, diminished testicular volume
Randomization of patients	No
Study quality	**3**
Reference	2131: Brauner R, Czernichow P, Cramer P, Schaison G, Rappaport R. Leydig-cell function in children after direct testicular irradiation for acute lymphoblastic leukemia. N Engl J Med. 1983 Jul 7;309(1):25–8.
Language	English

Compound	Radiation
Disease treated	Acute lymphoblastic leukemia (ALL) in childhood
Quantification of adverse effects	Hormones
No. of patients treated	11
Age group	Prepubertal
Dose	Testicular dose 2400 rad
Treatment consequences	Hormone levels, impairment
Efficacy	Stimulated FSH and LH levels increased, T basal and response to hCG low

Randomization of patients	No
Study quality	**3**
Reference	2128: Leiper AD, Grant DB, Chessells JM. The effect of testicular irradiation on Leydig cell function in prepubertal boys with acute lymphoblastic leukaemia. Arch Dis Child. 1983 Nov;58(11):906–10.
Language	English

Compound	Radiation
Disease treated	Acute lymphoblastic leukemia (ALL) in childhood
Quantification of adverse effects	Hormones
No. of patients treated	9
Age group	Prepubertal
Dose	1100–3000 rad
Treatment consequences	Hormone levels, impairment
Efficacy	At the age of 12 years, elevated basal and/or stimulated LH- and FSH values were elevated. T response to HCG test only in patients with gonadal dose of 1100 and 1500 rads. No response in doses of 2400 and 3000 rads.
Randomization of patients	No
Study quality	**3**
Reference	2132: Bramswig JH, Schellong G, Nieschlag E. Pituitary–gonadal function following therapy of testicular relapse in boys with acute lymphoblastic leukemia, Klin Padiatr. 1983 May–Jun;195(3):176–80.
Language	German

Compound	Radiation
Disease treated	Acute lymphoblastic leukemia (ALL) in childhood
Quantification of adverse effects	Hormones
No. of patients treated	7
Age group	Young
Dose	Testicular dose 2400 rad
Treatment consequences	Hormone levels, impairment
Efficacy	Three of four boys with bilateral lesion had delayed sexual maturation, elevated FSH and LH levels, and low testosterone levels.

Randomization of patients	No
Study quality	**3**
Reference	2125: Blatt J, Sherins RJ, Niebrugge D, Bleyer WA, Poplack DG. Leydig cell function in boys following treatment for testicular relapse of acute lymphoblastic leukemia. J Clin Oncol. 1985 Sep;3(9):1227–31.
Language	English

Compound	Radiation
Disease treated	Acute lymphoblastic leukemia (ALL) in childhood
Quantification of adverse effects	Hormones
No. of patients treated	7
Age group	Prepubertal
Dose	Testicular radiation
Treatment consequences	Hormone levels, impairment
Efficacy	Normal basal T levels , but T response to hCG low
Randomization of patients	No
Study quality	**3**
Reference	2126: Shalet SM, Horner A, Ahmed SR, Morris-Jones PH. Leydig cell damage after testicular irradiation for lymphoblastic leukaemia. Med Pediatr Oncol. 1985;13(2):65–8.
Language	English

Compound	Radiation
Disease treated	Cancer, brain, not including hypothalamo–hypophyseal region, in childhood
Quantification of adverse effects	Hormones
No. of patients treated	30
Age group	9 years (mean)
Treatment consequences	Hormone levels, impairment in age >18 years
Efficacy	FSH significantly higher than in controls, inhibin significantly lower, testicular volume lower
Randomization of patients	No
Study quality	**3**

Reference	2106: Schmiegelow M, Lassen S, Poulsen HS, Schmiegelow K, Hertz H, Andersson AM, Skakkebaek NE, Muller J. Gonadal status in male survivors following childhood brain tumors. J Clin Endocrinol Metab. 2001 Jun;86(6):2446–52.
Language	English

Compound	Radiation
Disease treated	Cancer, brain, not including hypothalamo–hypophyseal region, in childhood
Quantification of adverse effects	Hormones
No. of patients treated	13
Age group	Prepubertal
Dose	Cranial radiation
Treatment consequences	Hormone levels, impairment in puberty
Efficacy	FSH and LH levels increased, T levels normal
Randomization of patients	No
Study quality	**3**
Reference	2111: Lannering B, Jansson C, Rosberg S, Albertsson-Wikland K. Increased LH and FSH secretion after cranial irradiation in boys. Med Pediatr Oncol. 1997 Oct;29(4):280–7.
Language	English

Compound	Radiation
Disease treated	Nephroblastoma during childhood
Quantification of adverse effects	Semen
No. of patients treated	10
Age group	17–36 years
Dose	Testes: 268–983 rad
Treatment consequences	Sperm parameters, impairment
Efficacy	Eight men sperm count 0–5.6 million/ml, seven of whom had elevated FSH level.
Randomization of patients	No
Study quality	**3**
Reference	2078: Shalet SM, Beardwell CG, Jacobs HS, Pearson D. Testicular function following irradiation of the human prepubertal testis. Clin Endocrinol (Oxf). 1978 Dec;9(6):483–90.

2

Language	English

Compound	Radiation
Disease treated	Nephroblastoma during childhood
Quantification of adverse effects	Hormones
No. of patients treated	10
Age group	Prepubertal
Dose	Various
Treatment consequences	Hormone levels, impairment
Efficacy	Eight men had low sperm count (0–5.6 million/ml), seven had elevated FSH level. One man showed raised LH level and low T level.
Randomization of patients	No
Study quality	**3**
Reference	2138: Shalet SM, Beardwell CG, Jacobs HS, Pearson D. Testicular function following irradiation of the human prepubertal testis. Clin Endocrinol (Oxf). 1978 Dec;9(6):483–90.
Language	English

Compound	Radiation
Disease treated	Cancer, in childhood
Quantification of adverse effects	Semen
No. of patients treated	33; 66
Age group	Young
Dose	Various
Treatment consequences	Sperm parameters, impairment
Efficacy	Sperm count significantly lower than in controls, no differences in DNA integrity; FSH levels higher
Randomization of patients	No
Dose arms 1–3	Radiation; no radiation
Study quality	**2+**
Reference	2059: Thomson AB, Campbell AJ, Irvine DC, Anderson RA, Kelnar CJ, Wallace WH. Semen quality and spermatozoal DNA integrity in survivors of childhood cancer: a case-control study. Lancet. 2002 Aug 3;360(9330):361–7.

Language	English

Compound	Radiation
Disease treated	Cancer, in childhood
Quantification of adverse effects	Pubertal maturation
No. of patients treated	8
Age group	Prepubertal
Dose	Various
Treatment consequences	Pubertal stages, development
Efficacy	Mean adult standing height (167.5±9.9 cm) and mean adult leg length (80.8±6.2 cm) not significantly different from that in normal boys, but mean adult sitting height (86.7±4.8 cm) significantly less
Randomization of patients	No
Study quality	**3**
Reference	2114: Didi M, Morris-Jones PH, Gattamaneni HR, Shalet SM. Pubertal growth in response to testosterone replacement therapy for radiation-induced Leydig cell failure. Med Pediatr Oncol. 1994;22(4):250–4.
Language	English

Compound	Radiation
Disease treated	Nasopharyngeal radium irradiation for hypertrophic adenoid or otitis media serosa
Quantification of adverse effects	Fertility
No. of patients treated	5358; 5265
Age group	Young
Dose	2.75 Gy for nasopharynx
Treatment consequences	Fertility disorders, increased
Efficacy	Slightly more fertility disorders than men in the control group (OR: 1.4; 1.0–2.1)
Randomization of patients	No
Dose arms 1–3	Radiation; no radiation
Study quality	**2++**

Reference	2051: Ronckers CM, Verduijn PG, Land CE, Hayes RB, Stovall M, van Leeuwen FE. No convincing evidence for a causal relationship between childhood nasopharyngeal radium irradiation and head–neck tumors or hormone-related disorders later in life; a retrospective cohort study. Ned Tijdschr Geneeskd. 2004 Sep 4;148(36):1775–80.
Language	Dutch

L02	**Endocrine Therapy**
	Oestrogen-like Compounds
	Individual reports on diethylstibestrol when given during pregnancy of the mother as a cause of male subfertility are available. The association is far from being proven. **Overall level of evidence of adverse effects: D**

Compound	Diethylstibestrol in utero (L02AA01)
Disease treated	Abortion, threatening in the mother
Quantification of adverse effects	Testicular histology, chromosome synapsis
No. of patients treated	1
Age group	Young
Treatment period	n.g.
Dose	n.g.
Treatment consequences	Spermatogenesis, impairment
Efficacy	Meiotic dysruption
Study quality	**3**
Reference	357: Hembree WC, Nagler HM, Fang JS, Myles EL, Jagiello GM. Infertility in a patient with abnormal spermatogenesis and in utero DES exposure. Int J Fertil. 1988 May–Jun;33(3):173–7.
Language	English

Compound	Diethylstibestrol (L02AA01)
Disease treated	Abortion, threatening in the mother
Quantification of adverse effects	Genital malformations in the sons
Age group	Young
Treatment consequences	Testicular cancer, hypospadias, cryptorchidism

Efficacy	Significant increase
Randomization of patients	No
Study quality	**4 (review)**
Reference	798. Toppari J, Larsen JC, Christianse P et al. Male reproductive health and environmental xenoestrogens. Environ Health Perspect 1996;104 (Suppl 4), 741–803.
Language	English

L02 Endocrine Therapy

GnRH

Gonadotropin-releasing hormone (GnRH) was used for different purposes:

1. Stimulation of gonadotropin secretion from the pituitary gland in hypogonadism. In these cases, a pulsatile application was necessary in order to mimick the pulsatile secretion from the normal hypothalamus. The treatment of hypogonadism was effective in terms of gonadotropin secretion, testosterone secretion and maturation of spermatogenesis in nearly all cases; however, a treatment period of at least 3 months was necessary. The majority of patients (>50%) also became fertile and fathered children, if desired.

Overall level of evidence of positive effects: C
Overall level of evidence of adverse effects compromising effectiveness: D

2. Depression of gonadotropin secretion. Continuous application or application of long-acting agonists and antagonists inhibits gonadotropin seceretion and thus caused a decline in testosterone production and spermatogenic activity. Depression of testosterone secretion was successfully achieved in prostatic cancer. The depression impaired testosterone-dependent sexual functions and frequently caused gynaecomastia. Testosterone levels returned to normal within 10–12 months after cessation of treatment, but LH levels may remain increased. Long-term application of agonists and antagonists also depressed spermatogenesis. There were also trials for contraception, but azoospermia was achieved in only up to 70% of men. after application of bicalutamid, spermatogenesis was unexpectedly well preserved; organization of seminiferous tubules was normal, and mature spermatozoa were present.

Overall level of evidence of adverse effects: B

Based on these observations, it was expected that the depression by GnRH might prevent spermatogenesis against deleterious effects of cytotoxic treatment. This aim, however, could not be achieved in any of the studies.

Overall level of evidence of adverse effects: C

Adverse effects outside the hormonal system as described above were not observed.

Compound	GnRH (L02AE)+hCG
Disease treated	Idiopathic hypogonadotropic hypogonadism (IHH)
Quantification of dysfunction	Sperm, testicular volume
No. of patients treated	38
Age group	Young
Treatment period	12 months
Dose	2–20 µg GnRH puls
Treatment consequences	Gonadotropin levels, increase
Efficacy	In 35 of 38 patients
Randomization of patients	No
Study quality	**3**
Reference	257: Delemarre-Van de Waal HA. Induction of testicular growth and spermatogenesis by pulsatile, intravenous administration of gonadotrophin-releasing hormone in patients with hypogonadotrophic hypogonadism. Clin Endocrinol (Oxf). 1993 May;38(5):473–80.
Language	English

Compound	GnRH pulsatile (L02AE)
Disease treated	Idiopathic hypogonadotropic hypogonadism (IHH)
Quantification of dysfunction	Semen
No. of patients treated	23
Age group	Young
Treatment period	36 months
Dose	Various
Treatment consequences	Spermatogenesis, maturation

Efficacy	In 20 of 23 patients mature spermatozoa in semen
Randomization of patients	No
Study quality	**3**
Reference	400: Spratt DI, Finkelstein JS, O'Dea LS, Badger TM, Rao PN, Campbell JD, Crowley WF Jr. Long-term administration of gonadotropin-releasing hormone in men with idiopathic hypogonadotropic hypogonadism. A model for studies of the hormone's physiologic effects. Ann Intern Med. 1986 Dec;105(6):848–55.
Language	English

Compound	GnRH pulsatile (L02AE)
Disease treated	Idiopathic hypogonadotropic hypogonadism (IHH)
Quantification of dysfunction	Semen
No. of patients treated	11
Age group	Young
Treatment period	24 months
Dose	Various
Treatment consequences	Fertility
Efficacy	Pregnancy induced in 7 of 11 patients
Randomization of patients	No
Study quality	**3**
Reference	76: Christiansen P, Skakkebaek NE. Pulsatile gonadotropin-releasing hormone treatment of men with idiopathic hypogonadotropic hypogonadism. Horm Res. 2002;57(1–2):32–6.
Language	English

Compound	GnRH pulsatile (L02AE)
Disease treated	Idiopathic hypogonadotropic hypogonadism (IHH)
Quantification of dysfunction	Hormones
No. of patients treated	6
Age group	Young
Treatment period	74 weeks
Dose	Various
Treatment consequences	Spermatogenesis, maturation

Efficacy	In 3 of 6 patients
Randomization of patients	No
Study quality	**3**
Reference	398: Niles NL, McCorkell SJ, Woodhouse NJ. Male hypothalamic hypogonadism: induction of spermatogenesis by subcutaneous pulsatile gonadotrophin-releasing hormone. Horm Res. 1987;25(3):152–9.
Language	English

Compound	GnRH pulsatile (L02AE)
Disease treated	Idiopathic hypogonadotropic hypogonadism (IHH)
Quantification of dysfunction	Semen, hormones
No. of patients treated	6
Age group	Young
Treatment period	43 weeks
Dose	Various
Treatment consequences	Spermatogenesis, maturation
Efficacy	In all patients
Randomization of patients	No
Study quality	**3**
Reference	524: Hoffman AR, Crowley WF Jr. Induction of puberty in men by long-term pulsatile administration of low-dose gonadotropin-releasing hormone. N Engl J Med. 1982 Nov 11;307(20):1237–41.
Language	English

Compound	GnRH pulsatile (L02AE)
Disease treated	Idiopathic hypogonadotropic hypogonadism (IHH)
Quantification of dysfunction	Hormones
No. of patients treated	3
Age group	Young
Treatment period	6 months
Dose	Various
Treatment consequences	Spermatogenesis, maturation
Efficacy	In all patients after 161 days

Randomization of patients	No
Study quality	**3**
Reference	426: Klingmüller D, Schweikert HU. Maintenance of spermatogenesis by intranasal administration of gonadotropin-releasing hormone in patients with hypothalamic hypogonadism. J Clin Endocrinol Metab. 1985 Nov;61(5):868–72.
Language	English

Compound	GnRH pulsatile (L02AE)
Disease treated	Hypogonadism, secondary
Quantification of dysfunction	Semen
No. of patients treated	3
Age group	Young
Treatment period	250 days
Dose	Various
Treatment consequences	Fertility, improvement
Efficacy	Pregnancy induced in 2 of 3 patients after 181 days
Randomization of patients	No
Study quality	**3**
Reference	489: Skarin G, Nillius SJ, Wide L. Long-term subcutaneous pulsatile low dose LH–RH administration for treatment of infertile men with secondary hypogonadotrophic hypogonadism. Ups J Med Sci. 1984;89(1):81–90.
Language	English

Compound	GnRH pulsatile (L02AE)
Disease treated	Idiopathic hypogonadotropic hypogonadism (IHH)
Quantification of dysfunction	Semen
No. of patients treated	2
Age group	Young
Treatment period	6 months
Dose	Various
Treatment consequences	Spermatogenesis, maturation
Efficacy	After 42 days

Randomization of patients	No
Study quality	**3**
Reference	351: Blumenfeld Z, Makler A, Frisch L, Brandes JM. Induction of spermatogenesis and fertility in hypogonadotropic azoospermic men by intravenous pulsatile gonadotropin-releasing hormone (GnRH). Gynecol Endocrinol. 1988 Jun;2(2):151-64.
Language	English

Compound	GnRH pulsatile (L02AE)
Disease treated	Idiopathic hypogonadotropic hypogonadism (IHH)
Quantification of dysfunction	Hormones, pregnancy in the female partner
No. of patients treated	1
Age group	28
Treatment consequences	Spermatogenesis, maturation
Efficacy	Conception on day 162
Randomization of patients	No
Study quality	**3**
Reference	377: Oppermann D, Happ J, Mayr WR. Stimulation of spermatogenesis and biological paternity by intranasal (low dose) gonadotropin-releasing hormone (GnRH) in a male with Kallmann's syndrome: intraindividual comparison of GnRH and gonadotropins for stimulation of spermatogenesis. J Clin Endocrinol Metab. 1987 Nov;65(5):1060–6.
Language	English

Compound	GnRH pulsatile (L02AE)
Disease treated	Hypogonadism, traumatic
Quantification of dysfunction	Semen
No. of patients treated	1
Age group	36
Treatment period	15 months
Dose	Various
Treatment consequences	Spermatogenesis, recovery
Efficacy	Complete

Randomization of patients	No
Study quality	**3**
Reference	325: Fok AC, Tsakok FH, Sum CF, Cheah JS. Restoration of spermatogenesis with pulsatile gonadotrophin releasing hormone therapy in hypogonadotrophic hypogonadism of traumatic etiology. Aust N Z J Med. 1989 Aug;19(4):354–7.
Language	English

Compound	GnRH pulsatile (L02AE)
Disease treated	Infertility
Quantification of dysfunction	Semen
No. of patients treated	4
Age group	24–39 years
Treatment period	135 days
Dose	500 µg/day
Treatment consequences	Spermatogenesis, improvement
Efficacy	In 2 of 4 patients
Randomization of patients	No
Study quality	**3**
Reference	728: Schwarzstein L, Aparicio NJ, Turner D, Calamera JC, Mancini R, Schally AV. Use of synthetic luteinizing hormone-releasing hormone in treatment of oligospermic men: a preliminary report. Fertil Steril. 1975 Apr;26(4):331–6.
Language	English

Compound	GnRH agonist (L02AE)
Disease treated	Cancer, prostate
Quantification of adverse effects	Hormones
No. of patients treated	419
Age group	Old
Treatment period	6 months
Dose	Various
Treatment consequences	Hormone levels, impairment
Efficacy	T levels return to normal after cessation, LH levels remain increased

Randomization of patients	No
Study quality	**3**
Reference	2105: Shahidi M, Norman AR, Gadd J, Huddart RA, Horwich A, Dearnaley DP. Recovery of serum testosterone, LH and FSH levels following neoadjuvant hormone cytoreduction and radical radiotherapy in localized prostate cancer. Clin Oncol (R Coll Radiol). 2001;13(4):291–5.
Language	English

Compound	GnRH agonist (L02AE)
Disease treated	Cancer, prostate
Quantification of adverse effects	Hormones
No. of patients treated	276
Age group	Old
Treatment period	3 years
Dose	Various
Treatment consequences	Testosterone level, increase after cessation
Efficacy	97% recovered normal testosterone levels (10 nmol/l), and 93% recovered levels of at least 5 nmol/l. Median time to testosterone recovery was 10 months.
Randomization of patients	No
Dose arms 1–3	GnRH 1 month depot; GnRH 3 months depot
Study quality	**2+**
Reference	2103: Pickles T, Agranovich A, Berthelet E, Duncan GG, Keyes M, Kwan W, McKenzie MR, Morris WJ. British Columbia Cancer Agency, Prostate Cohort Outcomes Initiative. Testosterone recovery following prolonged adjuvant androgen ablation for prostate carcinoma. Cancer. 2002 Jan 15;94(2):362–7.
Language	English

Compound	GnRH agonist (L02AE)
Disease treated	Radiation therapy for seminoma
Quantification of dysfunction	Hormones, semen
No. of patients treated	20
Age group	Young
Treatment period	6 weeks

Dose	n.g.
Treatment consequences	Gonadotropin levels, decrease
Efficacy	Total suppression, recovery of spermatogenesis independent of GnRH treatment
Randomization of patients	No
Dose arms 1–3	GnRH agonist; no hormonal therapy
Study quality	**3**
Reference	230: Brennemann W, Brensing KA, Leipner N, Boldt I, Klingmuller D. Attempted protection of spermatogenesis from irradiation in patients with seminoma by D-tryptophan-6 luteinizing hormone releasing hormone. Clin Invest. 1994 Nov;72(11):838–42.
Language	English

Compound	GnRH agonist (L02AE)
Disease treated	Cancer, prostate
Quantification of adverse effects	Testicular histology
No. of patients treated	16
Age group	Old
Treatment period	10 months
Dose	n.g.
Treatment consequences	Spermatogenesis, impairment and maturation arrest
Efficacy	In all patients
Randomization of patients	No
Study quality	**3**
Reference	371: Lunglmayr G, Girsch E, Meixner EM, Viehberger G, Bieglmayer C. Effects of long term GnRH analogue treatment on hormone levels and spermatogenesis in patients with carcinoma of the prostate. Urol Res. 1988;16(4):315–9.
Language	English

Compound	GnRH agonist (L02AE)
Disease treated	Cancer, prostate
Quantification of adverse effects	T production in vitro
No. of patients treated	14

Age group	Old
Treatment period	6 months
Dose	3×600 µg/day
Treatment consequences	Testosterone production, decrease
Efficacy	By 94%
Randomization of patients	No
Study quality	**3**
Reference	378: Huhtaniemi I, Nikula H, Parvinen M, Rannikko S. Pituitary–testicular function of prostatic cancer patients during treatment with a gonadotropin-releasing hormone agonist analog. II. Endocrinology and histology of the testis. J Androl. 1987 Nov–Dec;8(6):363–73.
Language	English

Compound	GnRH agonist (L02AE)
Disease treated	Cancer, prostate
Quantification of adverse effects	Testicular histology
No. of patients treated	7
Age group	Old
Treatment period	32 months
Dose	3 mg/3 weeks
Treatment consequences	Spermatogenesis, impairment
Efficacy	In all men
Randomization of patients	No
Study quality	**3**
Reference	370: Giberti C, Barreca T, Martorana G, Truini M, Franceschini R, Rolandi E, Giuliani L. Hormonal pattern and testicular histology in patients with prostatic cancer after long-term treatment with a gonadotropin-releasing hormone agonist analogue. Eur Urol. 1988;15(1–2):125–7.
Language	English

Compound	GnRH agonist (L02AE)
Disease treated	Contraception
Quantification of dysfunction	Semen
No. of patients treated	8

Age group	Young
Treatment period	10 weeks
Dose	n.g.
Treatment consequences	Sperm count, decrease
Efficacy	To 70% of basal sperm count
Randomization of patients	No
Study quality	**3**
Reference	553: Linde R, Doelle GC, Alexander N, Kirchner F, Vale W, Rivier J, Rabin D. Reversible inhibition of testicular steroidogenesis and spermatogenesis by a potent gonadotropin-releasing hormone agonist in normal men: an approach toward the development of a male contraceptive. N Engl J Med. 1981 Sep 17;305(12):663–7.
Language	English

Compound	GnRH agonist (L02AE)+T
Disease treated	Contraception
Quantification of dysfunction	Semen, hormones
No. of patients treated	8
Age group	Young
Treatment period	20 weeks
Dose	500 μg/day
Treatment consequences	Spermatogenesis, impairment
Efficacy	In all men
Randomization of patients	No
Study quality	**3**
Reference	472: Rabin D, Evans RM, Alexander AN, Doelle GC, Rivier J, Vale W, Liddle GW. Heterogeneity of sperm density profiles following 20-week therapy with high-dose LHRH analog plus testosterone. J Androl. 1984 May–Jun;5(3):176–80.
Language	English

Compound	GnRH agonist (L02AE)+T
Disease treated	Contraception
Quantification of dysfunction	Semen
No. of patients treated	7

2

Age group	Young
Treatment period	16 weeks
Dose	400 μg/day
Treatment consequences	Sperm count, decrease
Efficacy	By 93% in week 16
Randomization of patients	No
Study quality	**3**
Reference	383: Bhasin S, Yuan QX, Steiner BS, Swerdloff RS. Hormonal effects of gonadotropin-releasing hormone (GnRH) agonist in men: effects of long term treatment with GnRH agonist infusion and androgen. J Clin Endocrinol Metab. 1987 Sep;65(3):568–74.
Language	English

Compound	GnRH agonist (L02AE)+T
Disease treated	Contraception
Quantification of dysfunction	Semen
No. of patients treated	7
Age group	Young
Treatment period	16 weeks
Dose	200 μg/day
Treatment consequences	Sperm count, decrease
Efficacy	By 83%
Randomization of patients	No
Study quality	**3**
Reference	447: Bhasin S, Heber D, Steiner BS, Handelsman DJ, Swerdloff RS. Hormonal effects of gonadotropin-releasing hormone (GnRH) agonist in the human male. III. Effects of long term combined treatment with GnRH agonist and androgen. J Clin Endocrinol Metab. 1985 May;60(5):998–1003.
Language	English

Compound	GnRH agonist (L02AE)+T
Disease treated	Contraception
Quantification of dysfunction	Semen
No. of patients treated	6

Age group	Young
Treatment period	20 weeks
Dose	50 µg/day
Treatment consequences	Sperm count, decrease
Efficacy	From 76.7×10^6/ml) to a mean nadir of 12.3×10^6/ml
Randomization of patients	No
Study quality	**3**
Reference	498: Doelle GC, Alexander AN, Evans RM, Linde R, Rivier J, Vale W, Rabin D. Combined treatment with an LHRH agonist and testosterone in man. Reversible oligozoospermia without impotence. J Androl. 1983 Sep–Oct;4(5):298–302.
Language	English

Compound	GnRH antagonist (L02AE)+T
Disease treated	Contraception
Quantification of dysfunction	Azoospermia
No. of patients treated	19
Age group	Young
Treatment period	20 weeks
Treatment consequences	Azoospermia, induction
Efficacy	In 7 of 10 men
Randomization of patients	No
Dose arms 1–3	T 200 mg/week+GnRH 100 µg/kg day^{-1}; T alone
Study quality	**2–**
Reference	255: Bagatell CJ, Matsumoto AM, Christensen RB, Rivier JE, Bremner WJ. Comparison of a gonadotropin releasing-hormone antagonist plus testosterone (T) versus T alone as potential male contraceptive regimens. J Clin Endocrinol Metab. 1993 Aug;77(2):427–32.
Language	English

Compound	GnRH antagonist (L02AE)+T
Disease treated	Contraception
Quantification of dysfunction	Semen
No. of patients treated	15
Age group	21–41 years

Treatment period	24 weeks
Dose	T 100 mg/week+GnRH 10 mg/week
Treatment consequences	Azoospermia, induction
Efficacy	In 10 of 15 men
Randomization of patients	No
Study quality	**3**
Reference	148: Swerdloff RS, Bagatell CJ, Wang C, Anawalt BD, Berman N, Steiner B, Bremner WJ. Suppression of spermatogenesis in man induced by Nal–Glu gonadotropin releasing hormone antagonist and testosterone enanthate (TE) is maintained by TE alone. J Clin Endocrinol Metab. 1998 Oct;83(10):3527–33.
Language	English

Compound	GnRH antagonist (L02AE)
Disease treated	Contraception
Quantification of dysfunction	Semen, evaluation by CASA
No. of patients treated	6
Age group	Young
Treatment period	20 weeks
Dose	10 mg/day
Treatment consequences	Sperm motility, CASA parameters, alteration
Efficacy	No significant alteration of motility parameters
Randomization of patients	No
Study quality	**3**
Reference	256: Bastias MC, Kamijo H, Pavlou SN. sperm motion parameters after suppression of spermatogenesis with a gonadotropin-releasing hormone antagonist plus testosterone supplementation. Fertil Steril. 1993 Jun;59(6):1261–5.
Language	English

Compound	GnRH (L02AE)
Disease treated	Cancer
Quantification of dysfunction	Semen
Age group	Young

Treatment consequences	Spermatogenesis, recovery after cancer therapy
Efficacy	No improvement by GnRH
Study quality	**4 (review)**
Reference	162: Meistrich ML. Hormonal stimulation of the recovery of spermatogenesis following chemo- or radiotherapy. Review article. APMIS. 1998 Jan;106(1):37–45; discussion 45–6.
Language	English

Compound	Buserelin (L02AE01)
Disease treated	Cancer
Quantification of adverse effects	Semen
No. of patients treated	20
Age group	Young
Treatment period	7 days prior to cytotoxic therapy
Dose	Various
Treatment consequences	Azoospermia, induction
Efficacy	All but one similar to cytotoxic therapy alone
Randomization of patients	No
Study quality	**3**
Reference	329: Krause W, Pfluger KH. Treatment with the gonadotropin-releasing hormone agonist buserelin to protect spermatogenesis against cytotoxic treatment in young men. Andrologia. 1989 May–Jun;21(3):265–70.
Language	English

Compound	Buserelin (L02AE01)
Disease treated	Cancer, prostate
Quantification of adverse effects	Testicular histology
No. of patients treated	12
Age group	Old
Treatment period	138 months
Dose	n.g.
Treatment consequences	Spermatogenesis, impairment
Efficacy	In 50% SCOS, in 92% Leydig cell atrophy
Randomization of patients	No

Dose arms 1–3	Buserelin alone; buserelin+flutamide
Study quality	**2–**
Reference	381: Hadziselimovic F, Senn E, Bandhauer K. Effect of treatment with chronic gonadotropin releasing hormone agonist on human testis. J Urol. 1987 Oct;138(4 Pt 2):1048–50.
Language	English

Compound	Buserelin (L02AE01)
Disease treated	Cancer, prostate
Quantification of dysfunction	Testicular histology
No. of patients treated	12
Age group	53–78 years
Treatment period	96 weeks
Dose	1.2 mg/day
Treatment consequences	Spermatogenesis, impairment
Efficacy	11 of 12
Randomization of patients	No
Study quality	**3**
Reference	341: Properzi G, Francavilla S, Vicentini C, Cordeschi G, Galassi P, Paradiso Galatioto G, Miano L. Testicular changes after treatment with a GnRH analog (buserelin) in association with cyproterone acetate in men with prostatic cancer. Eur Urol. 1989;16(6):426–32.
Language	English

Compound	Buserelin (L02AE01)
Disease treated	Cancer, prostate
Quantification of adverse effects	Testicular histology
No. of patients treated	7
Age group	Old
Treatment period	6 months
Dose	1800 µg/day
Treatment consequences	Spermatogenesis, suppression
Efficacy	High in all patients
Randomization of patients	No

Study quality	**3**
Reference	44: Huhtaniemi I, Nikula H, Parvinen M, Rannikko S. Pituitary-testicular function of prostatic cancer patients during treatment with a gonadotropin-releasing hormone agonist analog. II. Endocrinology and histology of the testis. J Androl. 1987 Nov–Dec;8(6):363–73.
Language	English

Compound	Buserelin (L02AE01)
Disease treated	Contraception
Quantification of dysfunction	Semen
No. of patients treated	15
Age group	Young
Treatment period	5 months
Treatment consequences	Sperm count, decrease
Efficacy	In all men
Randomization of patients	Yes
Dose arms 1–3	3×50 μg/week; 3×100 μg/week; 3×200 μg/week+5 mg fluoxymesterone
Study quality	**1–**
Reference	416: Frick J, Aulitzky W. Effects of a potent LHRH-agonist on the pituitary gonadal axis with and without testosterone substitution. Urol Res. 1986;14(5):261–4.
Language	English

Compound	Buserelin (L02AE01)
Disease treated	Contraception
Quantification of dysfunction	Sperm
No. of patients treated	10
Age group	Young
Treatment period	30 weeks
Treatment consequences	Spermatogenesis, impairment
Efficacy	4× azoospermia in group with oral T
Randomization of patients	Yes
Dose arms 1–3	Buserelin depot+125 mg/month T i.m.; buserelin depot+120 mg/day T orally

2

Study quality	**1–**
Reference	399: Bouchard P, Garcia E. Influence of testosterone substitution on sperm suppression by LHRH agonists. Horm Res. 1987;28(2–4):175–80.
Language	English

Compound	Leuprolide (L02AE02)
Disease treated	Cancer, prostate
Quantification of adverse effects	Testicular histology
No. of patients treated	12
Age group	46–72 years
Treatment period	24 months
Dose	1–10 mg/day
Treatment consequences	Spermatogenesis, impairment; Leydig cell, hypoplasia
Efficacy	In all patients
Randomization of patients	No
Study quality	**2–**
Reference	49: Smith JA Jr, Urry RL. Testicular histology after prolonged treatment with a gonadotropin-releasing hormone analogue. J Urol. 1985 Apr;133(4):612–4.
Language	English

Compound	Leuprolide (L02AE02)
Disease treated	Cancer, prostate
Quantification of adverse effects	Testicular histology
No. of patients treated	4
Age group	Old
Treatment period	12 months
Dose	n.g.
Treatment consequences	Spermatogenesis, impairment; Leydig cell, hypoplasia
Efficacy	In all patients after 1 year of treatment
Randomization of patients	No
Study quality	**3**
Reference	461: Rajfer J, Swerdloff RS, Heber DM. Testicular histology following chronic gonadotropin-releasing hormone agonist treatment. Fertil Steril. 1984 Nov;42(5):765–71.
Language	English

Compound	Goserelin (L02AE03)
Disease treated	Cancer, prostate
Quantification of adverse effects	Testicular histology
No. of patients treated	16
Age group	Old
Treatment period	17 months
Dose	n.g.
Treatment consequences	Spermatogenesis, suppression
Efficacy	Tubular atrophy in all patients
Randomization of patients	No
Study quality	**3**
Reference	46: Johansen TE, Ogreid P, Kjellevold K, Blom P. Testicular histology after treatment with LH–RH analogue for carcinoma of the prostate. Br J Urol. 1990 Apr;65(4):376–8.
Language	English

L02 **Endocrine Therapy**

Tamoxifen, Raloxifen and Letrozole

The oestrogen-receptor antagonist tamoxifen was used:

1. In the treatment of gynaecomastia and breast pain which occurred during antiandrogenic treatment with good efficacy. The success was demonstrated also in RCTs. In terms of clinical and clinical–chemical data, no adverse effects were observed.
2. For the stimulation of spermatogenic activity via an increase of gonadotropin and testosterone secretion. Following uncontrolled studies reporting successful results, a significant increase of hormone levels was proven in RCTs, whereas a significant increase of sperm count could not be proven. Also the pregnancy rate after treatment of men did not increase significantly.

A treatment with Raloxifene also induced a significant increase of sex steroid hormone levels, but in the studies a decrease of osteocalcin and IGF-1 levels was reported as an adverse effect.

Overall level of evidence of positive effects: B
Overall level of evidence of adverse effects compromising effectiveness: C

2

There is only a single report available which describes the effect of the aromatase inhibitor letrozole on testicular function.

Overall level of evidence of adverse effects: D

Compound	Tamoxifen (L02BA01)
Disease treated	Cancer, prostate, treatment with bicalutamide
Quantification of dysfunction	Breast swelling
No. of patients treated	114
Age group	Old
Treatment period	48 weeks
Dose	20 mg/day
Treatment consequences	Gynaecomastia and breast pain, development
Efficacy	10% of men treated with tamoxifen+bicalutamide, 73% of placebo+bicalutamide
Side effects compromising effectiveness	No differences in sexual function
Randomization of patients	Yes
Dose arms 1–3	Tamoxifen 20 mg/day+bicalutamide 150 mg/day; astronazol 1 mg/day+bicalutamide 150 mg/day; placebo+bicalutamide 150 mg/day
Study quality	**1+**
Reference	931: Boccardo F, Rubagotti A, Battaglia M, Tonno P di, Selvaggi FP, Conti G, Comeri G, Bertaccini A, Martorana G, Galassi P, Zattoni F, Macchiarella A, Siragusa A, Muscas G, Durand F, Potenzoni D, Manganelli A, Ferraris V, Montefiore F. Evaluation of tamoxifen and anastrozole in the prevention of gynecomastia and breast pain induced by bicalutamide monotherapy of prostate cancer. J Clin Oncol. 2005 Feb 1;23(4):808–15.
Language	English

Compound	Tamoxifen (L02BA01)
Disease treated	Cancer, prostate, treatment with bicalutamide
Quantification of dysfunction	Breast swelling
No. of patients treated	107

Age group	Old
Treatment period	n.g.
Dose	20 mg/day
Treatment consequences	Gynaecomastia and breast pain, development
Efficacy	Reduction in tamoxifen co-treated groups
Randomization of patients	Yes
Dose arms 1–3	Tamoxifen 20 mg/day+bicalutamide 150 mg/day; astronazol 1 mg/day+bicalutamide 150 mg/day; placebo+bicalutamide 150 mg/day
Study quality	**1+**
Reference	930: Saltzstein D, Sieber P, Morris T, Gallo J. Prevention and management of bicalutamide-induced gynecomastia and breast pain: randomized endocrinologic and clinical studies with tamoxifen and anastrozole. Prostate Cancer Prostatic Dis. 2005;8(1):75–83.
Language	English

Compound	Tamoxifen (L02BA01)
Disease treated	Gynaecomastia
Quantification of dysfunction	Breast swelling
No. of patients treated	37
Age group	Young
Treatment period	n.g.
Dose	n.g.
Treatment consequences	Gynaecomastia, reduction
Efficacy	In all patients
Side effects compromising effectiveness	No side effects
Randomization of patients	No
Study quality	**3**
Reference	932: Derman O, Kanbur NO, Kutluk T. Tamoxifen treatment for pubertal gynecomastia. Int J Adolesc Med Health. 2003 Oct–Dec;15(4):359–63.
Language	English

2

Compound	Tamoxifen (L02BA01)
Disease treated	Liver cirrhosis
Quantification of dysfunction	Breast swelling
No. of patients treated	16
Age group	Old
Treatment period	1 month
Dose	2×20 mg/day
Treatment consequences	Gynaecomastia and breast pain, reduction
Efficacy	In 14 of 16 patients
Side effects compromising effectiveness	No side effects
Randomization of patients	Yes
Dose arms 1–3	Tamoxifen 2×20 mg/day; placebo
Study quality	**1–**
Reference	934: Li CP, Lee FY, Hwang SJ, Chang FY, Lin HC, Kuo BI, Chu CJ, Lee SD. Treatment of mastalgia with tamoxifen in male patients with liver cirrhosis: a randomized crossover study. Am J Gastroenterol. 2000 Apr;95(4):1051–5.
Language	English

Compound	Tamoxifen (L02BA01)
Disease treated	Gynaecomastia
Quantification of dysfunction	Serum lipids
No. of patients treated	15
Age group	Young
Treatment period	3 months
Dose	10 mg/day
Treatment consequences	Serum lipid proteins, alteration
Efficacy	None in all patients
Randomization of patients	No
Study quality	**3**
Reference	933: Novoa FJ, Boronat M, Carrillo A, Tapia M, Diaz-Cremades J, Chirino R. Effects of tamoxifen on lipid profile and coagulation parameters in male patients with pubertal gynecomastia. Horm Res. 2002;57(5–6):187–91.
Language	English

Compound	Tamoxifen (L02BA01)
Disease treated	Healthy
Quantification of dysfunction	Hormones
No. of patients treated	13
Age group	Young
Treatment period	6 weeks
Dose	20 mg/day
Treatment consequences	LH pulsatility, increase
Efficacy	Levels and pulse frequency
Randomization of patients	No
Study quality	**3**
Reference	900: Spijkstra JJ, Spinder T, Gooren L, van Kessel H. Divergent effects of the antiestrogen tamoxifen and of estrogens on luteinizing hormone (LH) pulse frequency, but not on basal LH levels and LH pulse amplitude in men. Clin Endocrinol Metab. 1988 Feb;66(2):355–60.
Language	English

Compound	Tamoxifen (L02BA01)
Disease treated	Healthy
Quantification of dysfunction	Hormones
No. of patients treated	7
Age group	Young
Treatment period	3 months
Dose	20 mg/day
Treatment consequences	Gonadotropin and testosterone levels, increase
Efficacy	In tamoxifen group
Randomization of patients	No
Dose arms 1–3	Tamoxifen; placebo
Study quality	**2–**
Reference	902: van Bergeijk L, Gooren LJ, van Kessel H, Sassen AM. Effects of continuous LHRH infusion on plasma levels of LH and FSH in males, before and after oestrogen or anti-oestrogen treatment. Horm Metab Res. 1986 Aug;18(8):558–64.
Language	English

Compound	Tamoxifen (L02BA01)
Disease treated	Cancer, prostate, treatment with flutamide
Quantification of dysfunction	Breast swelling
No. of patients treated	6
Age group	Old
Treatment period	1 months
Dose	20 mg/day
Treatment consequences	Gynaecomastia and breast pain, reduction
Efficacy	In 5 of 6 patients
Side effects compromising effectiveness	No side effects
Randomization of patients	No
Study quality	**3**
Reference	935: Staiman VR, Lowe FC. Tamoxifen for flutamide/finasteride-induced gynecomastia. Urology. 1997 Dec;50(6):929–33.
Language	English

Compound	Tamoxifen (L02BA01)
Disease treated	Gynaecomastia, idiopathic
Quantification of dysfunction	Breast swelling
No. of patients treated	6
Age group	Old
Treatment period	1 month
Dose	n.g.
Treatment consequences	Gynaecomastia and breast pain, reduction
Efficacy	In 5 of 6 patients
Side effects compromising effectiveness	No side effects
Randomization of patients	Yes
Dose arms 1–3	Tamoxifen; placebo
Study quality	**1–**
Reference	936: McDermott MT, Hofeldt FD, Kidd GS. Tamoxifen therapy for painful idiopathic gynecomastia. South Med J. 1990 Nov;83(11):1283–5.

Language	English

Compound	Tamoxifen (L02BA01)
Disease treated	Healthy
Quantification of dysfunction	Hormones
No. of patients treated	5
Age group	Young
Treatment period	Single dose
Dose	50 mg
Treatment consequences	Gonadotropin and testosterone levels, alteration
Efficacy	No consistent effects
Randomization of patients	No
Study quality	**3**
Reference	903: Fauser BC, Dony JM, Doesburg WH, Thomas CM, Rolland R. Short- and long-term hormonal effects of a single dose of 50 mg tamoxifen administered to normal males. Andrologia. 1984 Sep–Oct;16(5):465–70.
Language	English

Compound	Tamoxifen (L02BA01)
Disease treated	Androgen receptor pathology
Quantification of dysfunction	Fertility
No. of patients treated	1
Age group	Young
Treatment period	20 weeks
Dose	20 mg/day
Treatment consequences	Gonadotropin levels, increase
Efficacy	Each time after tamoxifen application
Randomization of patients	No
Study quality	**3**
Reference	327: Gooren L. Improvement of spermatogenesis after treatment with the antiestrogen tamoxifen in a man with the incomplete androgen insensitivity syndrome. J Clin Endocrinol Metab. 1989 Jun;68(6):1207–10.
Language	English

Compound	Tamoxifen (L02BA01)
Disease treated	Infertility
Quantification of dysfunction	Semen
No. of patients treated	212
Age group	Young
Treatment period	6 months
Dose	20 mg/day
Treatment consequences	Sperm parameters, improvement
Efficacy	Increase of sperm count and sperm motility in verum group, not in placebo group; pregnancies 33.9% in verum group, 10.3% in placebo Group
Side effects compromising effectiveness	None
Randomization of patients	Yes
Dose arms 1–3	Tamoxifen; placebo
Study quality	**1–**
Reference	166: Adamopoulos DA, Pappa A, Billa E, Nicopoulou S, Koukkou E, Michopoulos J. Effectiveness of combined tamoxifen citrate and testosterone undecanoate treatment in men with idiopathic oligozoospermia. Fertil Steril. 2003 Oct;80(4):914–20.
Language	English

Compound	Tamoxifen (L02BA01)
Disease treated	Infertility
Quantification of dysfunction	Semen
No. of patients treated	77
Age group	Young
Treatment period	6 months
Dose	20 mg/day
Treatment consequences	Sperm parameters, improvement
Efficacy	Sperm count increased, testosterone levels increased
Side effects compromising effectiveness	None

Randomization of patients	Yes
Dose arms 1–3	Tamoxifen; placebo
Study quality	**1–**
Reference	174: Krause W, Holland-Moritz H, Schramm P. Treatment of idiopathic oligozoospermia with tamoxifen: a randomized controlled study. Int J Androl. 1992 Feb;15(1):14–8.
Language	English

Compound	Tamoxifen (L02BA01)
Disease treated	Infertility
Quantification of dysfunction	Semen
No. of patients treated	56
Age group	Young
Treatment period	Long term
Dose	30 mg/day
Treatment consequences	Sperm parameters, improvement
Efficacy	32 of 56 patients reached normal sperm density
Randomization of patients	No
Study quality	**3**
Reference	171: Bartsch G, Scheiber K. Tamoxifen treatment in oligozoospermia. Eur Urol. 1981;7(5):283–7.
Language	English

Compound	Tamoxifen (L02BA01)
Disease treated	Spermatogenic dysfunction
Quantification of dysfunction	Semen
No. of patients treated	43
Age group	Young
Treatment period	6 months
Dose	20 mg/day
Treatment consequences	Spermatogenesis, improvement
Efficacy	Most pronounced in men with initial sperm count $<5\times10^6$
Randomization of patients	No

Study quality	**3**
Reference	554: Traub AI, Thompson W. The effect of tamoxifen on spermatogenesis in subfertile men. Andrologia. 1981 Sep–Oct;13(5):486–90.
Language	English

Compound	Tamoxifen (L02BA01)
Disease treated	Infertility
Quantification of dysfunction	Semen, hormones
No. of patients treated	33
Age group	Young
Treatment period	Long term
Dose	20 mg/day
Treatment consequences	Sperm parameters, improvement
Efficacy	Significant increase of sperm count, sperm motility and morphology
Randomization of patients	No
Study quality	**3**
Reference	173: Schill WB, Landthaler M. Tamoxifen treatment of oligozoospermia. Andrologia. 1980 Nov–Dec;12(6):546–8.
Language	English

Compound	Tamoxifen (L02BA01)
Disease treated	Infertility
Quantification of dysfunction	Semen
No. of patients treated	29
Age group	Young
Treatment period	3 months
Dose	20 mg/day
Treatment consequences	Sperm parameters, improvement
Efficacy	No significant improvement in seminal volume, sperm count, sperm motility, morphology, and of hamster-oocyte-penetration test results
Side effects compromising effectiveness	n.g.

Randomization of patients	No
Study quality	**3**
Reference	167: Sterzik K, Rosenbusch B, Mogck J, Heyden M, Lichtenberger K. Tamoxifen treatment of oligozoospermia: a re-evaluation of its effects including additional sperm function tests. Arch Gynecol Obstet. 1993;252(3):143–7.
Language	English

Compound	Tamoxifen (L02BA01)
Disease treated	Infertility
Quantification of dysfunction	Hormones
No. of patients treated	n.g.
Age group	Young
Treatment period	3 months
Dose	20 mg/day
Treatment consequences	Hormone levels, increase
Efficacy	LH, FSH, progesterone, 17 alpha-progesterone, testosterone and oestradiol-17 beta
Randomization of patients	No
Study quality	**3**
Reference	170: Damber JE, Abramsson L, Duchek M. Tamoxifen treatment of idiopathic oligozoospermia: effect on hCG-induced testicular steroidogenesis and semen variables. Scand J Urol Nephrol. 1989;23(4):241–6.
Language	English

Compound	Raloxifen (G02CB04)
Disease treated	Healthy
Quantification of dysfunction	Hormones
No. of patients treated	43
Age group	49–70 years
Treatment period	6 weeks
Treatment consequences	Sex steroid hormones, increase
Efficacy	By 11–13%

2

Side effects compromising effectiveness	Decrease of osteocalcin
Randomization of patients	Yes
Dose arms 1–3	Raloxifen 120 mg/day; placebo
Study quality	**1–**
Reference	898: Uebelhart B, Herrmann F, Pavo I, Draper MW, Rizzoli R. Raloxifene treatment is associated with increased serum estradiol and decreased bone remodeling in healthy middle-aged men with low sex hormone levels. J Bone Miner Res. 2004 Sep;19(9):1518–24.
Language	English

Compound	Raloxifen (G02CB04)
Disease treated	Healthy
Quantification of dysfunction	Hormones
No. of patients treated	30
Age group	60–70 years
Treatment period	3 months
Treatment consequences	Testosterone level, increase
Efficacy	By 20%
Side effects compromising effectiveness	Decrease of IGF-1
Randomization of patients	Yes
Dose arms 1–3	Raloxifen 120 mg/day; placebo
Study quality	**1–**
Reference	897: Duschek EJ, Gooren LJ, Netelenbos C. Comparison of effects of the rise in serum testosterone by raloxifene and oral testosterone on serum insulin-like growth factor-1 and insulin-like growth factor binding protein-3. Maturitas. 2005 Jul 16;51(3):286–93.
Language	English

Compound	Bicalutamide (L02BB03)
Disease treated	Cancer, prostate
Quantification of dysfunction	Gynaecomastia

No. of patients treated	102
Age group	Old
Treatment period	Various
Dose	150 mg/day
Treatment consequences	Gynaecomastia, breast pain, development
Efficacy	67% (no additional treatment), 8% (tamoxifen), 34% (radiotherapy)
Randomization of patients	No
Dose arms 1–3	Bicalutamide alone; b+tamoxifen 10 mg/day; b+radiation
Study quality	**1–**
Reference	2096: Lorenzo G di, Perdona S, Placido S di, D'Armiento M, Gallo A, Damiano R, Pingitore D, Gallo L, Sio M de, Autorino R. Gynecomastia and breast pain induced by adjuvant therapy with bicalutamide after radical prostatectomy in patients with prostate cancer: the role of tamoxifen and radiotherapy J Urol. 2005 Dec;174(6):2197–203.
Language	English

Compound	Bicalutamide (L02BB03)
Disease treated	Cancer, prostate
Quantification of adverse effects	Testicular histology
No. of patients treated	2
Age group	Old
Treatment period	4 years
Dose	50 mg/day
Treatment consequences	Testicular morphology, alterations
Efficacy	Unexpectedly well preserved; normal organization of seminiferous tubules, mature spermatozoa present
Randomization of patients	No
Study quality	**3**
Reference	45: Morgante E, Gradini R, Realacci M, Sale P, D'Eramo G, Perrone GA, Cardillo MR, Petrangeli E, Russo M, Silverio F di. Effects of long-term treatment with the anti-androgen bicalutamide on human testis: an ultrastructural and morphometric study. Histopathology. 2001 Mar;38(3):195–201.
Language	English

2

Compound	Letrozole (L02BG04)
Disease treated	Obesity, severe
Quantification of adverse effects	Hormones
No. of patients treated	10
Age group	48.2 years (mean)
Treatment period	6 weeks
Dose	7.5–17.5 mg/week
Treatment consequences	Testosterone level increase, SHBG level unaltered
Efficacy	In all men
Randomization of patients	No
Study quality	**3**
Reference	828: de Boer H, Verschoor L, Ruinemans-Koerts J, Jansen M. Letrozole normalizes serum testosterone in severely obese men with hypogonadotropic hypogonadism. Diabetes Obes Metab. 2005 May;7(3):211–5.
Language	English

L04 Immunosuppressive Agents

The are few reports on the impairment of spermatogenesis. No studies are available concerning the calcineurin antagonists cyclosporin, tacrolimus, pimecrolimus, but sirolimus appears to cause severe defects in spermatogenesis. Infliximab, a TNFα antibody, also impairs spermatogenesis, whereas azathioprine appears to be of limited effect. The RCTs are not available.

Overall level of evidence of adverse effects: C

Compound	Sirolimus (L04AA10)
Disease treated	Kidney transplantation
Quantification of adverse effects	Semen
No. of patients treated	1
Age group	Young
Treatment period	8 mg/day
Dose	8 years
Treatment consequences	Azoospermia, continuous

Efficacy	Increase after cessation
Study quality	**3**
Reference	928: Skrzypek J, Krause W. Sirolimus and spermatogenesis. Abstract DGA-Congress 2006 Düsseldorf, Germany.
Language	German

Compound	Infliximab (L04AA12)
Disease treated	Healthy
Quantification of adverse effects	Sperm in vitro
No. of patients treated	31
Age group	Young
Treatment period	In vitro
Dose	n.g.
Treatment consequences	Sperm motility, functional integrity of plasma membrane, and DNA fragmentation, decrease
Efficacy	Effect of TNFα diminished in the presence of infliximab
Randomization of patients	Yes
Study quality	**1–**
Reference	822: Said TM, Agarwal A, Falcone T, Sharma RK, Bedaiwy MA, Li L. Infliximab may reverse the toxic effects induced by tumor necrosis factor alpha in human spermatozoa: an in vitro model. Fertil Steril. 2005 Jun;83(6):1665–73.
Language	English

Compound	Infliximab (L04AA12)
Disease treated	Inflammatory bowel disease
Quantification of adverse effects	Sperm parameters
No. of patients treated	10
Age group	Young
Treatment period	2 weeks
Dose	n.g.
Treatment consequences	Sperm motility and morphology, impairment
Efficacy	In longer treatment with infliximab more pronounced decrease in sperm progression
Randomization of patients	Cross-over
Study quality	**1–**

Reference	823: Mahadevan U, Terdiman JP, Aron J, Jacobsohn S, Turek P. Infliximab and semen quality in men with inflammatory bowel disease. Inflamm Bowel Dis. 2005 Apr;11(4):395–9.
Language	English

Compound	Azathioprine (L04AX01)
Disease treated	Chronic aggressive hepatitis
Quantification of adverse effects	Semen
No. of patients treated	Few
Age group	Young
Treatment period	1720 days
Dose	Various
Treatment consequences	Spermatogenesis, impairment
Efficacy	None below a dose of 150 mg/day
Randomization of patients	No
Study quality	**3**
Reference	643: Lange D, Henning H, Schirren C. Andrologic study in immunosuppressive treatment of chronic aggressive hepatitis. Andrologia 1978 Sep–Oct;10(5):373–9.
Language	German

M01 Antiinflammatory and Antirheumatic Products

An uncontrolled study described positive effects on sperm parameters by treatment with rofecoxib.

Overall level of evidence of adverse effects: C

Compound	Cinnoxicam (M01AC)
Disease treated	Infertility
Quantification of adverse effects	Semen
No. of patients treated	155
Age group	Young
Treatment period	12 months
Dose	30 mg/4 days
Treatment consequences	Sperm parameters, improvement

Efficacy	At 2 m, best at 4 m, decline to baseline after cessation of treatment
Randomization of patients	Yes
Study quality	**2–**
Reference	2306: Cavallini G, Biagiotti G, Ferraretti AP, Gianaroli L, Vitali G. Medical therapy of oligoasthenospermia associated with left varicocele. BJU Int. 2003 Apr;91(6):513–8.
Language	English

Compound	Rofecoxib (M01AH02)
Disease treated	Infertility
Quantification of adverse effects	Semen
No. of patients treated	47
Age group	Young
Treatment period	30 days
Dose	25 mg/day
Treatment consequences	Sperm parameters, improvement
Efficacy	Sperm motility and morphology
Randomization of patients	No
Study quality	**3**
Reference	2198: Gambera L, Serafini F, Morgante G, Focarelli R, Leo V de, Piomboni P. Sperm quality and pregnancy rate after COX-2 inhibitor therapy of infertile males with abacterial leukocytospermia. Human Reprod. 2007;22(4):1047–51.
Language	English

M04 Antigout Preparations

There is a single report in the literature which describes a decrease of testosterone levels in patients treated with allopurinol. This observation has never been confirmed by other studies.

A case report indicates a reduction of sperm count in a patient treated with colchicine for Behçet's disease. Comparing studies did not confirm this effect. In particular, a comparison with the effect of cyclophosphamide on spermatogenesis, which is far more pronounced, is impressive in this respect (Fukutani et al. 1981).

Overall level of evidence of adverse effects: C

Compound	Allopurinol (M04AA01)
Disease treated	Nephrolithiasis
Quantification of adverse effects	Testosterone levels
No. of patients treated	n.g.
Age group	Young
Treatment period	n.g.
Dose	n.g.
Treatment consequences	Testosterone level, decrease
Efficacy	Significant
Randomization of patients	No
Study quality	**3**
Reference	917: Graef V, Zubrzycki Z, Jarrar K. The effect of allopurinol on testosterone metabolism. Arzneimittelforschung. 1984;34(12):1760–2.
Language	German

Compound	Colchicine (M04AC01)
Disease treated	Behçet's disease
Quantification of adverse effects	Clinical
No. of patients treated	62
Age group	Young
Treatment period	n.g.
Dose	n.g.
Treatment consequences	Spermatogenesis, impairment
Efficacy	23 of 67 patients (37.1%) had oligonecrozoospermia, 2 of 67 patients (3.2%) had azoospermia
Randomization of patients	No
Study quality	**3**
Reference	795: Sarica K, Suzer O, Gurler A et al. Urological evaluation of Behçet patients and the effect of colchicine on fertility. Eur Urol 1995;27: 39–42.
Language	English

Compound	Colchicine (M04AC01)
Disease treated	Behçet's disease
Quantification of adverse effects	Semen
No. of patients treated	27
Age group	Young
Treatment period	64 months
Dose	n.g.
Treatment consequences	Azoospermia, induction
Efficacy	13 of 17 patients receiving cyclophosphamide, none of patients receiving colchicine
Randomization of patients	No
Study quality	**2–**
Reference	560: Fukutani K, Ishida H, Shinohara M, Minowada S, Niijima T, Hijikata K, Izawa Y. Suppression of spermatogenesis in patients with Behcet's disease treated with cyclophosphamide and colchicine. Fertil Steril. 1981 Jul;36(1):76–80.
Language	English

Compound	Colchicine (M04AC01)
Disease treated	Behçet's disease
Quantification of adverse effects	Semen
No. of patients treated	1
Age group	Young
Treatment period	n.g.
Dose	2 grains
Treatment consequences	Azoospermia, induction
Efficacy	With treatment; normal sperm count without treatment
Study quality	**3**
Reference	802. Merlin HE: Azoospermia caused by colchicines. A case report. Fertil Steril. 1972;23:180–181.
Language	English

Compound	Colchicine (M04AC01)
Disease treated	Behçet's disease
Quantification of adverse effects	Semen

No. of patients treated	131
Age group	Young
Treatment consequences	Spermatogenesis, impairment
Efficacy	No effect
Randomization of patients	No
Remarks	In prospective studies no effect of colchicine on spermatogenesis
Study quality	**4 (review)**
Reference	158: Haimov-Kochman R, Ben-Chetrit E. The effect of colchicine treatment on sperm production and function: a review. Hum Reprod. 1998 Feb;13(2):360–2.
Language	English

N01	**Anaesthetics**

Only few studies have investigated the effects on sperm production, and no significant alterations have been described.

A special drug of this group is cocaine; in only one study was the use of cocaine shown to increase the risk of low sperm count.

Overall level of evidence of adverse effects: B

Compound	Anaesthetics, general (N01A)
Disease treated	Healthy
Quantification of adverse effects	Sperm morphology, epididymis
No. of patients treated	46
Age group	Young
Treatment period	Professionals
Treatment consequences	Sperm abnormalities, increase
Efficacy	No effect
Randomization of patients	No
Study quality	**2–**
Reference	175: Wyrobek AJ, Brodsky J, Gordon L, Moore DH 2nd, Watchmaker G, Cohen EN. Sperm studies in anesthesiologists. Anesthesiology. 1981;55(5):527–32.

Language	English

Compound	Halothane (N01AB01)
Disease treated	Anaesthesia
Quantification of adverse effects	Semen
No. of patients treated	17
Age group	Young
Treatment period	Single dose
Dose	Various
Treatment consequences	Spermatogenesis, impairment
Efficacy	No effect
Randomization of patients	No
Study quality	**3**
Reference	283: Andersen BN, Mortensen JT, Hansen P, Jakobsen J, Johansen JP. The influence of halothane on spermatogenesis in surgical patients. Acta Anaesthesiol Scand. 1992 Feb;36(2):125–7.
Language	English

Compound	Cocaine (N01BC01)
Disease treated	Cocaine abuse
Quantification of adverse effects	Semen
No. of patients treated	39
Age group	31–35 years
Treatment period	2–5 years
Dose	>1 dose/month
Treatment consequences	Sperm count, impairment
Efficacy	OR 2.3 (95% CI 1.0–5.4) in comparison with non-users
Randomization of patients	Yes
Study quality	**2+**
Reference	2026: Bracken MB, Eskenazi B, Sachse K, McSharry JE, Hellenbrand K, Leo-Summers L. Association of cocaine use with sperm concentration, motility, and morphology. Fertil Steril. 1990 Feb;53(2):315–22.
Language	English

2

N02	Analgesics
	There are controversy reports on the effects of intrathecal injection of opioids on testosterone levels and sexual functions. **Overall level of evidence of adverse effects: C** Aspirin in healthy men had an inhibiting effect on the function pituitary gonadotrophs and of Leydig cell. **Overall level of evidence of adverse effects: B**

Compound	Opioids intrathecally (N02A)
Disease treated	Intractable pain
Quantification of adverse effects	Hormones
No. of patients treated	29
Age group	49.2 years (mean)
Treatment period	26 months
Dose	Various
Treatment consequences	FSH, LH, testosterone levels, alteration
Efficacy	Levels unaltered, hormone substitution not necessary
Randomization of patients	No
Study quality	**2–**
Reference	857: Abs R, Verhelst J, Maeyaert J, Van Buyten JP, Opsomer F, Adriaensen H, Verlooy J, Van Havenbergh T, Smet M, Van Acker K. Endocrine consequences of long-term intrathecal administration of opioids. J Clin Endocrinol Metab. 2000 Jun;85(6):2215–22.
Language	English

Compound	Opioids intrathecally (N02A)
Disease treated	Intractable pain
Quantification of adverse effects	Hormones
No. of patients treated	6
Age group	Middle-aged
Treatment period	Continuous
Dose	Various

Treatment consequences	Testosterone level, decline
Efficacy	Decrease of libido and sexual functions
Randomization of patients	No
Study quality	**3**
Reference	858: Paice JA, Penn RD, Ryan WG. Altered sexual function and decreased testosterone in patients receiving intraspinal opioids. J Pain Symptom Manage. 1994 Feb;9(2):126–31.
Language	English

Compound	Aspirin (N02BA01)
Disease treated	Healthy
Quantification of adverse effects	Hormones
No. of patients treated	16
Age group	Young
Treatment period	2 weeks
Dose	n.g.
Treatment consequences	Steroid hormone, response to hCG, decrease
Efficacy	Significant
Randomization of patients	Yes
Dose arms 1–3	Aspirin; placebo
Study quality	**1–**
Reference	921: Conte D, Romanelli F, Fillo S, Guidetti L, Isidori A, Franceschi F, Latini M, Luigi L di. Aspirin inhibits androgen response to chorionic gonadotropin in humans. Am J Physiol. 1999 Dec;277(6 Pt 1):E1032–7.
Language	English

Compound	Aspirin (N02BA01)
Disease treated	Healthy
Quantification of adverse effects	LH response to naloxon
No. of patients treated	16
Age group	20–38 years
Treatment period	Single dose
Dose	650 mg
Treatment consequences	Stimulatory activity of naloxone on LH release, inhibited

Efficacy	By 80%
Randomization of patients	Yes
Dose arms 1–3	Aspirin; placebo
Study quality	**1–**
Reference	948: Conte D, Nordio M, Fillo S, Giorgio G de, Isidori A, Romanelli F. Aspirin inhibition of naloxone-induced luteinizing hormone secretion in man. J Clin Endocrinol Metab. 1996 May;81(5):1772–5.
Language	English

N03	**Antiepileptics**

The effects of antiepileptics on male sexual hormones and spermatogenesis are moderate. Most of the drugs use depress testosterone levels and increase SHBG levels, thus leading to a decrease in androgenicity. There are no RCTs available; most of the data originate from case-control studies or from investigations during continuous antiepileptic treatment.

Phenobarbital impaired gonadotropin secretion from the pituitary, but not all studies confirmed also an alteration of testosterone levels. Since the hormonal changes were independent of the epileptic syndrome, it is likely that they indeed represent adverse effects of the drugs.

During phenytoin therapy, an impaired spermatogenesis and various alterations of sexual steroid level were found; thus, a direct cytotoxic effect on spermatogenesis is likely.

Carbamazepine application increased testosterone levels in several studies. There are, however, also studies which report contrary results. In healthy persons it induced a depression of sexual function, although the testosterone levels increased. The increase in SHBG levels resulted in a negative correlation between free testosterone levels and circulating carbamazepine levels.

During treatment with valproate testosterone levels remained unaltered or decreased, and sperm motility diminished in some studies.

Overall level of evidence of adverse effects: C

Compound	Antiepileptics (N03A)
Disease treated	Epilepsy
Quantification of adverse effects	Hormones

No. of patients treated	275
Age group	36 mean
Treatment period	Continuous
Treatment consequences	Testosterone level, decrease; LH level, increase
Efficacy	Mean values, also without treatment, especially in temporal lobe epilepsy
Study quality	**3**
Reference	967: Bauer J, Blumenthal S, Reuber M, Stoffel-Wagner B. Epilepsy syndrome, focus location, and treatment choice affect testicular function in men with epilepsy. Neurology. 2004 Jan 27;62(2):243–6.
Language	English

Compound	Antiepileptics (N03A)
Disease treated	Epilepsy
Quantification of adverse effects	Hormones
No. of patients treated	140
Age group	Young
Treatment period	Continuous
Dose	Various
Treatment consequences	Testosterone level, decrease; SHBG level, increase
Efficacy	Mean values
Randomization of patients	No
Dose arms 1–3	Valproate; carbamazepine; age-matched controls
Study quality	**2–**
Reference	1366: Mikkonen K, Tapanainen P, Pakarinen AJ, Paivansalo M, Isojarvi JI, Vainionpaa LK. Serum androgen levels and testicular structure during pubertal maturation in male subjects with epilepsy. Epilepsia. 2004 Jul;45(7):769–76.
Language	English

Compound	Antiepileptics (N03A)
Disease treated	Epilepsy
Quantification of adverse effects	Hormones
No. of patients treated	70
Age group	Young
Treatment period	2 years

Dose	Various
Treatment consequences	Testosterone level, unaltered; SHBG level, decrease
Efficacy	Mean values
Randomization of patients	No
Dose arms 1–3	Valproate; carbamazepine; age-matched controls
Study quality	**2–**
Reference	1365: Roste LS, Tauboll E, Morkrid L, Bjornenak T, Saetre ER, Morland T, Gjerstad L. Antiepileptic drugs alter reproductive endocrine hormones in men with epilepsy. Eur J Neurol. 2005 Feb;12(2):118–24.
Language	English

Compound	**Antiepileptics (N03A)**
Disease treated	Epilepsy
Quantification of adverse effects	Pubertal development
No. of patients treated	57
Age group	Pubertal
Treatment period	Continuous
Dose	Various
Treatment consequences	Puberty stage II earlier, in puberty stage III lower FSH levels
Efficacy	Mean values
Randomization of patients	No
Study quality	**2–**
Reference	1377: Nalin A, Galli V, Ciccarone V, Grandi F, Baraldi E, Carani C. Antiepileptic drugs and puberty. Brain Dev. 1988;10(3):192–4.
Language	English

Compound	**Antiepileptics (N03A)**
Disease treated	Epilepsy
Quantification of adverse effects	Hormones
No. of patients treated	16
Age group	Young
Treatment period	Continuous
Dose	Various

Treatment consequences	Testosterone level, increase; SHBG level, increased
Efficacy	Mean values
Randomization of patients	No
Study quality	**3**
Reference	1379: Barragry JM, Makin HL, Trafford DJ, Scott DF. Effect of anticonvulsants on plasma testosterone and sex hormone binding globulin levels. J Neurol Neurosurg Psychiatry. 1978 Oct;41(10):913–4.
Language	English

Compound	Phenobarbital (N03AA02)
Disease treated	Epilepsy
Quantification of adverse effects	Hormones
No. of patients treated	70
Age group	Young
Treatment period	Continuous
Dose	Various
Treatment consequences	LH response to GnRH, decrease
Efficacy	Significant changes in SHBG, testosterone, androstendione independent of the epileptic syndrome
Randomization of patients	No
Study quality	**2–**
Reference	1374: Murialdo G, Galimberti CA, Fonzi S, Manni R, Costelli P, Parodi C, Torre F, Solinas GP, Polleri A, Tartara A. Sex hormones, gonadotropins and prolactin in male epileptic subjects in remission: role of the epileptic syndrome and of antiepileptic drugs. Neuropsychobiology. 1994;30(1):29–36.
Language	English

Compound	Phenobarbital (N03AA02)
Disease treated	Epilepsy
Quantification of adverse effects	Hormones
No. of patients treated	35
Age group	Young
Treatment period	Continuous
Dose	Various

Treatment consequences	Sex steroid hormones and LH pulsatility, low response to GnRH
Efficacy	Significant
Randomization of patients	No
Study quality	**3**
Reference	876: Murialdo G, Galimberti CA, Fonzi S, Manni R, Costelli P, Parodi C, Torre F, Solinas GP, Polleri A, Tartara A. Sex hormones, gonadotropins and prolactin in male epileptic subjects in remission: role of the epileptic syndrome and of antiepileptic drugs. Neuropsychobiology. 1994;30(1):29–36.
Language	English

Compound	Phenobarbital (N03AA02)
Disease treated	Healthy
Quantification of adverse effects	Hormones
No. of patients treated	18
Age group	Young
Treatment period	7 days
Dose	100 mg/day
Treatment consequences	Testosterone level, alteration
Efficacy	None
Randomization of patients	No
Study quality	**2–**
Reference	877: Bammel A, van der Mee K, Ohnhaus EE, Kirch W. Divergent effects of various enzyme-inducing agents on endogenous and exogenous testosterone. Eur J Clin Pharmacol. 1992;42(6):641–4.
Language	English

Compound	Phenobarbital (N03AA02)
Disease treated	Epilepsy
Quantification of adverse effects	Hormones
No. of patients treated	8
Age group	Young
Treatment period	Continuous
Dose	Various
Treatment consequences	GnRH-induced LH release

Efficacy	Blunted in comparison with control subjects
Randomization of patients	No
Study quality	**2–**
Reference	881: Murialdo G, Manni R, Maria A de, Bonura ML, Polleri A, Tartara A. Luteinizing hormone pulsatile secretion and pituitary response to gonadotropin releasing hormone and to thyrotropin releasing hormone in male epileptic subjects on chronic phenobarbital treatment. J Endocrinol Invest. 1987 Feb;10(1):27–31.
Language	English

Compound	Phenytoin (N03AB02)
Disease treated	Epilepsy
Quantification of adverse effects	Semen, hormones
No. of patients treated	55; 28
Age group	Young
Treatment period	12 months
Dose	Various
Treatment consequences	Spermatogenesis, impairment
Efficacy	Not significant
Randomization of patients	No
Dose arms 1–3	Phenytoin; no phenytoin
Study quality	**2–**
Reference	244: Taneja N, Kucheria K, Jain S, Maheshwari MC. Effect of phenytoin on semen. Epilepsia. 1994 Jan–Feb;35(1):136–40.
Language	English

Compound	Phenytoin (N03AB02)
Disease treated	Epilepsy
Quantification of adverse effects	Semen, hormones
No. of patients treated	55
Age group	Young
Treatment period	Continuous
Dose	Various
Treatment consequences	Spermatogenesis, impairment; testosterone levels, decrease
Efficacy	Clearly

Randomization of patients	No
Study quality	**3**
Reference	939: Taneja N, Kucheria K, Jain S, Maheshwari MC. Effect of phenytoin on semen. Epilepsia. 1994 Jan–Feb;35(1):136–40.
Language	English

Compound	Phenytoin (N03AB02)
Disease treated	Epilepsy
Quantification of adverse effects	Hormones
No. of patients treated	41
Age group	Young
Treatment period	Continuous
Dose	Various
Treatment consequences	Oestradiol levels, increase; SHBG levels, increase
Efficacy	Significant
Randomization of patients	No
Dose arms 1–3	Phenytoin; placebo
Study quality	**2–**
Reference	945: Heroz AG, Levesque LA, Drislane FW, Ronthal M, Schomer DL. Phenytoin-induced elevation of serum estradiol and reproductive dysfunction in men with epilepsy. Epilepsia. 1991 Jul–Aug;32(4):550–3.
Language	English

Compound	Phenytoin (N03AB02)
Disease treated	Epilepsy
Quantification of adverse effects	Hormones
No. of patients treated	35
Age group	Young
Treatment period	Continuous
Dose	Various
Treatment consequences	Sex steroid hormones and LH pulsatility, decrease; SHBG levels, increase
Efficacy	Significant
Randomization of patients	No

Study quality	**3**
Reference	876: Murialdo G, Galimberti CA, Fonzi S, Manni R, Costelli P, Parodi C, Torre F, Solinas GP, Polleri A, Tartara A. Sex hormones, gonadotropins and prolactin in male epileptic subjects in remission: role of the epileptic syndrome and of antiepileptic drugs. Neuropsychobiology. 1994;30(1):29–36.
Language	English

Compound	Phenytoin (N03AB02)
Disease treated	Epilepsy
Quantification of adverse effects	Hormones
No. of patients treated	29
Age group	Young
Treatment period	Continuous
Dose	Various
Treatment consequences	Testosterone level, increase; SHBG level, increase
Efficacy	Lower androgenicity due to increased SHBG levels
Randomization of patients	No
Study quality	**2–**
Reference	969: Brunet M, Rodamilans M, Martinez-Osaba MJ, Santamaria J, To-Figueras J, Torra M, Corbella J, Rivera F. Effects of long-term antiepileptic therapy on the catabolism of testosterone. Pharmacol Toxicol. 1995 Jun;76(6):371–5.
Language	English

Compound	Phenytoin (N03AB02)
Disease treated	Epilepsy
Quantification of adverse effects	Hormones
No. of patients treated	13
Age group	32 years (mean)
Treatment period	Continuous
Dose	Various
Treatment consequences	Hormone levels, alteration
Efficacy	Increased SHBG levels
Randomization of patients	No
Study quality	**2–**

Reference	970: Macphee GJ, Larkin JG, Butler E, Beastall GH, Brodie MJ. Circulating hormones and pituitary responsiveness in young epileptic men receiving long-term antiepileptic medication. Epilepsia. 1988 Jul–Aug;29(4):468–75.
Language	English

Compound	Carbamazepine (N03AF01)
Disease treated	Epilepsy
Quantification of adverse effects	Hormones
No. of patients treated	93
Age group	Young
Treatment period	Continuous
Dose	Various
Treatment consequences	Testosterone level, increase; DHEA level, decrease; SHBG level, decrease
Efficacy	Negative correlation between free T and circulating carbamazepine levels
Randomization of patients	No
Study quality	**2–**
Reference	970: Macphee GJ, Larkin JG, Butler E, Beastall GH, Brodie MJ. Circulating hormones and pituitary responsiveness in young epileptic men receiving long-term antiepileptic medication. Epilepsia. 1988 Jul–Aug;29(4):468–75.
Language	English

Compound	Carbamazepine (N03AF01)
Disease treated	Epilepsy
Quantification of adverse effects	Hormones
No. of patients treated	70
Age group	Young
Treatment period	Continuous
Dose	Various
Treatment consequences	LH response to GnRH, decreased
Efficacy	Significant
Randomization of patients	No
Study quality	**3**

Reference	952: Murialdo G, Galimberti CA, Fonzi S, Manni R, Costelli P, Parodi C, Torre F, Solinas GP, Polleri A, Tartara A. Sex hormones, gonadotropins and prolactin in male epileptic subjects in remission: role of the epileptic syndrome and of antiepileptic drugs. Neuropsychobiology. 1994;30(1):29–36.
Language	English

Compound	Carbamazepine (N03AF01)
Disease treated	Epilepsy
Quantification of adverse effects	Hormones
No. of patients treated	65
Age group	Young
Treatment period	Continuous
Dose	Various
Treatment consequences	Testosterone level, unaltered; SHBG level, increase
Efficacy	Significant
Randomization of patients	No
Study quality	**3**
Reference	968: Rattya J, Turkka J, Pakarinen AJ, Knip M, Kotila MA, Lukkarinen O, Myllyla VV, Isojarvi JI. Reproductive effects of valproate, carbamazepine, and oxcarbazepine in men with epilepsy. Neurology. 2001 Jan 9;56(1):31–6.
Language	English

Compound	Carbamazepine (N03AF01)
Disease treated	Epilepsy
Quantification of adverse effects	Hormones
No. of patients treated	35
Age group	Young
Treatment period	Continuous
Dose	Various
Treatment consequences	Sex steroid hormones, LH pulsatility and response to GnRH, lower
Efficacy	Significant
Randomization of patients	No
Study quality	**3**

Reference	876: Murialdo G, Galimberti CA, Fonzi S, Manni R, Costelli P, Parodi C, Torre F, Solinas GP, Polleri A, Tartara A. Sex hormones, gonadotropins and prolactin in male epileptic subjects in remission: role of the epileptic syndrome and of antiepileptic drugs. Neuropsychobiology. 1994;30(1):29–36.
Language	English

Compound	Carbamazepine (N03AF01)
Disease treated	Epilepsy
Quantification of adverse effects	Hormones
No. of patients treated	28
Age group	Young
Treatment period	Continuous
Dose	Various
Treatment consequences	Testosterone level, increase; SHBG level, increase
Efficacy	Lower androgenicity due to increased SHBG levels
Randomization of patients	No
Study quality	**3**
Reference	969: Brunet M, Rodamilans M, Martinez-Osaba MJ, Santamaria J, To-Figueras J, Torra M, Corbella J, Rivera F. Effects of long-term antiepileptic therapy on the catabolism of testosterone. Pharmacol Toxicol. 1995 Jun;76(6):371–5.
Language	English

Compound	Carbamazepine (N03AF01)
Disease treated	Epilepsy
Quantification of adverse effects	Hormones
No. of patients treated	21
Age group	Young
Treatment period	2 months
Dose	Various
Treatment consequences	Oestradiol levels, increase, PRL response to metoclopramide, increase
Efficacy	Significant
Randomization of patients	No
Study quality	**3**

Reference	950: Isojarvi JI, Pakarinen AJ, Myllyla VV. Effects of carbamazepine on the hypothalamic–pituitary–gonadal axis in male patients with epilepsy: a prospective study. Epilepsia. 1989 Jul–Aug;30(4):446–52.
Language	English

Compound	Carbamazepine (N03AF01)
Disease treated	Epilepsy
Quantification of adverse effects	Hormones
No. of patients treated	18
Age group	29 years (mean)
Treatment period	Continuous
Dose	Various
Treatment consequences	Hormone levels, alteration
Efficacy	LH and prolactin levels enhanced
Randomization of patients	No
Study quality	**2–**
Reference	970: Macphee GJ, Larkin JG, Butler E, Beastall GH, Brodie MJ. Circulating hormones and pituitary responsiveness in young epileptic men receiving long-term antiepileptic medication. Epilepsia. 1988 Jul–Aug;29(4):468–75.
Language	English

Compound	Carbamazepine (N03AF01)
Disease treated	Epilepsy
Quantification of adverse effects	Sperm motility, hormones
No. of patients treated	15
Age group	Young
Treatment period	Long term
Dose	Various
Treatment consequences	DHEA levels, decrease; sperm motility, decrease
Efficacy	Significant
Randomization of patients	No
Study quality	**3**

Reference	746: Isojarvi JI, Lofgren E, Juntunen KS, Pakarinen AJ, Paivansalo M, Rautakorpi I, Tuomivaara L. Effect of epilepsy and antiepileptic drugs on male reproductive health. Neurology. 2004 Jan 27;62(2):247–53.
Language	English

Compound	Carbamazepine (N03AF01)
Disease treated	Healthy
Quantification of adverse effects	Sexual function scale; hormones
No. of patients treated	6
Age group	Young
Treatment period	21 days
Dose	400 mg
Treatment consequences	Sexual function, depression; testosterone level, increase
Efficacy	Various
Randomization of patients	No
Study quality	**2–**
Reference	978: Connell JM, Rapeport WG, Beastall GH, Brodie MJ. Changes in circulating androgens during short term carbamazepine therapy. Br J Clin Pharmacol. 1984 Mar;17(3):347–51.
Language	English

Compound	Valproate (N03AG01)
Disease treated	Epilepsy
Quantification of adverse effects	Hormones
No. of patients treated	115
Age group	Young
Treatment period	Continuous
Dose	Various
Treatment consequences	Testosterone level, decrease; SHBG level, unaltered
Efficacy	Moderate
Randomization of patients	No
Study quality	**3**

Reference	968: Rattya J, Turkka J, Pakarinen AJ, Knip M, Kotila MA, Lukkarinen O, Myllyla VV, Isojarvi JI. Reproductive effects of valproate, carbamazepine, and oxcarbazepine in men with epilepsy. Neurology. 2001 Jan 9;56(1):31–6.
Language	English

Compound	Valproate (N03AG01), lamotrigine
Disease treated	Epilepsy
Quantification of adverse effects	Hormones
No. of patients treated	76
Age group	Young
Treatment period	Continuous
Dose	Various
Treatment consequences	Testosterone level, alteration; gonadotropin level, alteration
Efficacy	None
Randomization of patients	No
Study quality	**2–**
Reference	976: Stephen LJ, Kwan P, Shapiro D, Dominiczak M, Brodie MJ. Hormone profiles in young adults with epilepsy treated with sodium valproate or lamotrigine monotherapy. Epilepsia. 2001 Aug;42(8):1002–6.
Language	English

Compound	Valproate (N03AG01), carbamazepine
Disease treated	Epilepsy
Quantification of adverse effects	Sperm motility
No. of patients treated	36
Age group	Young
Treatment period	>2 years
Dose	Various
Treatment consequences	Sperm motility, alteration; testicular volume, decrease
Efficacy	Significant
Randomization of patients	No
Study quality	**2–**

Reference	747: Roste LS, Tauboll E, Haugen TB, Bjornenak T, Saetre ER, Gjerstad L. Alterations in semen parameters in men with epilepsy treated with valproate or carbamazepine monotherapy. Eur J Neurol. 2003 Sep;10(5):501–6.
Language	English

Compound	**Valproate (N03AG01)**
Disease treated	Epilepsy
Quantification of adverse effects	Sperm motility
No. of patients treated	27
Age group	Young
Treatment period	Long term
Dose	Various
Treatment consequences	Androstendione levels, increase; sperm motility, decreased
Efficacy	Significant
Randomization of patients	No
Study quality	**2–**
Reference	746: Isojarvi JI, Lofgren E, Juntunen KS, Pakarinen AJ, Paivansalo M, Rautakorpi I, Tuomivaara L. Effect of epilepsy and antiepileptic drugs on male reproductive health. Neurology. 2004 Jan 27;62(2):247–53.
Language	English

Compound	**Valproate (N03AG01)**
Disease treated	Epilepsy
Quantification of adverse effects	Hormones
No. of patients treated	10
Age group	23 years (mean)
Treatment period	Continuous
Dose	Various
Treatment consequences	Hormone levels, alteration
Efficacy	No difference to control groups
Randomization of patients	No
Study quality	**2–**

Reference	970: Macphee GJ, Larkin JG, Butler E, Beastall GH, Brodie MJ. Circulating hormones and pituitary responsiveness in young epileptic men receiving long-term antiepileptic medication. Epilepsia. 1988 Jul–Aug;29(4):468–75.
Language	English

Compound	Valproate (N03AG01)
Disease treated	Terminal renal insufficiency
Quantification of adverse effects	Hormones
No. of patients treated	5
Age group	Young
Treatment period	2 weeks
Dose	Various
Treatment consequences	Gonadotropin levels, unaltered; response to GnRH, increase
Efficacy	Significant
Randomization of patients	No
Study quality	**2–**
Reference	947: Elias AN, Pahl M, Stone S, Vaziri ND, Valenta LJ. Modulatory role of gamma-aminobutyric acid (GABA) in the regulation of gonadotropin secretion in patients with chronic renal failure. Int J Artif Organs. 1982 Jan;5(1):13–6.
Language	English

N04 Antiparkinson Drugs (Dopamine Agonists)

Treatment with L-DOPA improved spermatogenesis in more than half of men in an uncontrolled study. This observation has not been confirmed by other studies.

Bromocriptine treatment for hyperprolactinaemia did not alter gonadotropin levels and sperm parameters. Since in some men spermatogenic dysfunction is associated with hyperprolactinaemia, an improvement of sperm parameters with bromocriptine was expected, similar to the improvement of ovulation function in female hyperprolactinaemia. The treatment in males, however, had no effect also in prospective, randomized studies. A Cochrane review from Vandekerckhove et al. (2000) confirmed these observations.

Overall level of evidence of adverse effects: B

2

Compound	L-DOPA (N04BA02)
Disease treated	Infertility
Quantification of dysfunction	Semen
No. of patients treated	39
Age group	Young
Treatment period	2 months
Treatment consequences	Spermatogenesis, improvement
Efficacy	14 of 25 patients in group 1; 8 of 14 patients in group 2
Randomization of patients	No
Dose arms 1–3	500 mg/day; 750 mg/day
Study quality	**1–**
Reference	653: Lavieri JC, Pierini AA. L-dopa and oligozoospermia. Andrologia. 1978 Jan–Feb;10(1):74–9.
Language	English

Compound	Bromocriptine (N04BC01)
Disease treated	Infertility
Quantification of adverse effects	Semen
No. of patients treated	50
Age group	Young
Treatment period	n.g.
Dose	n.g.
Treatment consequences	Sperm parameters, alteration; pregnancy rate, increase
Efficacy	No effect
Randomization of patients	No
Study quality	**1–**
Reference	2187: Lunglmayr G, Maier U, Spona J. [Therapy of idiopathic oligozoospermia with bromicriptine. Results of a prospective controlled study] Andrologia. 1983;15 Spec No:548–53.
Language	English

Compound	Bromocriptine (N04BC01)
Disease treated	Infertility
Quantification of adverse effects	Semen

No. of patients treated	42
Age group	Young
Treatment period	n.g.
Dose	n.g.
Treatment consequences	Sperm parameters, alteration
Efficacy	No effect
Randomization of patients	No
Study quality	**3**
Reference	2189: Szollosi J, Szilagyi I, Sas M. Parlodel treatment of patients with pathospermia. Int Urol Nephrol. 1982;14(3):307–12.
Language	English

Compound	Bromocriptine (N04BC01)
Disease treated	Infertility
Quantification of adverse effects	Semen
No. of patients treated	40
Age group	Young
Treatment period	12 weeks
Dose	n.g.
Treatment consequences	Sperm parameters, alteration
Efficacy	No significant effect over placebo on sperm volume, motility and morphology
Side effects	Yes
Randomization of patients	
Dose arms 1–3	Bromocriptine; placebo
Study quality	**1–**
Reference	2192: Hovatta O, Koskimies AI, Ranta T, Stenman UH, Seppala M. Bromocriptine treatment of oligospermia: a double blind study. Clin Endocrinol (Oxf). 1979 Oct;11(4):377–82.
Language	English

Compound	Bromocriptine (N04BC01)
Disease treated	Infertility
Quantification of adverse effects	Semen

2

No. of patients treated	21
Age group	Young
Treatment period	6 months
Dose	2.5 mg/day
Treatment consequences	Sperm parameters, alteration
Efficacy	No effect
Randomization of patients	No
Study quality	**3**
Reference	2184: Merino G, Carranza-Lira S, Martinez-Chequer JC, Barahona E, Moran C, Bermudez JA. Hyperprolactinemia in men with asthenozoospermia, oligozoospermia, or azoospermia. Arch Androl. 1997 May–Jun;38(3):201–6.
Language	English

Compound	Bromocriptine (N04BC01)
Disease treated	Infertility
Quantification of adverse effects	Semen
No. of patients treated	17
Age group	Young
Treatment period	4 months
Dose	5 mg/day
Treatment consequences	Sperm parameters, alteration; pregnancy rate, increase
Efficacy	No effect
Randomization of patients	Yes
Dose arms 1–3	Bromocriptine; placebo
Study quality	**1–**
Reference	2188: AinMelk Y, Belisle S, Kandalaft N, McClure D, Tetreault L, Elhilali M. Bromocriptine therapy in oligozoospermic infertile men. Arch Androl. 1982 Mar;8(2):135–41.
Language	English

Compound	Bromocriptine (N04BC01)
Disease treated	Uraemia
Quantification of adverse effects	Hormones, semen
No. of patients treated	14
Age group	Young

Treatment period	3 months
Dose	2.5 mg/day
Treatment consequences	Gonadotropin levels, alteration
Efficacy	Normalization of spermatogenesis
Randomization of patients	No
Study quality	**3**
Reference	420: Ermolenko VM, Kukhtevich AV, Dedov II, Bunatian AF, Melnichenko GA, Gitel EP. Parlodel treatment of uremic hypogonadism in men. Nephron. 1986;42(1):19–22.
Language	English

Compound	Bromocriptine (N04BC01)
Disease treated	Prolactinoma
Quantification of adverse effects	Semen, hormones
No. of patients treated	10
Age group	Young
Treatment period	n.g.
Dose	Various
Treatment consequences	Testosterone level, alteration; sperm parameters; alteration
Efficacy	No alteration of hormone and semen parameters
Randomization of patients	No
Study quality	**3**
Reference	126: Nishimura K, Matsumiya K, Tsuboniwa N, Yamanaka M, Koga M, Miura H, Tsujimura A, Uchida K, Kondoh N, Kitamura M, Okuyama A. Bromocriptine for infertile males with mild hyperprolactinemia: hormonal and spermatogenic effects. Arch Androl. 1999 Nov–Dec;43(3):207–13.
Language	English

Compound	Bromocriptine (N04BC01)
Disease treated	Infertility
Quantification of adverse effects	Semen
No. of patients treated	9
Age group	Young
Treatment period	6 months

Dose	7.5 mg/day
Treatment consequences	Sperm parameters, alteration
Efficacy	Significant increase of sperm count
Randomization of patients	Yes
Dose arms 1–3	Bromocriptine; placebo
Study quality	**3**
Reference	2186: Mancini A, Guitelman A, Levalle O, Aparicio N, Aszenmil G. Bromocriptine in the management of infertile men after surgery of prolactin secreting adenomas. J Androl. 1984 Jul–Aug;5(4):294–6.
Language	English

Compound	Bromocriptine (N04BC01)
Disease treated	Infertility
Quantification of adverse effects	Semen
No. of patients treated	4
Age group	Young
Treatment period	90 days
Dose	n.g.
Treatment consequences	Sperm parameters, alteration
Efficacy	No effect
Randomization of patients	No
Study quality	**3**
Reference	2191: Madsen H, Andersen O, Hansen P. Bromocriptine treatment for male infertility. Andrologia. 1980 Jul–Aug;12(4):379–80.
Language	English

Compound	Bromocriptine (N04BC01)
Disease treated	Infertility
Quantification of adverse effects	Semen
No. of patients treated	3
Age group	Young
Treatment period	16 weeks
Dose	2.5–7.5 mg/day

Treatment consequences	Sperm parameters, alteration
Efficacy	Increase in sperm motility
Randomization of patients	No
Study quality	**3**
Reference	2190: Laufer N, Yaffe H, Margalioth EJ, Livshin J, Ben-David M, Schenker JG. Effect of bromocriptine treatment on male infertility associated with hyperprolactinemia. Arch Androl. 1981 Jun;6(4):343–6.
Language	English

Compound	Bromocriptine (N04BC01)
Disease treated	Infertility
Quantification of adverse effects	Semen
No. of patients treated	3
Age group	Young
Treatment period	10 months
Dose	n.g.
Treatment consequences	Sperm parameters, alteration
Efficacy	No effect
Randomization of patients	No
Study quality	**3**
Reference	2185: Okada H, Iwamoto T, Fujioka H, Shirakawa T, Tatsumi N, Kanzaki M, Minayoshi K, Ohya K, Fujisawa M, Arakawa S, Kamidono S, Ishigami J. Hyperprolactinaemia among infertile patients and its effect on sperm functions. Andrologia. 1996 Jul–Aug;28(4):197–202.
Language	English

Compound	Bromocriptine (N04BC01)
Disease treated	Prolactinoma
Quantification of adverse effects	Semen
No. of patients treated	1
Age group	23
Treatment period	120 days
Dose	5 mg/day

Treatment consequences	Spermatogenesis, recovery
Efficacy	After normalization of prolactin levels
Study quality	**3**
Reference	588: Fraioli F, Paolucci D, Dondero F, Spera G, Isidori A. Prolactin secreting adenoma in man and the role of prolactin in spermatogenesis. J Endocrinol Invest. 1980 Apr–Jun;3(2):155–61.
Language	English

Compound	Bromocriptine (N04BC01)
Disease treated	Healthy
Quantification of dysfunction	Hormones
No. of patients treated	n.g.
Age group	Young
Treatment period	3 days
Dose	2.5 mg/day
Treatment consequences	Testosterone level and response to hCG, increase
Efficacy	Significant
Randomization of patients	No
Study quality	**2–**
Reference	896: Nakagawa K, Obara T, Matsubara M, Kubo M. Relationship of changes in serum concentrations of prolactin and testosterone during dopaminergic modulation in males. Clin Endocrinol (Oxf). 1982 Oct;17(4):345–52.
Language	English

Compound	Bromocriptine (N04BC01)
Disease treated	Infertility
Quantification of adverse effects	Semen
Age group	Young
Treatment consequences	Sperm parameters, alteration; pregnancy rate, increase
Efficacy	No effect, OR for pregnancy rate 0.70 (95% CI 0.15–3.24)
Side effects	Yes
Study quality	**1+ (Cochrane review)**

Reference	2182: Vandekerckhove P, Lilford R, Vail A, Hughes E. Bromocriptine for idiopathic oligo/asthenospermia. Cochrane Database Syst Rev. 2000;(2):CD000152.
Language	English

N05 Psycholeptics

A number of studies have investigated the effect of thioridazine, trifluoperazine, chlorpromazine and sulpiride on gonadotropin and testosterone secretion. No differences between treated and untreated men could be detected. In one case, a slow development of gynaecomastia was described.

Also in studies which have investigated the effect of lithium on testicular function, no alteration of testosterone levels or spermatogenic activity was found.

In diazepam addicts, the number of spermatozoa with chromosomal abnormalities was increased.

The clearance of zolpidem was found to be influenced by endogenous testosterone levels.

Overall level of evidence of adverse effects: C

Compound	Thioridazine (N05AC02), trifluoperazine, chlorpromazine
Disease treated	Schizophrenia
Quantification of adverse effects	Hormones
No. of patients treated	42
Age group	Young
Treatment period	Continuous
Dose	n.g.
Treatment consequences	Testosterone level, decrease; LH level, decrease
Efficacy	Lower in thioridazine patients
Randomization of patients	No
Study quality	**2–**
Reference	972: Brown WA, Laughren TP, Williams B. Differential effects of neuroleptic agents on the pituitary–gonadal axis in men. Arch Gen Psychiatry. 1981 Nov;38(11):1270–2.
Language	English

2

Compound	Haloperidol (N05AD01)
Disease treated	Schizophrenia
Quantification of adverse effects	Hormones
No. of patients treated	62
Age group	19–62 years
Treatment period	30 days
Dose	6 mg/day
Treatment consequences	Gonadotropin and 17-keto-steroid urinary excretion, increase
Efficacy	As compared with subnormal levels before treatment
Randomization of patients	No
Study quality	**3**
Reference	951: Brambilla F, Guerrini A, Guastalla A, Rovere C, Riggi F. Neuroendocrine effects of haloperidol therapy in chronic schizophrenia. Psychopharmacologia. 1975 Oct 14;44(1):17–22.
Language	English

Compound	Haloperidol (N05AD01)
Disease treated	Schizophrenia
Quantification of adverse effects	Hormones
No. of patients treated	30
Age group	Young
Treatment period	4+4 weeks
Dose	15–60 mg/day
Treatment consequences	Testosterone level, alteration
Efficacy	Decrease with higher dose of haloperidol
Randomization of patients	No
Study quality	**2–**
Reference	817: Rinieris P, Hatzimanolis J, Markianos M, Stefanis C. Effects of treatment with various doses of haloperidol on the pituitary–gonadal axis in male schizophrenic patients. Neuropsychobiology. 1989;22(3):146–9.
Language	English

Compound	Sulpiride (N05AL01)
Disease treated	Healthy
Quantification of adverse effects	Hormones
No. of patients treated	8
Age group	Young
Treatment period	14 days
Dose	150 mg/day
Treatment consequences	Gonadotropins and response to GnRH, alteration
Efficacy	No effect
Randomization of patients	No
Study quality	**2–**
Reference	892: Nakano R, Yagi S, Nishi T. Pituitary and testicular response to luteinizing hormone releasing hormone in normal and sulpiride-induced hyperprolactinaemic men. Exp Clin Endocrinol. 1988 May;91(2):191–6.
Language	English

Compound	Sulpiride (N05AL01)
Disease treated	Healthy
Quantification of adverse effects	Hormones
No. of patients treated	7
Age group	Young
Treatment period	14 days
Dose	150 mg/day
Treatment consequences	Testosterone level and response to hCG, increase
Efficacy	Significant
Randomization of patients	No
Study quality	**2–**
Reference	895: Bernini GP, Gasperi M, Franchi F, Luisi M. Effects of sulpiride induced hyperprolactinemia on testosterone secretion and metabolism before and after HCG in normal men. J Endocrinol Invest. 1983 Aug;6(4):287–91.
Language	English

Compound	Sulpiride (N05AL01)
Disease treated	Healthy
Quantification of adverse effects	Hormones
No. of patients treated	6
Age group	Young
Treatment period	Single dose
Dose	200 mg
Treatment consequences	Gonadotropin levels, alteration; sex steroid levels, alteration
Efficacy	None
Randomization of patients	Yes
Study quality	**1–**
Reference	890: Bahr C von, Wiesel FA, Movin G, Eneroth P, Jansson P, Nilsson L, Ogenstad S. Neuroendocrine responses to single oral doses of remoxipride and sulpiride in healthy female and male volunteers. Psychopharmacology (Berl). 1991;103(4):443–8.
Language	English

Compound	Sulpiride (N05AL01)
Disease treated	Healthy
Quantification of adverse effects	Hormones
No. of patients treated	5
Age group	Young
Treatment period	64 days
Dose	300 mg/day
Treatment consequences	Testosterone level and response to hCG, alteration
Efficacy	No consistent effects
Randomization of patients	No
Study quality	**3**
Reference	891: Oseko F, Oka N, Furuya H, Morikawa K. Effects of chronic sulpiride-induced hyperprolactinemia on plasma testosterone and its responses to hCG in normal men. J Androl. 1988 Jul–Aug;9(4):231–3.
Language	English

Compound	Sulpiride (N05AL01)
Disease treated	Psychosis
Quantification of adverse effects	Breast swelling
No. of patients treated	1
Age group	38
Treatment period	5 months
Dose	100 mg/day
Treatment consequences	Gynaecomastia
Efficacy	Slow development
Study quality	**3**
Reference	929: Kaneda Y, Fujii A. Gynecomastia with sulpiride. J Clin Pharm Ther. 2002 Feb;27(1):75–7.
Language	English

Compound	Sulpiride (N05AL01)
Disease treated	Healthy
Quantification of adverse effects	Hormones
No. of patients treated	n.g.
Age group	Young
Treatment period	3 days
Dose	50 mg/day
Treatment consequences	Testosterone level and response to hCG, alteration
Efficacy	No effect
Randomization of patients	No
Study quality	**2–**
Reference	896: Nakagawa K, Obara T, Matsubara M, Kubo M. Relationship of changes in serum concentrations of prolactin and testosterone during dopaminergic modulation in males. Clin Endocrinol (Oxf). 1982 Oct;17(4):345–52.
Language	English

Compound	Remoxipiride (N05AL04)
Disease treated	Healthy
Quantification of adverse effects	Hormones

No. of patients treated	6
Age group	Young
Treatment period	Single dose
Dose	100 mg
Treatment consequences	Gonadotropin levels, alteration; sex steroid levels, alteration
Efficacy	None
Randomization of patients	Yes, cross-over
Remarks	Remoxipiride; placebo
Study quality	**1–**
Reference	890: Bahr C von, Wiesel FA, Movin G, Eneroth P, Jansson P, Nilsson L, Ogenstad S. Neuroendocrine responses to single oral doses of remoxipride and sulpiride in healthy female and male volunteers. Psychopharmacology (Berl). 1991;103(4):443–8.
Language	English

Compound	Lithium (N05AN01)
Disease treated	Depression
Quantification of adverse effects	Sperm functions
No. of patients treated	36
Age group	Young
Treatment period	3 weeks
Dose	25 µm
Treatment consequences	Sperm motility, alteration
Efficacy	None
Randomization of patients	No
Study quality	**3**
Reference	755: Levin RM, Amsterdam JD, Winokur A, Wein AJ. Effects of psychotropic drugs on human sperm motility. Fertil Steril. 1981 Oct;36(4):503–6.
Language	English

Compound	Lithium (N05AN01)
Disease treated	Bipolar psychosis
Quantification of adverse effects	Hormones
No. of patients treated	14

Age group	Young
Treatment period	Various
Dose	Below 1 mmol Li+
Treatment consequences	Testosterone level, alteration
Efficacy	None
Randomization of patients	No
Dose arms 1–3	Drug-free mania; lithium
Study quality	**2–**
Reference	974: Hunter R, Christie JE, Whalley LJ, Bennie J, Carroll S, Dick H, Goodwin GM, Wilson H, Fink G. Luteinizing hormone responses to luteinizing hormone releasing hormone (LHRH) in acute mania and the effects of lithium on LHRH and thyrotrophin releasing hormone tests in volunteers. Psychol Med. 1989 Feb;19(1):69–77.
Language	English

Compound	Lithium (N05AN01)
Disease treated	Psychosis
Quantification of adverse effects	Semen
No. of patients treated	10
Age group	Young
Treatment period	10 weeks
Dose	Various
Treatment consequences	Spermatogenesis, impairment
Efficacy	No effect
Randomization of patients	No
Study quality	**3**
Reference	337: Tollefson G, Garvey MJ. Spermatogenesis during extended lithium treatment. Hillside J Clin Psychiatry. 1989;11(1):35–41.
Language	English

Compound	Lithium (N05AN01)
Disease treated	Bipolar psychosis
Quantification of adverse effects	Hormones
No. of patients treated	n.g.

Age group	16–24 years
Treatment period	3 months
Dose	n.g.
Treatment consequences	Testosterone level, alteration
Efficacy	None
Randomization of patients	No
Study quality	**3**
Reference	953: Sheard MH, Marini JL, Giddings SS. The effect of lithium on luteinizing hormone and testosterone in man. Dis Nerv Syst. 1977 Oct;38(10):765–9.
Language	English

Compound	Lithium (N05AN01)
Disease treated	Healthy
Quantification of adverse effects	Hormones
No. of patients treated	n.g.
Age group	Young
Treatment period	1 month
Dose	900 mg/day
Treatment consequences	Testosterone level, alteration; oestradiol level, alteration
Efficacy	None
Randomization of patients	No
Dose arms 1–3	Lithium 900 mg/day; placebo
Study quality	**2–**
Reference	973: Baptista T, Alastre T, Contreras Q, Martinez JL, Araujo de Baptista E, Burguera JL, de Burguera M, Hernandez L. Effects of lithium carbonate on reproductive hormones in healthy men: relationship with body weight regulation: a pilot study. Prog Neuropsychopharmacol Biol Psychiatry. 1997 Aug;21(6):937–50.
Language	English

Compound	Diazepam (N05BA01)
Disease treated	Diazepam addiction
Quantification of adverse effects	Sperm chromosomes
No. of patients treated	2

Age group	Young
Treatment period	6 months
Dose	0.3 mg/kg day^{-1}
Treatment consequences	Sperm aneuploidy
Efficacy	Sperm number with disomy 13, disomy X, and total sex-chromosomal disomies enhanced as compared with controls
Randomization of patients	No
Study quality	**3**
Reference	805: Baumgartner A, Schmid TE, Schuetz CG, Adler ID. Detection of aneuploidy in rodent and human sperm by multicolor FISH after chronic exposure to diazepam. Mutat Res. 2001 Jan 25;490(1):11–9.
Language	English

Compound	Diazepam (N05BA01)
Disease treated	Diazepam addiction
Quantification of adverse effects	DNA probes specific for certain chromosomes
No. of patients treated	n.g.
Age group	Young
Treatment period	In vitro
Dose	Various
Treatment consequences	Sperm chromosomes
Efficacy	Aberrations as analysed by FISH
Randomization of patients	No
Study quality	**3**
Reference	870: Adler ID, Schmid TE, Baumgartner A. Induction of aneuploidy in male mouse germ cells detected by the sperm-FISH assay: a review of the present data base. Mutat Res. 2002 Jul 25;504(1–2):173–82.
Language	English

Compound	Zolpidem (N05CF02)
Disease treated	Healthy
Quantification of adverse effects	Clearence of zolpidem as influenced by testosterone
No. of patients treated	16
Age group	61–85 years

Treatment period	Single dose
Dose	5 mg
Treatment consequences	Clearance of zolpidem
Efficacy	Decreased in elderly men, greater relative contribution of serum testosterone than age
Randomization of patients	No
Study quality	**2–**
Reference	905: Olubodun JO, Ochs HR, Moltke LL von, Roubenoff R, Hesse LM, Harmatz JS, Shader RI, Greenblatt DJ. Pharmacokinetic properties of zolpidem in elderly and young adults: possible modulation by testosterone in men. Br J Clin Pharmacol. 2003 Sep;56(3):297–304.
Language	English

N06	**Psychoanaleptics**
	Only marginal effects of psychoanaleptics on testosterone secretion and spermatogenesis have been described. The RCTs are not available. **Overall level of evidence of adverse effects: D**

Compound	Imipramine (N06AA02)
Disease treated	Depression
Quantification of adverse effects	Sperm functions
No. of patients treated	n.g
Age group	Young
Treatment period	3 weeks
Dose	In vitro
Treatment consequences	Sperm vitality, decrease
Efficacy	Significant
Randomization of patients	No
Study quality	**3**
Reference	755: Levin RM, Amsterdam JD, Winokur A, Wein AJ. Effects of psychotropic drugs on human sperm motility. Fertil Steril. 1981 Oct;36(4):503–6.
Language	English

Compound	Amitryptilin (N06AA09)
Disease treated	Infertility
Quantification of adverse effects	Sperm parameters
No. of patients treated	20
Age group	Young
Treatment period	n.g.
Dose	n.g.
Treatment consequences	Sperm count and sperm morphology, increase
Efficacy	After treatment
Randomization of patients	No
Study quality	**3**
Reference	919: Padron RS, Nodarse M. Effects of amitriptyline on semen of infertile men. Br J Urol. 1980 Jun;52(3):226–8.
Language	English

Compound	Venlafaxine (N06AX16)
Disease treated	Paraphilia
Quantification of adverse effects	Hormones
No. of patients treated	1
Age group	26
Treatment period	13 weeks
Dose	112 mg/day
Treatment consequences	Testosterone level, decreased
Efficacy	Increase after cessation
Study quality	**3**
Reference	975: Bell S, Shipman M. Reduced testosterone level in a venlafaxine treated patient. Ann Clin Psychiatry. 2000 Sep;12(3):171–3.
Language	English

Compound	Oxcarbazepine (not listed)
Disease treated	Epilepsy
Quantification of adverse effects	Hormones
No. of patients treated	29
Age group	Young

Treatment period	Continuous
Dose	<900 mg/day
Treatment consequences	Testosterone level, alteration; SHBG level, alteration
Efficacy	None
Randomization of patients	No
Study quality	**2–**
Reference	968: Rattya J, Turkka J, Pakarinen AJ, Knip M, Kotila MA, Lukkarinen O, Myllyla VV, Isojarvi JI. Reproductive effects of valproate, carbamazepine, and oxcarbazepine in men with epilepsy. Neurology. 2001 Jan 9;56(1):31–6.
Language	English

Compound	Oxcarbazepine (not listed)
Disease treated	Epilepsy
Quantification of adverse effects	Semen, hormones, testicular volume
No. of patients treated	18
Age group	Young
Treatment period	Continuous
Dose	Various
Treatment consequences	DHEA levels alteration, abnormal sperm alteration, testicular volume alteration
Efficacy	None
Randomization of patients	No
Study quality	**3**
Reference	984: Isojarvi JI, Lofgren E, Juntunen KS, Pakarinen AJ, Paivansalo M, Rautakorpi I, Tuomivaara L. Effect of epilepsy and antiepileptic drugs on male reproductive health. Neurology. 2004 Jan 27;62(2):247–53.
Language	English

N07	**Other Nervous System Drugs**
	Nicotine
	Nicotine is not a drug for treating diseases, but it is a drug in the sense of the definition given by Goodman–Gilman (see above). Herein it has to be considered that adverse effects of smoking may not be due to nicotine alone.

The effects of smoking on spermatogenesis have been found to be surprisingly mild to moderate. A large number of studies have described no differences between sperm parameters including DNA content of spermatozoa found in smokers, ex-smokers and non-smokers; however, higher levels of DNA strand breaks and of the frequency of aneuploidy have been found in spermatozoa of smokers than in non-smokers. Some other studies have described a decrease in sperm count, viability and motility in smokers, and a negative correlation of these parameters with the dose of smoking (pack-years or daily use). In particular, the function of sperm motility appeared to be sensitive against the toxins from tobacco smoke. This could also be demonstrated by in-vitro exposition of spermatozoa of non-smokers to the seminal plasma of smokers. Leukocyte count and ROS were found to be significantly higher in smokers than in non-smokers.

Even in groups with reduced sperm parameters, the fertilization rate appears to be unaffected.

Overall level of evidence of adverse effects: B

Compound	Nicotine (N07BA01)
Disease treated	Infertility
Quantification of adverse effects	Semen
No. of patients treated	1104
Age group	Young
Treatment period	Continuous
Dose	Various
Treatment consequences	Sperm parameters, decrease
Efficacy	No differences between non-smokers and ex-smokers
Randomization of patients	No
Study quality	**2+**
Reference	28: Trummer H, Habermann H, Haas J, Pummer K. The impact of cigarette smoking on human semen parameters and hormones. Hum Reprod. 2002 Jun;17(6):1554–9.
Language	English

Compound	Nicotine (N07BA01)
Disease treated	Infertility
Quantification of adverse effects	IVF outcome

No. of patients treated	462 cycles
Age group	Young
Treatment period	Continuous
Dose	Various
Treatment consequences	Sperm parameters, impairment
Efficacy	Significant reduction of sperm count, fertilization rate unaffected
Randomization of patients	No
Dose arms 1–3	smokers; non–smokers;
Study quality	**2–**
Reference	2022: Hughes EG, Yeo J, Claman P, YoungLai EV, Sagle MA, Daya S, Collins JA. Cigarette smoking and the outcomes of in vitro fertilization: measurement of effect size and levels of action. Fertil Steril. 1994 Oct;62(4):807–14.
Language	English

Compound	**Nicotine (N07BA01)**
Disease treated	Infertility
Quantification of adverse effects	Semen
No. of patients treated	350
Age group	Young
Treatment period	Continuous
Dose	Various
Treatment consequences	Sperm parameters, impairment
Efficacy	No statistically significant differences in any aspect of sperm quality including DNA distribution between non-smokers, moderate smokers and heavy smokers
Randomization of patients	No
Dose arms 1–3	Smokers; non-smokers
Study quality	**2+**
Reference	2027: Oldereid NB, Rui H, Clausen OP, Purvis K. Cigarette smoking and human sperm quality assessed by laser-Doppler spectroscopy and DNA flow cytometry. J Reprod Fertil. 1989 Jul;86(2):731–6.
Language	English

Compound	Nicotine (N07BA01)
Disease treated	Infertility
Quantification of adverse effects	Semen
No. of patients treated	333
Age group	19–40 years
Treatment period	Continuous
Dose	Various
Treatment consequences	Sperm parameters, impairment
Efficacy	No statistically significant effect of smoking habits on sperm density, motility or morphological features
Randomization of patients	No
Dose arms 1–3	Smokers; non-smokers
Study quality	**2+**
Reference	2030: Vogt HJ, Heller WD, Borelli S. Sperm quality of healthy smokers, ex-smokers, and never-smokers. Fertil Steril. 1986 Jan;45(1):106–10.
Language	English

Compound	Nicotine (N07BA01)
Disease treated	Infertility
Quantification of adverse effects	Semen
No. of patients treated	191; 110
Age group	Young
Treatment period	Continuous
Dose	Various
Treatment consequences	Sperm parameters, impairment
Efficacy	Sperm density, viability and motility in smokers than in the non-smokers and negatively correlated with pack-years.
Randomization of patients	No
Dose arms 1–3	Smokers; non-smokers
Study quality	**2+**
Reference	2009: Zhang JP, Meng QY, Wang Q, Zhang LJ, Mao YL, Sun ZX. Effect of smoking on semen quality of infertile men in Shandong, China. Asian J Androl. 2000 Jun;2(2):143–6.
Language	English

Compound	Nicotine (N07BA01)
Disease treated	Infertility
Quantification of adverse effects	Semen
No. of patients treated	290
Age group	Young
Treatment period	Continuous
Dose	Various
Treatment consequences	Sperm parameters, impairment
Efficacy	Heavy smokers showed sperm motility decrease
Randomization of patients	No
Dose arms 1–3	Heavy smokers; light smokers
Study quality	**2–**
Reference	2003: Ozgur K, Isikoglu M, Seleker M, Donmez L. Semen quality of smoking and non-smoking men in infertile couples in a Turkish population. Arch Gynecol Obstet. 2005 Feb;271(2):109–12. Epub 2003 18 Dec. Turkey.
Language	English

Compound	Nicotine (N07BA01)
Disease treated	Infertility
Quantification of adverse effects	Semen
No. of patients treated	252
Age group	Young
Treatment period	Continuous
Dose	Various
Treatment consequences	Sperm parameters, impairment
Efficacy	No association with smoking habits
Randomization of patients	No
Dose arms 1–3	Smokers; non-smokers
Study quality	**2–**
Reference	2024: Oldereid NB, Rui H, Purvis K. Life styles of men in barren couples and their relationship to sperm quality. Int J Fertil. 1992 Nov–Dec;37(6):343–9.
Language	English

Compound	Nicotine (N07BA01)
Disease treated	Healthy
Quantification of adverse effects	Semen
No. of patients treated	238
Age group	Young
Treatment period	Continuous
Dose	Various
Treatment consequences	Sperm parameters, impairment
Efficacy	Morphological abnormalities did not differ significantly between smokers and non-smokers.
Randomization of patients	No
Dose arms 1–3	Smokers; non-smokers
Study quality	**2+**
Reference	2031: Kulikauskas V, Blaustein D, Ablin RJ. Cigarette smoking and its possible effects on sperm. Fertil Steril. 1985 Oct;44(4):526–8.
Language	English

Compound	Nicotine (N07BA01)
Disease treated	Infertility
Quantification of adverse effects	Semen
No. of patients treated	225
Age group	Young
Treatment period	Continuous
Dose	Various
Treatment consequences	Sperm parameters, impairment
Efficacy	No significant changes in the spermiogram
Randomization of patients	No
Dose arms 1–3	Smokers; non-smokers
Study quality	**2–**
Reference	2025: Gerhard I, Lenhard K, Eggert-Kruse W, Runnebaum B. Clinical data which influence semen parameters in infertile men. Hum Reprod. 1992 Jul;7(6):830–7.
Language	English

Compound	Nicotine (N07BA01)
Disease treated	Infertility
Quantification of adverse effects	Semen
No. of patients treated	223
Age group	Young
Treatment period	Continuous
Dose	Various pack-years
Treatment consequences	Sperm parameters, impairment
Efficacy	Smoking is negatively correlated with sperm motility, not with sperm count and morphology
Randomization of patients	No
Dose arms 1–3	Smokers; non-smokers
Study quality	**2–**
Reference	2000: Hassa H, Yildirim A, Can C, Turgut M, Tanir HM, Senses T, Sahin-Mutlu F. Effect of smoking on semen parameters of men attending an infertility clinic. Clin Exp Obstet Gynecol. 2006;33(1):19–22.
Language	English

Compound	Nicotine (N07BA01)
Disease treated	Healthy
Quantification of adverse effects	Semen
No. of patients treated	201
Age group	Young
Treatment period	Continuous
Dose	Various
Treatment consequences	Sperm parameters, impairment
Efficacy	Smoking associated with poorer morphology
Randomization of patients	No
Dose arms 1–3	Smokers; non-smokers
Study quality	**2+**
Reference	2017: Figa-Talamanca I, Cini C, Varricchio GC, Dondero F, Gandini L, Lenzi A, Lombardo F, Angelucci L, Grezia R di, Patacchioli FR. Effects of prolonged autovehicle driving on male reproduction function: a study among taxi drivers. Am J Ind Med. 1996 Dec;30(6):750–8.
Language	English

Compound	Nicotine (N07BA01)
Disease treated	Infertility
Quantification of adverse effects	Semen
No. of patients treated	58; 101
Age group	31 years (mean)
Treatment period	Continuous
Dose	Various
Treatment consequences	Sperm parameters, impairment
Efficacy	Sperm count, motility, morphology not different between smokers and non-smokers
Randomization of patients	No
Dose arms 1–3	Smokers; non-smokers
Study quality	2-
Reference	2033: Rodriguez-Rigau LJ, Smith KD, Steinberger E. Cigarette smoking and semen quality. Fertil Steril. 1982 Jul;38(1):115–6.
Language	English

Compound	Nicotine (N07BA01)
Disease treated	Healthy
Quantification of adverse effects	Semen
No. of patients treated	119
Age group	Young
Treatment period	Continuous
Dose	Various
Treatment consequences	Sperm parameters, impairment
Efficacy	No significant differences in hormones and sperm count, but significantly lower motility (67 as compared with 72%), lower number of total oval sperm (120 as compared with 251×10^6) in smokers as compared with non-smokers
Randomization of patients	No
Dose arms 1–3	Smokers; non-smokers
Study quality	**2+**
Reference	2032: Handelsman DJ, Conway AJ, Boylan LM, Turtle JR. Testicular function in potential sperm donors: normal ranges and the effects of smoking and varicocele. Int J Androl. 1984 Oct;7(5):369–82.

Language	English

Compound	Nicotine (N07BA01)
Disease treated	Infertility
Quantification of adverse effects	Semen
No. of patients treated	115
Age group	Young
Treatment period	Continuous
Dose	Various
Treatment consequences	Sperm parameters, impairment
Efficacy	Insignificantly higher proportion of smokers in group with poor semen quality
Randomization of patients	No
Dose arms 1–3	Smokers; non-smokers
Study quality	**2–**
Reference	2020: Goverde HJ, Dekker HS, Janssen HJ, Bastiaans BA, Rolland R, Zielhuis GA. Semen quality and frequency of smoking and alcohol consumption: an explorative study. Int J Fertil Menopausal Stud. 1995 May–Jun;40(3):135–8.
Language	English

Compound	Nicotine (N07BA01)
Disease treated	Infertility
Quantification of adverse effects	Semen
No. of patients treated	110
Age group	Young
Treatment period	Continuous
Dose	Various
Treatment consequences	Sperm parameters, impairment
Efficacy	Non-smokers' sperm count 74.3, motility 65%; smokers' sperm count 67, motility 62% (significantly lower); sperm morphology: no difference
Randomization of patients	No
Dose arms 1–3	Smokers; non-smokers
Study quality	**2–**

Reference	2029: Rantala ML, Koskimies AI. Semen quality of infertile couples: comparison between smokers and non-smokers. Andrologia. 1987 Jan–Feb;19(1):42–6.
Language	English

Compound	Nicotine (N07BA01)
Disease treated	Infertility
Quantification of adverse effects	Semen
No. of patients treated	90
Age group	Young
Treatment period	Continuous
Dose	Various
Treatment consequences	Sperm parameters, impairment
Efficacy	Percentages of DNA fragmentation in spermatozoa were not statistically different in the heavy smokers (12.11%), light smokers (11.66%) and non-smokers (20.41%).
Randomization of patients	No
Dose arms 1–3	Smokers; non-smokers
Study quality	**2–**
Reference	2010: Sergerie M, Ouhilal S, Bissonnette F, Brodeur J, Bleau G. Lack of association between smoking and DNA fragmentation in the spermatozoa of normal men. Hum Reprod. 2000 Jun;15(6):1314–21.
Language	English

Compound	Nicotine (N07BA01)
Disease treated	Healthy
Quantification of adverse effects	Semen
No. of patients treated	86
Age group	18–35 years
Treatment period	Continuous
Dose	Various
Treatment consequences	Sperm parameters, impairment
Efficacy	No significant effect on sperm nuclear size, shape or chromatin texture
Randomization of patients	No

Dose arms 1–3	Smokers; non-smokers
Study quality	**2+**
Reference	2016: Vine MF, Setzer RW Jr, Everson RB, Wyrobek AJ. Human sperm morphometry and smoking, caffeine, and alcohol consumption. Reprod Toxicol. 1997 Mar–Jun;11(2–3):179–84.
Language	English

Compound	Nicotine (N07BA01)
Disease treated	Infertility
Quantification of adverse effects	Semen
No. of patients treated	43; 43
Age group	Young
Treatment period	Continuous
Dose	Various
Treatment consequences	Sperm parameters, impairment
Efficacy	Higher percentage of abnormal forms in smokers
Randomization of patients	No
Dose arms 1–3	Smokers; non-smokers
Study quality	**2+**
Reference	2034: Evans HJ, Fletcher J, Torrance M, Hargreave TB. sperm abnormalities and cigarette smoking. Lancet. 1981 Mar 21;1(8221):627–9.
Language	English

Compound	Nicotine (N07BA01)
Disease treated	Infertility
Quantification of adverse effects	Semen
No. of patients treated	49; 28
Age group	Young
Treatment period	Continuous
Dose	Various
Treatment consequences	Sperm parameters, impairment
Efficacy	No significant differences in semen volume and sperm count, significantly lower motility, morphology, and hamster-oocyte-penetration test

Randomization of patients	No
Dose arms 1–3	Smokers; non-smokers
Study quality	**2–**
Reference	2019: Sofikitis N, Miyagawa I, Dimitriadis D, Zavos P, Sikka S, Hellstrom W. Effects of smoking on testicular function, semen quality and sperm fertilizing capacity. J Urol. 1995 Sep;154(3):1030–4.
Language	English

Compound	Nicotine (N07BA01)
Disease treated	Infertility
Quantification of adverse effects	Semen
No. of patients treated	20; 45
Age group	Young
Treatment period	Continuous
Dose	Various
Treatment consequences	Sperm parameters, impairment
Efficacy	Leukocyte count and ROS significantly higher in smokers. Differences in standard sperm variables and DNA damage indices not significant
Randomization of patients	No
Dose arms 1–3	Smokers; non-smokers
Study quality	**2–**
Reference	2005: Saleh RA, Agarwal A, Sharma RK, Nelson DR, Thomas AJ Jr. Effect of cigarette smoking on levels of seminal oxidative stress in infertile men: a prospective study. Fertil Steril. 2002 Sep;78(3):491–9.
Language	English

Compound	Nicotine (N07BA01)
Disease treated	Smoking
Quantification of adverse effects	Semen
No. of patients treated	25; 20
Age group	25–35 years
Treatment period	Continuous
Dose	>20 cigarettes/day

Treatment consequences	Sperm motility, decrease
Efficacy	Significant as compared with that of non-smokers
Randomization of patients	No
Dose arms 1–3	Smokers; non-smokers
Study quality	**2–**
Reference	991: Shaarawy M, Mahmoud KZ. Endocrine profile and semen characteristics in male smokers. Fertil Steril. 1982 Aug;38(2):255–7.
Language	English

Compound	Nicotine (N07BA01)
Disease treated	Infertility
Quantification of adverse effects	Semen
No. of patients treated	31
Age group	Young
Treatment period	Continuous
Dose	Various
Treatment consequences	Sperm parameters, impairment
Efficacy	No significant differences in semen parameters or in age across groups. The frequency of disomy 13 was significantly higher in light and heavy smokers than in non-smokers.
Randomization of patients	No
Dose arms 1–3	Smokers; non-smokers
Study quality	**2–**
Reference	2008: Shi Q, Ko E, Barclay L, Hoang T, Rademaker A, Martin R. Cigarette smoking and aneuploidy in human sperm. Mol Reprod Dev. 2001 Aug;59(4):417–21.
Language	English

Compound	Nicotine (N07BA01)
Disease treated	Healthy
Quantification of adverse effects	Semen
No. of patients treated	10; 15
Age group	Exactly 18 years
Treatment period	Continuous
Dose	Various

Treatment consequences	Sperm parameters, impairment
Efficacy	Sperm count and motility significantly lower; elevated frequencies of sperm aneuploidy in smokers
Randomization of patients	No
Dose arms 1–3	Smokers; non-smokers
Study quality	**2–**
Reference	2014: Rubes J, Lowe X, Moore D 2nd, Perreault S, Slott V, Evenson D, Selevan SG, Wyrobek AJ. Smoking cigarettes is associated with increased sperm disomy in teenage men. Fertil Steril. 1998 Oct;70(4):715–23.
Language	English

Compound	Nicotine (N07BA01)
Disease treated	Infertility
Quantification of adverse effects	Semen
No. of patients treated	n.g.
Age group	Young
Treatment period	In vitro
Dose	Spermatozoa of non-smokers in seminal plasma of smokers
Treatment consequences	sperm parameters, impairment
Efficacy	By exposure to seminal plasma from smokers
Randomization of patients	No
Dose arms 1–3	smokers; non–smokers;
Study quality	**2–**
Reference	2001: Arabi M, Moshtaghi H. Influence of cigarette smoking on spermatozoa via seminal plasma. Andrologia. 2005 Aug;37(4):119–24.
Language	English

Compound	Nicotine (N07BA01)
Disease treated	Infertility
Quantification of adverse effects	Semen
No. of patients treated	n.g.
Age group	Young
Treatment period	Continuous
Dose	Various

Treatment consequences	Sperm parameters, impairment
Efficacy	Higher levels of DNA strand breaks in spermatozoa of smokers
Randomization of patients	No
Dose arms 1–3	Smokers; non-smokers
Study quality	**2–**
Reference	2013: Potts RJ, Newbury CJ, Smith G, Notarianni LJ, Jefferies TM. Sperm chromatin damage associated with male smoking. Mutat Res. 1999 Jan 25;423(1–2):103–11.
Language	English

N07	**Other Nervous System Drugs**
	Opiates
	In opiate addicts, independent of the drug used, the following alterations were observed: decrease of seminal volume, impairment of sperm parameters, but no alteration of testosterone levels. The improvement of symptoms after cessation of abuse was not described. There are no RCTs available. **Overall level of evidence of adverse effects: C**

Compound	Narcomania (N07BB)
Disease treated	Spermatogenic dysfunction
Quantification of adverse effects	FISH analysis
No. of patients treated	45
Age group	19–35 years
Treatment period	Continuous
Dose	Various
Treatment consequences	Sperm aneuploidy of XX18 and YY18, increase
Efficacy	Significant
Randomization of patients	No
Study quality	**3**

Reference	799: Robbins WA, Vine MF, Truong KY, Everson RB. Use of fluorescence in situ hybridization (FISH) to assess effects of smoking, caffeine, and alcohol on aneuploidy load in sperm of healthy men. Environ Mol Mutagen. 1997;30(2):175–83.
Language	English

Compound	Methadone (N07BC02), heroin
Disease treated	Opiate addiction
Quantification of adverse effects	Semen, hormones
No. of patients treated	80
Age group	Young
Treatment period	Continuous
Dose	Various
Treatment consequences	Spermatogenesis, impairment; testosterone levels, alteration
Efficacy	All men
Randomization of patients	No
Dose arms 1–3	Heroin; methadone
Study quality	**2–**
Reference	941: Ragni G, Lauretis L de, Bestetti O, Sghedoni D, Gambaro V. Gonadal function in male heroin and methadone addicts. Int J Androl. 1988 Apr;11(2):93–100.
Language	English

Compound	Methadone (N07BC02)
Disease treated	Opiate addiction
Quantification of adverse effects	Sexual function
No. of patients treated	29
Age group	Young
Treatment period	Continuous
Dose	n.g.
Treatment consequences	Sexual function, alteration
Efficacy	Ejaculate volume reduced by over 50%
Randomization of patients	No
Study quality	**3**

Reference	979: Cicero TJ, Bell RD, Wiest WG, Allison JH, Polakoski K, Robins E. Function of the male sex organs in heroin and methadone users. N Engl J Med. 1975 Apr 24;292(17):882–7.
Language	English

Compound	Methadone (N07BC02)
Disease treated	Opiate addiction
Quantification of adverse effects	Hormones
No. of patients treated	25
Age group	Young
Treatment period	2 months
Dose	30 mg/day
Treatment consequences	Gonadotropin levels, decrease; sex steroid levels, increase
Efficacy	Significant
Randomization of patients	No
Study quality	**3**
Reference	942: Lafisca S, Bolelli G, Franceschetti F, Filicori M, Flamigni C, Marigo M. Hormone levels in methadone-treated drug addicts. Drug Alcohol Depend. 1981 Nov;8(3):229–34.
Language	English

Compound	Methadone (N07BC02), heroin
Disease treated	Heroin addiction
Quantification of adverse effects	Sperm functions
No. of patients treated	n.g.
Age group	Young
Treatment period	Continuous
Dose	Various
Treatment consequences	Sperm parameters, deterioration
Efficacy	Clearly
Randomization of patients	No
Study quality	**3**
Reference	756: Ragni G, Lauretis L de, Gambaro V, Pietro R di, Bestetti O, Recalcati F, Papetti C. Semen evaluation in heroin and methadone addicts. Acta Eur Fertil. 1985 Jul–Aug;16(4):245–9.

Language	English

Compound	Methadone (N07BC02), heroin
Disease treated	Opiate addiction
Quantification of adverse effects	Hormones
No. of patients treated	n.g.
Age group	Young
Treatment period	7 days
Dose	45 mg/day
Treatment consequences	Testosterone level, alteration; cortisol level, alteration
Efficacy	Also after change to methadone
Randomization of patients	No
Dose arms 1–3	Heroin; methadone
Study quality	**2–**
Reference	943: Mendelson JH, Meyer RE, Ellingboe J, Mirin SM, McDougle M. Effects of heroin and methadone on plasma cortisol and testosterone. J Pharmacol Exp Ther. 1975 Nov;195(2):296–302.
Language	English

N07 Other Nervous System Drugs

Tetrahydrocannabinol (THC)

Clinical studies which investigate the effect of THC on spermatogenesis and testicular function are not available. The compound inhibits sperm motility in vitro.

Overall level of evidence of adverse effects: C

Compound	Tetrahydrocannabinol (not listed)
Disease treated	Healthy
Quantification of adverse effects	Sperm motility and acrosome reaction
No. of patients treated	87
Age group	Sperm in vitro
Treatment period	Single time
Dose	4.8 μmol maximally

Treatment consequences	Sperm motility and acrosome reaction, reduction
Efficacy	Dose dependent
Randomization of patients	No
Study quality	**2–**
Reference	779: Whan LB, West MC, McClure N, Lewis SE. Effects of delta-9-tetrahydrocannabinol, the primary psychoactive cannabinoid in marijuana, on human sperm function in vitro. Fertil Steril. 2006 Mar;85(3):653–60.
Language	English

P01	**Antiprotozoals**
	There is a case report on impairment of sperm parameters in a male infected with malaria. **Overall level of evidence of adverse effects: D**

Compound	Malaria toxin (not listed)
Disease treated	Malaria
Quantification of adverse effects	Semen
No. of patients treated	1
Age group	33
Treatment period	n.g.
Treatment consequences	Azoospermia or oligo-astheno-teratozoospermia, induction
Efficacy	During 2 years
Study quality	**3**
Reference	379: Singer R, Segenreich E, Sagiv M, Shohat B, Livni E, Bartoov B, Zukerman Z, Leiba S, Servadio C. Decreased semen quality in a male infected with malaria. Int J Androl. 1987 Oct;10(5):685–9.
Language	English

P02	Anthelmintics
	A report on the impairment of sperm parameters in bilharziasis described improvement after cessation of therapy.
	Overall level of evidence of adverse effects: D

Compound	Niridazol (P02BX02)
Disease treated	Bilharziasis
Quantification of adverse effects	Semen
No. of patients treated	20
Age group	Young
Treatment period	n.g.
Dose	n.g.
Treatment consequences	Sperm parameters, impairment
Efficacy	All, recovery 3 months after therapy
Randomization of patients	No
Study quality	**3**
Reference	531: El-Beheiry AH, Kamel MN, Gad A. Niridazole and fertility in bilharzial men. Arch Androl. 1982 Jun;8(4):297–300.
Language	English

P03	Ectoparasiticides
	Lindane is accumulated in the testis, followed by a decreased production of testosterone and impairment spermatogenesis.
	Overall level of evidence of adverse effects: D

Compound	Lindane (P03AB02)
Disease treated	Genital malformation
Quantification of adverse effects	Malformation
Age group	Mammals

Treatment consequences	Azoospermia, induction
Efficacy	In 94.8% of exposed men
Randomization of patients	No
Remarks	Lindane accumulates in the testis. It induces hypoproduction of testosterone and impairs spermatogenesis.
Study quality	**4 (review)**
Reference	52: Pages N, Sauviat MP, Bouvet S, Goudey-Perriere F. Reproductive toxicity of lindane. J Soc Biol. 2002;196(4):325–38.
Language	French

R05	**Cough and Cold Preparations**
	N-acetyl-cysteine in vitro inhibited ROS production in vitro. Studies on the clinical use of the compound in male infertility have been scheduled but have not yet been completed. In healthy volunteers, no alteration of sperm parameters was observed. **Overall level of evidence of adverse effects: D**

Compound	N-acetyl-cysteine (R05CB01)
Disease treated	Sperm in vitro
Quantification of adverse effects	Chemiluminescent signal of the oxidation of luminol
No. of patients treated	n.g.
Age group	Young
Treatment period	In vitro
Dose	1.0 mg/ml
Treatment consequences	ROS in sperm, decrease
Efficacy	Significant
Study quality	**2–**
Reference	915: Oeda T, Henkel R, Ohmori H, Schill WB. Scavenging effect of N-acetyl-L-cysteine against reactive oxygen species in human semen: A possible therapeutic modality for male factor infertility? Andrologia. 1997 May–Jun;29(3):125–31.
Language	English

Compound	N-acetyl-cysteine (R05CB01)
Disease treated	Infertility
Quantification of adverse effects	Sperm parameters
No. of patients treated	27
Age group	Young
Treatment period	Not mentioned
Dose	Various
Treatment consequences	Sperm parameters, alteration; ROS, decrease; acrosome reaction, increase
Efficacy	No alteration, decrease, increase
Randomization of patients	No
Study quality	**3**
Reference	911: Comhaire FH, Christophe AB, Zalata AA, Dhooge WS, Mahmoud AM, Depuydt CE. The effects of combined conventional treatment, oral antioxidants and essential fatty acids on sperm biology in subfertile men. Prostaglandins Leukot Essent Fatty Acids. 2000 Sep;63(3):159–65.
Language	English

R06 Antihistamines for Systemic Use

In testicular histology of infertile patients with poor sperm parameters, often mast cells surrounding or infiltrating the seminiferous tubules are demonstrable. From this observation, the benefit of antihistamine treatment has been suggested. Results of clinical studies, however, have been disappointing.

Overall level of evidence of adverse effects: C

Compound	Antihistamines for systemic use (R06A)
Disease treated	Healthy
Quantification of adverse effects	Histamine-induced rise of sperm Ca
No. of patients treated	Not mentioned
Age group	Sperm in vitro
Dose	Not mentioned
Treatment consequences	Sperm Ca^{2+}, histamin induced rise, no prevention by famotidine

Efficacy	Significant
Randomization of patients	No
Study quality	**2–**
Reference	759: Gupta A, Khosla R, Gupta S, Tiwary AK. Influence of histamine and H1-receptor antagonists on ejaculated human spermatozoa: role of intrasperm Ca2+. Indian J Exp Biol. 2004 May;42(5):481–5.
Language	English

Compound	Ketotifen (R06AX17)
Disease treated	Leukocytospermia
Quantification of dysfunction	Sperm parameters
No. of patients treated	55
Age group	Young
Treatment period	12 weeks
Dose	2 mg/day
Treatment consequences	Sperm parameters, improvement; leucocyte count, decrease
Efficacy	During treatment
Randomization of patients	No
Study quality	**3**
Reference	827: Oliva A, Multigner L. Ketotifen improves sperm motility and sperm morphology in male patients with leukocytospermia and unexplained infertility. Fertil Steril. 2006 Jan;85(1):240–3.
Language	English

Compound	Ebastine (R06AX22)
Disease treated	Infertility
Quantification of adverse effects	Semen
No. of patients treated	15
Age group	Young
Treatment period	3 months
Dose	10 mg/day
Treatment consequences	Sperm parameters, improvement
Efficacy	In 9 of 15 patients

Randomization of patients	No
Study quality	**3**
Reference	115: Matsuki S, Sasagawa I, Suzuki Y, Yazawa H, Tateno T, Hashimoto T, Nakada T, Saito H, Hiroi M. The use of ebastine, a mast cell blocker, for treatment of oligozoospermia. Arch Androl. 2000 Mar–Apr;44(2):129–32.
Language	English

Compound	Fexofenadine (R06AX26)
Disease treated	Infertility, testicular histology with mast cells
Quantification of adverse effects	Semen
No. of patients treated	16
Age group	Young
Treatment period	9 months
Dose	180 mg/day
Treatment consequences	Sperm parameters, improvement
Efficacy	No significant effect
Randomization of patients	No
Study quality	**2–**
Reference	111: Cayan S, Apa DD, Akbay E. Effect of fexofenadine, a mast cell blocker, in infertile men with significantly increased testicular mast cells. Asian J Androl. 2002 Dec;4(4):291–4.
Language	English

Compound	Fexofenadine (R06AX26)
Disease treated	Infertility
Quantification of dysfunction	Semen
No. of patients treated	2
Age group	35, 44 years
Treatment period	Continuous
Dose	120 mg/day
Treatment consequences	Sperm motility, decrease
Efficacy	Improvement after cessation
Randomization of patients	No

Study quality	**3**
Reference	107: Hayashi T, Yoshida S, Ohno R, Ishii N, Terao T, Yamada T. Asthenospermia in hay fever patients improved by stopping treatment with histamine H1 receptor antagonists. Int J Urol. 2006 Jul;13(7):1028–30.
Language	English

Compound	Tranilast (not listed)
Disease treated	Infertility
Quantification of dysfunction	Semen
No. of patients treated	50
Age group	Young
Treatment period	12 weeks
Dose	300 mg/day
Treatment consequences	Sperm parameters, improvement
Efficacy	Significantly in verum group
Randomization of patients	Yes
Dose arms 1–3	Tranilast; placebo
Study quality	**1–**
Reference	113: Yamamoto M, Hibi H, Miyake K. New treatment of idiopathic severe oligozoospermia with mast cell blocker: results of a single-blind study. Fertil Steril. 1995 Dec;64(6):1221–3.
Language	English

Compound	Tranilast (not listed)
Disease treated	Infertility
Quantification of dysfunction	Semen
No. of patients treated	17
Age group	Young
Treatment period	12 weeks
Dose	300 mg/day
Treatment consequences	Sperm count, increase
Efficacy	In 41% of patients
Randomization of patients	No

Study quality	**3**
Reference	100: Hibi H, Kato K, Mitsui K, Taki T, Yamada Y, Honda N, Fukatsu H, Yamamoto M. The treatment with tranilast, a mast cell blocker, for idiopathic oligozoospermia. Arch Androl. 2001 Apr–Jun;47(2):107–11.
Language	English

Compound	Tranilast (not listed)
Disease treated	Infertility
Quantification of dysfunction	Semen
No. of patients treated	1
Age group	Young
Treatment period	1 year
Dose	300 mg/day
Treatment consequences	Spermatogenesis, recovery
Efficacy	After azoospermia
Study quality	**3**
Reference	237: Yamamoto M, Hibi H, Miyake K. Appearance of spermatozoon after administration of mast cell blocker to a patient with azoospermia. Hinyokika Kiyo. 1994 Jun;40(6):541–3.
Language	English

V03 All Other Therapeutic Products – Alcohol

Long-term abuse of larger doses of alcohol impaired spermatogenesis and sperm parameters in semen. This has been particularly proven by histological examination of the testicular tissue in men who died from alcohol diseases. On the other hand, some studies describe that moderate alcohol consumption is associated with a better profile of sperm parameter, or that there is an apparent protective effect of moderate alcohol drinking on sperm parameters or at least no significant influence. The difference may be explained by the alcohol doses used by the population studied. If the dose was below 160 g/week, no alteration of sperm parameters was observed; however, in groups with doses >100 g/day, a significant deterioration of sperm parameters and spermatogenesis was demonstrable, clearly dependent on the daily dose and the life-time dose.

2

The extent of spermatogenic dysfunction was found to be dependent on the glutathione S-transferase-M1 (GSTM) genotype, but not on the cytochrome genotype.

Overall level of evidence of adverse effects: B

Compound	Alcohol (V03AZ01)
Disease treated	Alcohol disease
Quantification of adverse effects	Glutathione S-transferase-M1 (GSTM) genotype
No. of patients treated	271
Age group	Young
Treatment period	Continuous
Dose	Various
Treatment consequences	Alcohol-induced impairment of spermatogenesis
Efficacy	Of 212 men with mean daily alcohol consumption >80 g, 21.2% had normal spermatogenesis; of these, 27 (60%) men had GST M1 'null' genotype (OR 2.7; 95% CI 1.0–4.0, compared with those with disorders of spermatogenesis).
Randomization of patients	No
Study quality	**2+**
Reference	198: Pajarinen J, Savolainen V, Perola M, Penttila A, Karhunen PJ. Glutathione S-transferase-M1 'null' genotype and alcohol-induced disorders of human spermatogenesis. Int J Androl. 1996 Jun;19(3):155–63.
Language	English

Compound	Alcohol (V03AZ01)
Disease treated	Infertility
Quantification of dysfunction	Semen
No. of patients treated	258
Age group	Young
Treatment period	Continuous
Dose	Various
Treatment consequences	Sperm parameters, impairment
Efficacy	No significant association between alcohol consumption and any semen parameter
Randomization of patients	No

Dose arms 1–3	Various doses of alcohol
Study quality	**2–**
Reference	2043: Dunphy BC, Barratt CL, Cooke ID. Male alcohol consumption and fecundity in couples attending an infertility clinic. Andrologia. 1991 May–Jun;23(3):219–21.
Language	English

Compound	Alcohol (V03AZ01)
Disease treated	Alcohol disease
Quantification of adverse effects	Amount per lifetime
No. of patients treated	204
Age group	All ages
Treatment period	Continuous
Dose	Various
Treatment consequences	Cytochrome gene type, spermatogenesis, depression in alcohol disease
Efficacy	No association
Randomization of patients	No
Dose arms 1–3	Various genetic polymorphism
Study quality	**2–**
Reference	191: Pajarinen J, Savolainen V, Perola M, Penttila A, Karhunen PJ. Polymorphism in the cytochrome P450 2E1 gene and alcohol-induced disorders of human spermatogenesis. Int J Androl. 1996 Oct;19(5):314–22.
Language	English

Compound	Alcohol (V03AZ01)
Disease treated	Healthy
Quantification of adverse effects	Semen
No. of patients treated	201
Age group	Young
Treatment period	Continuous
Dose	Various
Treatment consequences	Sperm parameters, impairment
Efficacy	Moderate alcohol consumption associated with a better seminological profile
Randomization of patients	No

2

Dose arms 1–3	Alcohol; no alcohol
Study quality	**2–**
Reference	2042: Figa-Talamanca I, Cini C, Varricchio GC, Dondero F, Gandini L, Lenzi A, Lombardo F, Angelucci L, Grezia R di, Patacchioli FR. Effects of prolonged autovehicle driving on male reproduction function: a study among taxi drivers. Am J Ind Med. 1996 Dec;30(6):750–8.
Language	English

Compound	Alcohol (V03AZ01)
Disease treated	Alcohol disease
Quantification of adverse effects	Testicular histology
No. of patients treated	195
Age group	36–69 years
Treatment period	Continuous
Dose	Various
Treatment consequences	Spermatogenesis, impairment
Efficacy	Significantly dependent on daily dose
Randomization of patients	No
Dose arms 1–3	<40 g; 40–80 g; 80–160 g
Study quality	**2–**
Reference	200: Pajarinen J, Karhunen PJ, Savolainen V, Lalu K, Penttila A, Laippala P. Moderate alcohol consumption and disorders of human spermatogenesis. Alcohol Clin Exp Res. 1996 Apr;20(2):332–7.
Language	English

Compound	Alcohol (V03AZ01)
Disease treated	Alcohol disease
Quantification of adverse effects	Semen, hormones
No. of patients treated	66; 30
Age group	All ages
Treatment period	1 year
Dose	>180 ml/day
Treatment consequences	Semen parameters, impairment
Efficacy	Significant for sperm count, motility, normal sperm

Randomization of patients	No
Dose arms 1–3	Alcohol, non-smokers; non-exposed
Study quality	**2–**
Reference	19. Muthusami KR, Chinnaswamy P. Effect of chronic alcoholism on male fertility hormones and semen quality. Fertil Steril. 2005 Oct;84(4):919–24.
Language	English

Compound	Alcohol (V03AZ01)
Disease treated	Alcohol disease
Quantification of adverse effects	Semen
No. of patients treated	38; 19
Age group	39 years (mean)
Treatment period	Continuous
Dose	100–350 g/day
Treatment consequences	Spermatogenesis, impairment
Efficacy	39.4% of patients reduced sperm count, 44.7% reduced morphology, 50% reduced motility; correlation with lifetime dose of alcohol
Randomization of patients	No
Dose arms 1–3	Alcohol; no alcohol
Study quality	**2–**
Reference	186: Villalta J, Ballesca JL, Nicolas JM, Martinez de Osaba MJ, Antunez E, Pimentel C. Testicular function in asymptomatic chronic alcoholics: relation to ethanol intake. Alcohol Clin Exp Res. 1997 Feb;21(1):128–33.
Language	English

Compound	Alcohol (V03AZ01)
Disease treated	Alcohol disease
Quantification of adverse effects	Testicular histology of corpses
No. of patients treated	50
Age group	18–35 years
Treatment period	Lifelong
Dose	Various
Treatment consequences	Spermatogenesis, impairment

Efficacy	Depression of cell count in chronic alcohol intoxication
Randomization of patients	No
Dose arms 1–3	Chronic intoxication; chronic illness
Study quality	**2–**
Reference	39: Dmitrieva OA. Morphological changes in genesial system of men: medico-legal aspects. Leg Med (Tokyo). 2003 Mar;5 Suppl 1:S228–32.
Language	English

Compound	Alcohol (V03AZ01)
Disease treated	Infertility
Quantification of adverse effects	Semen
No. of patients treated	34
Age group	Young
Treatment period	Continuous
Dose	Various
Treatment consequences	Sperm parameters, impairment
Efficacy	Non-significant reduction in sperm concentration, motility, viability, and normal morphology in men with drinking habits
Randomization of patients	No
Dose arms 1–3	Alcohol; no alcohol
Study quality	**2–**
Reference	2038: Stutz G, Zamudio J, Santillan ME, Vincenti L, Cuneo MF de, Ruiz RD. The effect of alcohol, tobacco, and aspirin consumption on seminal quality among healthy young men. Arch Environ Health. 2004 Nov;59(11):548–52.
Language	English

Compound	Alcohol (V03AZ01)
Disease treated	Healthy
Quantification of adverse effects	Hormones
No. of patients treated	16
Age group	Young
Treatment period	Acute intoxication
Dose	Single dose
Treatment consequences	Hormone levels, alteration

Efficacy	At peak blood alcohol levels (109±4.6 mg/100 ml) T levels were significantly depressed and LH levels significantly increased. During descending phase of the blood-alcohol curve, T levels remained depressed and LH levels decreased again.
Study quality	**3**
Reference	2144: Mendelson JH, Mello NK, Ellingboe J. Effects of acute alcohol intake on pituitary–gonadal hormones in normal human males. J Pharmacol Exp Ther. 1977 Sep;202(3):676–82.
Language	English

Compound	Alcohol (V03AZ01)
Disease treated	Infertility
Quantification of adverse effects	Semen
Age group	Young
Treatment period	Continuous
Dose	Various
Treatment consequences	Sperm parameters, impairment
Efficacy	Apparent protective effect of moderate alcohol drinking on sperm parameters
Study quality	**4 (review)**
Reference	2037: Marinelli D, Gaspari L, Pedotti P, Taioli E. Mini-review of studies on the effect of smoking and drinking habits on semen parameters. Int J Hyg Environ Health. 2004 Jul;207(3):185–92.
Language	English

Compound	Alcohol (V03AZ01)
Disease treated	Alcohol disease
Quantification of adverse effects	Hormones
Age group	All ages
Treatment consequences	Spermatogenesis, impairment
Efficacy	Recovery possible
Study quality	**4 (review)**
Reference	516: Gavaler JS, Urso T, Van Thiel DH. Ethanol: its adverse effects upon the hypothalamic–pituitary–gonadal axis. Subst Alcohol Actions Misuse. 1983;4(2–3):97–110.
Language	English

2

Medicinal Plants

There are some uncontrolled studies which report the improvement of spermatogenesis by medicinal plants.

Overall level of evidence of adverse effects: D

Compound	Kan Yang, Valeriana, Ginseng (not listed)
Disease treated	Infertility
Quantification of dysfunction	Semen
No. of patients treated	n.g.
Age group	Young
Treatment period	n.g.
Dose	n.g.
Treatment consequences	Spermatogenesis, improvement
Efficacy	n.g.
Randomization of patients	No
Remarks	Small effects in an accurate study
Study quality	**3**
Reference	1: Mkrtchyan A, Panosyan V, Panossian A, Wikman G, Wagner H. A phase I clinical study of Andrographis paniculata fixed combination Kan Jang versus ginseng and valerian on the semen quality of healthy male subjects. Phytomedicine. 2005 Jun;12(6–7):403–9.
Language	English

Compound	Lepidium meyenii
Disease treated	Infertility
Quantification of dysfunction	Semen
No. of patients treated	9
Age group	24–44 years
Treatment period	4 months
Dose	3000 mg/day
Treatment consequences	Sperm count, increase
Efficacy	Increase of sperm count not related to dose of Maca
Randomization of patients	No
Study quality	**3**

Reference 992: Gonzales GF, Cordova A, Gonzales C, Chung A, Vega K, Villena A. Lepidium meyenii (Maca) improved semen parameters in adult men Asian J Androl. 2001 Dec;3(4):301–3.

Language English

Environmental Toxicants

A number of chemicals which are pollutants to the human environment were suspected to cause spermatogenic failure. The evidence of declining male fertility in the general population as a consequence of concrete substances is scarce; in particular, the "endocrine disruptor hypothesis" is unproven, although testicular function per se as an integrated biological model is well suited to assess these effect.

There are, however, some well-conducted studies which gave evidence for a deleterious effects in workplace expositions.

Men being exposed to *alachlor*, a pesticide, had a higher risk of impairment of sperm parameters when they had higher urinary concentrations (OR 30.0 in the highest concentration as compared to non-exposed men).

Butadiene, on the other hand, had no detrimental effects on spermatogenesis.

The decrease in fertility related to *boron* and of *bromine* has not been proven in humans.

Carbon disulfide induces impairment of sexual functions in general. The OR of conception was found to be 0.57 in comparison with that of unexposed men.

The exposure to *chlorpyrifos*, an herbicide, was associated with a significant increase in sperm DNA damage.

The most interesting compound is *dibromochloropropane* (DBCP). An impairment of spermatogenesis in men exposed to DBCP has been clearly demonstrated in several studies since the early 1970s, and the number of exposed men having azoospermia has been significantly greater than that of non-exposed men. A recovery after cessation of exposure was possible but lasted up to 8 years. The gender rate of the offspring was shown to be unaltered, and genital malformation in the children was not more likely than in the children fathered by non-exposed men.

A workplace with exposure to *fungicides* enhances the risk of alteration of sperm parameters.

The extent of impairment of spermatogenesis in men exposed to *glycol ethers* has not been correlated to the urinary excretion.

Heavy metals also impair spermatogenesis but only together with severe toxic effects to other organs.

The pesticide *isopropoxy-4-methylpyrimidinol* impairs sperm parameters. Poor sperm parameters are more likely in men with higher urinary concentrations (OR 16.7 as compared with unexposed men).

A large body of evidence is available for the influence of *lead*. Impairment of spermatogenesis appears to occur if the levels in organic lead are >40 μg/day in blood. In these men, an increased frequency of asthenozoospermia, oligozoospermia and teratozoospermia has been found; however, in another study the birth rate was found to be unaltered.

Phthalates, polybromobisphenyl (PBB) and *polychlorinated bisphenyls* (PCB) have been shown to have various toxic effects on gonadal function in animal experiments. At present, however, there is no evidence of the effects in human.

No significant association between paternal or maternal exposure to styrene, toluene, xylene, tetrachloroethylene, trichloroethylene and 1,1,1-trichloroethane has been found in terms of abortion rate.

Overall level of evidence of adverse effects: C

Compound	Environmental toxicants in general
Disease treated	Paternal exposure to toxicants
Quantification of adverse effects	Gonadal dysfunction
Age group	Young
Treatment consequences	The father's role in abnormal reproductive outcomes
Efficacy	(a) Insufficient number of functional sperm; (b) transmitted genetic defects; (c) non-mutational changes of DNA; (d) possible source of toxic or infectious agents that negatively affect pregnancy; (e) postnatal toxic exposure of the offspring; (f) bridging biomarkers for comparisons between exposed men and laboratory animals, i.e. biomarkers that can be measured in men and animals in response to damaging agents.
Randomization of patients	No
Study quality	**4 (review)**
Reference	2048: Wyrobek AJ. Methods and concepts in detecting abnormal reproductive outcomes of paternal origin. Reprod Toxicol. 1993;7 Suppl 1:3–16.
Language	English

Compound	Environmental toxicants in general
Disease treated	Spermatogenic dysfunction
Quantification of adverse effects	Semen
Age group	Young
Treatment consequences	Spermatogenesis, impairment
Efficacy	As an indicator of toxicants
Randomization of patients	No
Study quality	**4 (expert opinion)**
Reference	504: Wyrobek AJ, Gordon LA, Burkhart JG, Francis MW, Kapp RW Jr, Letz G, Malling HV, Topham JC, Whorton MD. An evaluation of human sperm as indicators of chemically induced alterations of spermatogenic function. A report of the U.S. Environmental Protection Agency Gene-Tox Program. Mutat Res. 1983 May;115(1):73–148.
Language	English

Compound	Endocrine disruptors (not listed)
Disease treated	Spermatogenesis
Quantification of adverse effects	Histology, semen
Age group	Young
Treatment consequences	Spermatogenesis, impairment
Efficacy	As an effect of endocrine disruptors in the environment
Remarks	The "endocrine disruptor hypothesis" is unproven
Study quality	**4 (review)**
Reference	151: Spira A, Multigner L. The effect of industrial and agricultural pollution on human spermatogenesis. Hum Reprod. 1998 Aug;13(8):2041–2.
Language	English

Compound	Endocrine disruptors (not listed)
Disease treated	Genital malformation
Quantification of adverse effects	Methods of homeostasis
Age group	Testis in vitro
Treatment consequences	Genital malformation

Efficacy	Various modes of action and points of effect
Remarks	Testicular function as an integrated biologic read-out is well suited to assess the effects
Study quality	**4 (review)**
Reference	136: Ben-Jonathan N, Cooper RL, Foster P, Hughes CL, Hoyer PB, Klotz D, Kohn M, Lamb DJ, Stancel GM. An approach to the development of quantitative models to assess the effects of exposure to environmentally relevant levels of endocrine disruptors on homeostasis in adults. Environ Health Perspect. 1999 Aug;107 Suppl 4:605–11.
Language	English

Compound	Alachlor (not listed)
Disease treated	Infertility
Quantification of adverse effects	Semen
No. of patients treated	25; 25
Age group	Young
Treatment period	Continuous
Dose	Quantified by urinary excretion
Treatment consequences	Sperm parameters, impairment
Efficacy	In higher urinary concentrations more likely (OR 6.3 and 30.0)
Randomization of patients	No
Study quality	**2+**
Reference	176: Swan SH. Semen quality in fertile US men in relation to geographical area and pesticide exposure. Int J Androl. 2006 Feb;29(1):62–8; discussion 105–8.
Language	English

Compound	Butadiene (not listed)
Disease treated	Healthy, HPRT mutant frequency
Quantification of adverse effects	Molecular biology
No. of patients treated	38
Age group	Young
Treatment period	n.g.
Dose	n.g.
Treatment consequences	Sperm parameters, alteration

Efficacy	No significant differences between gene types
Randomization of patients	No
Study quality	**2–**
Reference	800: Tates AD, van Dam JJ, de Zwart FA et al. Biological effect monitoring in industrial workers from the Czech Republic exposed to low levels of butadiens. Toxicology 1996;113: 91–99.
Language	English

Compound	Butadiene (not listed)
Disease treated	Infertility
Quantification of adverse effects	Spermatogenesis
Age group	Young
Treatment period	320–380 ppm exposure time
Treatment consequences	Spermatogonial cytogenesis, alteration
Efficacy	None
Remarks	Categories for germ cell mutagens of the MAK
Study quality	**4 (review)**
Reference	106: Adler ID. spermatogenesis and mutagenicity of environmental hazards: extrapolation of genetic risk from mouse to man. Andrologia. 2000 Sep;32(4–5):233–7.
Language	English

Compound	Butadiene (not listed)
Disease treated	Poisoning
Quantification of adverse effects	Germinal cell DNA
Age group	Young
Treatment consequences	Genotoxic effect
Efficacy	None
Study quality	**4 (review)**
Reference	775: Adler ID, Cochrane J, Osterman-Golkar S, Skopek TR, Sorsa M, Vogel E. 1,3-butadiene working group report. Mutat Res. 1995 Aug;330(1–2):101–14.
Language	English

Compound	Butadiene, organic solvents (not listed)
Disease treated	Infertility
Quantification of adverse effects	Progeny outcome
Age group	Young
Treatment consequences	Alteration of number and quality of progeny
Efficacy	No effect
Study quality	**4 (review)**
Reference	2044: Hales BF, Robaire B. Paternal exposure to drugs and environmental chemicals: effects on progeny outcome. J Androl. 2001 Nov–Dec;22(6):927–36.
Language	English

Compound	Boron (not listed)
Disease treated	Poisoning
Quantification of adverse effects	Concentration of boron
Age group	All
Treatment consequences	Fertility, decrease
Efficacy	In wild rodents; in humans not proven
Remarks	No further references
Study quality	**4 (review)**
Reference	231: Moseman RF. Chemical disposition of boron in animals and humans. Environ Health Perspect. 1994 Nov;102 Suppl 7:113–7.
Language	English

Compound	Bromine vapor (not listed)
Disease treated	Poisoning
Quantification of adverse effects	Semen
No. of patients treated	8
Age group	Young
Treatment period	Accidental
Dose	n.g.
Treatment consequences	Spermatogenesis, impairment
Efficacy	No alteration
Randomization of patients	No

Study quality	**3**
Reference	285: Potashnik G, Carel R, Belmaker I, Levine M. Spermatogenesis and reproductive performance following human accidental exposure to bromine vapor. Reprod Toxicol. 1992;6(2):171–4.
Language	English

Compound	Carbon disulfide (not listed)
Disease treated	Infertility
Quantification of adverse effects	Time to pregnacy (TTP)
No. of patients treated	2585
Age group	Young
Treatment period	Workplace
Treatment consequences	Spermatogenesis, impairment
Efficacy	OR of conception 0.57 as compared with low-exposed men
Randomization of patients	No
Dose arms 1–3	40 µg/month; 40–80; >80
Study quality	**2–**
Reference	114: Dejmek J, Jelinek R, Solansky' I, Benes I, Sram RJ. Fecundability and parental exposure to ambient sulfur dioxide. Environ Health Perspect. 2000 Jul;108(7):647–54.
Language	English

Compound	Chlorpyrifos (not listed)
Disease treated	Infertility
Quantification of adverse effects	Sperm parameters
No. of patients treated	260
Age group	Young
Treatment period	Continuous
Dose	Various
Treatment consequences	Sperm parameters, impairment
Efficacy	Significant increase in DNA damages
Randomization of patients	No
Study quality	**3**

Reference	2002: Meeker JD, Singh NP, Ryan L, Duty SM, Barr DB, Herrick RF, Bennett DH, Hauser R. Urinary levels of insecticide metabolites and DNA damage in human sperm. Hum Reprod. 2004 Nov;19(11):2573–80.
Language	English

Compound	Dibromochloropropane (not listed)
Disease treated	Infertility
Quantification of adverse effects	Semen
No. of patients treated	142
Age group	Young
Treatment period	Workplace
Dose	n.g.
Treatment consequences	Azoospermia, induction
Efficacy	13%, 2.9% in control group
Randomization of patients	No
Dose arms 1–3	exposed; nonexposed;
Study quality	**2–**
Reference	626: Whorton D, Milby TH, Krauss RM, Stubbs HA. Testicular function in DBCP exposed pesticide workers. J Occup Med. 1979 Mar;21(3):161–6.

Compound	Dibromochloropropane (not listed)
Disease treated	Poisoning
Quantification of adverse effects	Semen
No. of patients treated	47
Age group	Young
Treatment period	18 months
Dose	High/low
Treatment consequences	Spermatogenesis, recovery after cessation
Efficacy	Complete
Randomization of patients	No
Dose arms 1–3	Various jobs with DBCP
Study quality	**2–**

Reference	308: Olsen GW, Lanham JM, Bodner KM, Hylton DB, Bond GG. Determinants of spermatogenesis recovery among workers exposed to 1,2-dibromo-3-chloropropane. J Occup Med. 1990 Oct;32(10):979–84.
Language	English

Compound	Dibromochloropropane (not listed)
Disease treated	Offspring of exposed fathers
Quantification of adverse effects	Gender ratio
No. of patients treated	30
Age group	Young
Treatment period	Workplace
Dose	n.g.
Treatment consequences	Offspring, gender rate (boys:girls)
Efficacy	52.9% boys in non-exposed vs 35.2% in exposed period
Randomization of patients	No
Study quality	**2–**
Reference	471: Potashnik G, Goldsmith J, Insler V. Dibromochloropropane-induced reduction of the sex-atio in man. Andrologia. 1984 May–Jun;16(3):213–8.
Language	English

Compound	Dibromochloropropane (not listed)
Disease treated	Poisoning
Quantification of adverse effects	Semen
No. of patients treated	15
Age group	Young
Treatment period	Workplace
Treatment consequences	Spermatogenesis, recovery
Efficacy	After up to 8 years
Randomization of patients	No
Study quality	**3**
Reference	393: Potashnik G, Yanai-Inbar I. Dibromochloropropane (DBCP): an 8-year reevaluation of testicular function and reproductive performance. Fertil Steril. 1987 Feb;47(2):317–23.

Language	English

Compound	Dibromochloropropane (not listed)
Disease treated	Infertility
Quantification of adverse effects	Semen
No. of patients treated	6
Age group	Young
Treatment period	Workplace
Dose	n.g.
Treatment consequences	Spermatogenesis, impairment
Efficacy	In 2 of 6 men
Randomization of patients	No
Study quality	**3**
Reference	639: Potashnik G, Ben-Aderet N, Israeli R, Yanai-Inbar I, Sober I. Suppressive effect of 1,2-dibromo-3-chloropropane on human spermatogenesis. Fertil Steril. 1978 Oct;30(4):444–7.
Language	English

Compound	Dibromochloropropane (not listed)
Disease treated	Infertility
Quantification of adverse effects	Semen
No. of patients treated	n.g.
Age group	Young
Treatment period	Workplace
Treatment consequences	Spermatogenesis, impairment
Efficacy	Most
Randomization of patients	No
Study quality	**3**
Reference	607: Sandifer SH, Wilkins RT, Loadholt CB, Lane LG, Eldridge JC. Spermatogenesis in agricultural workers exposed to dibromochloropropane (DBCP). Bull Environ Contam Toxicol. 1979 Nov;23(4–5):703–10.
Language	English

Compound	Dibromochloropropane (not listed)
Disease treated	Infertility
Quantification of adverse effects	Semen
No. of patients treated	n.g.
Age group	Young
Treatment period	Workplace
Dose	n.g.
Treatment consequences	Spermatogenesis, impairment
Efficacy	Most, associated with duration of exposition
Randomization of patients	No
Study quality	**3**
Reference	627: Glass RI, Lyness RN, Mengle DC, Powell KE, Kahn E. Sperm count depression in pesticide applicators exposed to dibromochloropropane. Am J Epidemiol. 1979 Mar;109(3):346–51.
Language	English

Compound	Dibromochloropropane (not listed)
Disease treated	Infertility
Quantification of adverse effects	Testicular histology
No. of patients treated	n.g.
Age group	Young
Treatment period	Workplace
Dose	n.g.
Treatment consequences	Spermatogenesis, impairment
Efficacy	Most
Randomization of patients	No
Study quality	**3**
Reference	635: Biava CG, Smuckler EA, Whorton D. The testicular morphology of individuals exposed to dibromochloropropane. Exp Mol Pathol. 1978 Dec;29(3):448–58.
Language	English

Compound	Dibromochloropropane (not listed)
Disease treated	Offspring of exposed fathers
Quantification of dysfunction	Health
No. of patients treated	n.g.
Age group	Young
Treatment period	Workplace
Dose	n.g.
Treatment consequences	Children fathered; genital malformation
Efficacy	None
Randomization of patients	No
Study quality	**3**
Reference	444: Potashnik G, Abeliovich D. Chromosomal analysis and health status of children conceived to men during or following dibromochloropropane-induced spermatogenic suppression. Andrologia. 1985 May–Jun;17(3):291–6.
Language	English

Compound	Fungicides (not listed)
Disease treated	Infertility
Quantification of adverse effects	Semen
No. of patients treated	92; 73
Age group	34.4 years (mean)
Treatment period	Workplace
Dose	n.g.
Treatment consequences	Oligozoospermia
Efficacy	OR 8.3 (95% CI 1.0–71.0) as compared with non-exposed men, p=0.02
Randomization of patients	No
Study quality	**2–**
Reference	2177: Wong WY, Zielhuis GA, Thomas CM, Merkus HM, Steegers-Theunissen RP. New evidence of the influence of exogenous and endogenous factors on sperm count in man. Eur J Obstet Gynecol Reprod Biol. 2003 Sep 10;110(1):49–54.
Language	English

Compound	Glycol ethers (not listed)
Disease treated	Poisoning
Quantification of adverse effects	Semen
No. of patients treated	1019; 475
Age group	Young
Treatment period	Workplace
Dose	n.g.
Treatment consequences	Spermatogenesis, impairment
Efficacy	No correlation to urinary excretion
Randomization of patients	No
Study quality	**2–**
Reference	267: Veulemans H, Steeno O, Masschelein R, Groeseneken D. Exposure to ethylene glycol ethers and spermatogenic disorders in man: a case-control study. Br J Ind Med. 1993 Jan;50(1):71–8.
Language	English

Compound	Heavy metals (not listed)
Disease treated	Infertility
Quantification of adverse effects	Semen
No. of patients treated	92; 73
Age group	34.4 years (mean)
Treatment period	Workplace
Dose	Various
Treatment consequences	Oligozoospermia
Efficacy	OR 2.6 (95% CI 1.1–6.2) as compared with non-exposed men, p=0.03
Randomization of patients	No
Study quality	**2–**
Reference	2177: Wong WY, Zielhuis GA, Thomas CM, Merkus HM, Steegers-Theunissen RP. New evidence of the influence of exogenous and endogenous factors on sperm count in man. Eur J Obstet Gynecol Reprod Biol. 2003 Sep 10;110(1):49–54.
Language	English

Compound	Heavy metals (not listed)
Disease treated	Infertility
Quantification of adverse effects	Semen
No. of patients treated	37
Age group	Young
Treatment period	Workplace
Dose	n.g.
Treatment consequences	Spermatogenesis, impairment
Efficacy	Improvement by gonadotropins
Randomization of patients	No
Dose arms 1–3	Lead; hydrargirum; copper
Remarks	No data on kind and duration of exposure; no data on disturbances of other organs
Study quality	**3**
Reference	667: Ruse M, Suciu L, Zegreanu O. Participation of gonads in chronic poisonings with heavy metals. Z Gesamte Inn Med. 1977 Sep 15;32(18):469–70.
Language	German

Compound	Heavy metals (not listed)
Disease treated	Infertility
Quantification of adverse effects	Progeny outcome
Age group	Young
Treatment consequences	Alteration of number and quality of progeny
Efficacy	No effect
Study quality	**4 (review)**
Reference	2044: Hales BF, Robaire B. Paternal exposure to drugs and environmental chemicals: effects on progeny outcome. J Androl. 2001 Nov–Dec;22(6):927–36.
Language	English

Compound	Isopropoxy-4-methylpyrimidinol (not listed)
Disease treated	Infertility
Quantification of adverse effects	Semen
No. of patients treated	25; 25
Age group	Young

Treatment period	Continuous
Dose	Estimated from urinary excretion
Treatment consequences	Sperm parameters, impairment
Efficacy	In higher urinary concentrations more likely (OR 10 and 16.7)
Randomization of patients	No
Study quality	**2+**
Reference	176: Swan SH. Semen quality in fertile US men in relation to geographical area and pesticide exposure. Int J Androl. 2006 Feb;29(1):62–8; discussion 105–8.
Language	English

Compound	Lead (not listed)
Disease treated	Infertility
Quantification of adverse effects	Birth rate
No. of patients treated	1349
Age group	<60 years
Treatment period	Workplace
Dose	38.9 μg/ml
Treatment consequences	Birth rate, alteration
Efficacy	None
Randomization of patients	No
Dose arms 1–3	Lead
Study quality	**2–**
Reference	169: Bonde JP, Kolstad H. Fertility of Danish battery workers exposed to lead. Int J Epidemiol. 1997 Dec;26(6):1281–8.
Language	English

Compound	Lead (not listed)
Disease treated	Lead exposure
Quantification of adverse effects	Semen
No. of patients treated	150
Age group	Young
Treatment period	Workplace
Dose	n.g.

Treatment consequences	Spermatogenesis, impairment
Efficacy	Increased frequency of asthenospermia, hypospermia and teratospermia as compared with non-exposed men
Randomization of patients	No
Dose arms 1–3	Lead exposed; not lead exposed
Study quality	**2–**
Reference	2036: Lancranjan I, Popescu HI, GAvanescu O, Klepsch I, Serbanescu M. Reproductive ability of workmen occupationally exposed to lead. Arch Environ Health. 1975 Aug;30(8):396–401.
Language	English

Compound	Lead (not listed)
Disease treated	Lead exposure
Quantification of adverse effects	Semen, genotype
No. of patients treated	134
Age group	<60 years
Treatment period	Workplace
Dose	n.g.
Treatment consequences	Spermatogenesis, impairment
Efficacy	Lead in blood per gene type
Randomization of patients	No
Study quality	**2–**
Reference	165: Alexander BH, Checkoway H, Costa-Mallen P, Faustman EM, Woods JS, Kelsey KT, van Netten C, Costa LG. Interaction of blood lead and delta-aminolevulinic acid dehydratase genotype on markers of heme synthesis and sperm production in lead smelter workers. Environ Health Perspect. 1998 Apr;106(4):213–6.
Language	English

Compound	Lead (not listed)
Disease treated	Poisoning
Quantification of adverse effects	Semen
No. of patients treated	38
Age group	Young

Treatment period	Workplace
Dose	n.g.
Treatment consequences	Spermatogenesis, impairment
Efficacy	Correlation to uptake of lead
Randomization of patients	No
Study quality	**3**
Reference	288: Lerda D. Study of sperm characteristics in persons occupationally exposed to lead. Am J Ind Med. 1992;22(4):567–71.
Language	English

Compound	Lead (not listed)
Disease treated	Lead exposure
Quantification of adverse effects	Semen
No. of patients treated	36
Age group	Young
Treatment period	Workplace
Dose	n.g.
Treatment consequences	Spermatogenesis, impairment
Efficacy	Lower sperm count in lead exposed
Randomization of patients	No
Dose arms 1–3	Lead exposed; not lead exposed
Study quality	**2–**
Reference	401: Assennato G, Paci C, Baser ME, Molinini R, Candela RG, Altamura BM, Giorgino R. Sperm count suppression without endocrine dysfunction in lead-exposed men. Arch Environ Health. 1986 Nov–Dec;41(6):387–90.
Language	English

Compound	Lead (not listed)
Disease treated	Infertility
Quantification of adverse effects	Fertility
Age group	Young
Treatment period	Lifelong
Dose	>40 ug/ml blood

2

Treatment consequences	Spermatogenesis, impairment
Efficacy	If inorganic lead >40 μg/day in blood
Study quality	**4 (review)**
Reference	149: Apostoli P, Kiss P, Porru S, Bonde JP, Vanhoorne M. Male reproductive toxicity of lead in animals and humans. ASCLEPIOS Study Group. Occup Environ Med. 1998 Jun;55(6):364–74.
Language	English

Compound	Phthalates (not listed)
Disease treated	Genital malformation
Quantification of adverse effects	Malformation
Dose	Default reference dose of 66 μg/kg day^{-1}
Treatment consequences	Monoesters of DBP humans, low risk of malformation
Efficacy	Calculation of reference dose
Study quality	**4 (review)**
Reference	796: Foster PMD, Cattley RC, Mylchrest E. Effects of di-n-butyl phthalate (DBP) on male reproductive development in the rat: implication for human risk assessment. Food Chem Toxicol 2000;38 (Suppl 1): S97–S99.
Language	English

Compound	Polybromobisphenyl (PBB) (not listed)
Disease treated	Poisoning
Quantification of adverse effects	Semen
No. of patients treated	104
Age group	Young
Treatment period	Workplace
Dose	n.g.
Treatment consequences	Spermatogenesis, impairment
Efficacy	No difference between exposed and control men
Randomization of patients	No
Dose arms 1–3	Exposed; nonexposed
Remarks	No further references
Study quality	**2–**

Reference	617: Rosenman KD, Anderson HA, Selikoff IJ, Wolff MS, Holstein E. spermatogenesis in men exposed to polybrominated biphenyl (PBB). Fertil Steril. 1979 Aug;32(2):209–13.
Language	English

Compound	Polychlorinated bisphenyls (not listed)
Disease treated	Healthy
Quantification of adverse effects	Semen
No. of patients treated	29
Age group	Young
Treatment period	Workplace
Dose	n.g.
Treatment consequences	Sperm count, decrease
Efficacy	No significant difference between groups
Randomization of patients	No
Dose arms 1–3	Exposed; nonexposed
Study quality	**2–**
Reference	22. Hauser R, Altshul L, Chen Z, Ryan L, Overstreet J, Schiff I, Christiani DC. Environmental organochlorines and semen quality: results of a pilot study. Environ Health Perspect. 2002 Mar;110(3):229–33.
Language	English

Compound	Polychlorinated bisphenyls (not listed)
Disease treated	Infertility
Quantification of adverse effects	Progeny outcome
Age group	Young
Treatment consequences	Alteration of number and quality of progeny
Efficacy	Reduced fecundity
Study quality	**4 (review)**
Reference	2044: Hales BF, Robaire B. Paternal exposure to drugs and environmental chemicals: effects on progeny outcome. J Androl. 2001 Nov–Dec;22(6):927–36.
Language	English

Compound	Polypropylene mesh (not listed)
Disease treated	Hernia inguinalis, herniorrhaphy
Quantification of adverse effects	Semen
No. of patients treated	14
Age group	35.5 years (mean)
Treatment period	6.3 years after surgery
Treatment consequences	Azoospermia
Efficacy	Obstruction after herniorraphy
Randomization of patients	No
Study quality	**3**
Reference	2174: Shin D, Lipshultz LI, Goldstein M, Barme GA, Fuchs EF, Nagler HM, McCallum SW, Niederberger CS, Schoor RA, Brugh VM III, Honig SC. Herniorrhaphy with polypropylene mesh causing inguinal vasal obstruction: a preventable cause of obstructive azoospermia. Ann Surg. 2005 Apr;241(4):553–8.
Language	English

Compound	Stainless steel, welding (not listed)
Disease treated	Infertility
Quantification of adverse effects	Offspring health
No. of patients treated	23,264
Age group	Young
Treatment period	Workplace
Treatment consequences	Childhood malignancies in the offspring
Efficacy	The overall incidence of childhood malignancies was equal to national rates (RR 0.97, 95% CI 0.63–1.42)
Randomization of patients	No
Dose arms 1–3	Exposed; non-exposed
Study quality	**2++**
Reference	2152: Bonde JP, Olsen JH, Hansen KS. Adverse pregnancy outcome and childhood malignancy with reference to paternal welding exposure. Scand J Work Environ Health. 1992 Jun;18(3):169–77.
Language	English

Compound	Stainless steel, welding (not listed)
Disease treated	Infertility
Quantification of adverse effects	Semen
No. of patients treated	430
Age group	Young
Treatment period	Workplace
Treatment consequences	Sperm count, impairment
Efficacy	Median sperm density for welders 56×10^6/ml and 52.5×10^6/ml, and 50.0×10^6/ml in two reference groups
Randomization of patients	No
Dose arms 1–3	Exposed; non-exposed
Study quality	**2–**
Reference	2148: Hjollund NH, Bonde JP, Jensen TK, Ernst E, Henriksen TB, Kolstad HA, Giwercman A, Skakkebaek NE, Olsen J. Semen quality and sex hormones with reference to metal welding. Reprod Toxicol. 1998 Mar–Apr;12(2):91–5.
Language	English

Compound	Stainless steel, welding (not listed)
Disease treated	Infertility
Quantification of adverse effects	Conceptions
No. of patients treated	430
Age group	Young
Treatment period	Workplace
Treatment consequences	Fecundity, decreased
Efficacy	Fecundability of male exposure to welding OR of 0.86 (95% CI 0.58–1.28)
Randomization of patients	No
Dose arms 1–3	Exposed; non-exposed
Study quality	**2–**
Reference	2149: Hjollund NH, Bonde JP, Jensen TK, Henriksen TB, Kolstad HA, Ernst E, Giwercman A, Pritzl G, Skakkebaek NE, Olsen J. A follow-up study of male exposure to welding and time to pregnancy. Reprod Toxicol. 1998 Jan–Feb;12(1):29–37.
Language	English

Compound	Stainless steel, welding (not listed)
Disease treated	Infertility
Quantification of adverse effects	Abortion rate after IVF
No. of patients treated	319
Age group	Young
Treatment period	Workplace
Treatment consequences	Proportion of pregnancies terminated by spontaneous abortion before gestational week 28
Efficacy	18% in pregnancies with paternal exposure to stainless steel welding, 25% with mild steel welding, 28% in reference group
Randomization of patients	No
Dose arms 1–3	Stainless steel welding ; mild steel welding; reference group
Study quality	**2+**
Reference	2146: Hjollund NH, Bonde JP, Ernst E, Lindenberg S, Andersen AN, Olsen J. Spontaneous abortion in IVF couples: a role of male welding exposure. Hum Reprod. 2005 Jul;20(7):1793–7.
Language	English

Compound	Stainless steel, welding (not listed)
Disease treated	Infertility
Quantification of adverse effects	Abortion rate after spontaneous conception
No. of patients treated	245
Age group	Young
Treatment period	Workplace
Treatment consequences	Risk of spontaneous abortion, increased
Efficacy	With paternal exposure to stainless steel welding, RR 3.5 (95% CI 1.3–9.1)
Randomization of patients	No
Dose arms 1–3	Exposed; non-exposed
Study quality	**2–**
Reference	2147: Hjollund NH, Bonde JP, Jensen TK, Henriksen TB, Andersson AM, Kolstad HA, Ernst E, Giwercman A, Skakkebaek NE, Olsen J. Male-mediated spontaneous abortion among spouses of stainless steel welders. Scand J Work Environ Health. 2000 Jun;26(3):187–92. Denmark. akh-hhjol@aaa.dk

Language	English

Compound	**Stainless steel, welding (not listed)**
Disease treated	Healthy
Quantification of adverse effects	Semen
No. of patients treated	77
Age group	Young
Treatment period	Workplace
Treatment consequences	Chromium in urine, increase; semen parameters, impairment
Side effects	No association of semen parameters with increasing level of internal exposure to chromium
Randomization of patients	No
Dose arms 1–3	Exposed; non-exposed
Study quality	**2–**
Reference	2151: Bonde JP, Ernst E. Sex hormones and semen quality in welders exposed to hexavalent chromium. Hum Exp Toxicol. 1992 Jul;11(4):259–63.
Language	English

Compound	**Stainless steel, welding (not listed)**
Disease treated	Healthy
Quantification of adverse effects	Semen
No. of patients treated	53
Age group	Young
Treatment period	Workplace; after 3 weeks break of exposure
Treatment consequences	Semen parameters, improvement
Efficacy	No consistent alteration
Randomization of patients	No
Dose arms 1–3	Exposed; non-exposed
Study quality	**2–**
Reference	2153: Bonde JP. Semen quality in welders before and after three weeks of non-exposure. Br J Ind Med. 1990 Aug;47(8):515–8.
Language	English

Compound	Styrene, toluene, xylene, tetrachloroethylene, trichloroethylene, and 1,1,1-trichloroethane (not listed)
Disease treated	Infertility
Quantification of adverse effects	Pregnancy induction
No. of patients treated	n.g.
Age group	Young
Treatment period	Workplace
Dose	n.g.
Treatment consequences	Abortion rate, increase
Efficacy	No significant association between different degrees of paternal or maternal exposure
Randomization of patients	Case control
Dose arms 1–3	Exposed; unexposed
Study quality	**2–**
Reference	322: Taskinen H, Anttila A, Lindbohm ML, Sallmen M, Hemminki K. Spontaneous abortions and congenital malformations among the wives of men occupationally exposed to organic solvents. Scand J Work Environ Health. 1989 Oct;15(5):345–52.
Language	English

Renal Dialysis and Renal Transplantation

Spermatogenesis is impaired in men with terminal renal insufficiency. After renal transplantation sperm parameters, such as sperm count and sperm motility, as well as testosterone levels, improve and may return to normal values, independent of the immune suppression applied. It is unclear, however, whether the renal insufficiency itself or the dialysis causes the impairment.

Overall level of evidence of adverse effects: D

Compound	Renal transplantation
Disease treated	In renal insufficiency
Quantification of adverse effects	Semen
No. of patients treated	30
Age group	Young

Treatment period	3 months
Treatment consequences	Sperm parameters, improvement
Efficacy	Significant increase of sperm motility
Randomization of patients	No
Study quality	**3**
Reference	129: Akbari F, Alavi M, Esteghamati A, Mehrsai A, Djaladat H, Zohrevand R, Pourmand G. Effect of renal transplantation on sperm quality and sex hormone levels. BJU Int. 2003 Aug;92(3):281–3.
Language	English

Compound	Renal transplantation
Disease treated	Renal insufficiency
Quantification of adverse effects	Semen, hormones
No. of patients treated	19
Age group	22–41 years
Treatment period	6 months
Treatment consequences	Sperm parameters, improvement
Efficacy	After renal transplantation, testosterone and LH levels returned to normal in most patients, while FSH levels became normal in only two patients. Semen quality improved in 13 patients, and the improvement in sperm density and motility was statistically significant.
Randomization of patients	No
Study quality	**3**
Reference	2196: Prem AR, Punekar SV, Kalpana M, Kelkar AR, Acharya VN. Male reproductive function in uraemia: efficacy of haemodialysis and renal transplantation. Br J Urol. 1996 Oct;78(4):635–8.
Language	English

Compound	Renal transplantation
Disease treated	In renal insufficiency
Quantification of adverse effects	Semen
No. of patients treated	18
Age group	22–41 years

Treatment period	3 months
Treatment consequences	Sperm parameters, improvement
Efficacy	In 13 patients, for sperm density and motility being significant
Randomization of patients	No
Study quality	**3**
Reference	130: Prem AR, Punekar SV, Kalpana M, Kelkar AR, Acharya VN. Male reproductive function in uraemia: efficacy of haemodialysis and renal transplantation. Br J Urol. 1996 Oct;78(4):635–8.
Language	English

Compound	Renal dialysis
Disease treated	Renal insufficiency
Quantification of adverse effects	Hormones
No. of patients treated	13
Age group	Young
Treatment period	6 months
Treatment consequences	hCG-induced rise of testosterone levels, impairment
Efficacy	Significant as compared with normal men
Randomization of patients	No
Study quality	**3**
Reference	2197: Bundschu HD, Rager K, Heller S, Hayduk K, Pfeiffer EH, Luders G, Liebau G. Effects of long-term HCG administration on testicular function in hemodialysis patients. Klin Wochenschr. 1976 Nov 1;54(21):1039–46.
Language	German

Compound	Renal transplantation in adolescence
Disease treated	Renal insufficiency
Quantification of adverse effects	Semen
No. of patients treated	7
Age group	13–19 years
Treatment consequences	Spermatogenesis, maturation

Efficacy	Only one patient had normal sperm parameters, and 6 of 7 had oligo-astheno-teratozoospermia.
Randomization of patients	No
Study quality	**3**
Reference	990: Inci K, Duzova A, Aki FT, Bilginer Y, Erkan I, Tasar C, Bakkaloglu A, Bakkaloglu M. Semen variables and hormone profiles after kidney transplantation during adolescence. Transplant Proc. 2006 Mar;38(2):541–2.
Language	English

Compound	Renal transplantation
Disease treated	Renal insufficiency
Quantification of adverse effects	Semen
No. of patients treated	7
Age group	Young
Treatment consequences	Spermatogenesis, impairment
Efficacy	Improvement after renal transplantation
Randomization of patients	No
Study quality	**3**
Reference	663: Baumgarten SR, Lindsay GK, Wise GJ. Fertility problems in the renal transplant patient. J Urol. 1977 Dec;118(6):991–3.
Language	English

Compound	Renal transplantation
Disease treated	Renal insufficiency
Quantification of adverse effects	Semen
No. of patients treated	5
Age group	Young
Treatment period	3 months
Treatment consequences	Spermatogenesis, impairment
Efficacy	Return to normal values after transplantation
Randomization of patients	No
Study quality	**3**

2

Reference	110: Xu LG, Shi SF, Qi XP, Huang XF, Xu HM, Song QZ, Wang XH, Shao ZF, Zhang JR. Morphological characteristics of spermatozoa before and after renal transplantation. Asian J Androl. 2005 Mar;7(1):81–5.
Language	English

Compound	Renal transplantation
Disease treated	Renal insufficiency
Quantification of adverse effects	Semen
No. of patients treated	5
Age group	Young
Treatment consequences	Sperm parameters, improvement
Efficacy	After renal transplantation, most of the spermatozoa became normal.
Randomization of patients	No
Study quality	**3**
Reference	2194: Xu LG, Shi SF, Qi XP, Huang XF, Xu HM, Song QZ, Wang XH, Shao ZF, Zhang JR. Morphological characteristics of spermatozoa before and after renal transplantation. Asian J Androl. 2005 Mar;7(1):81–5.
Language	English

Compound	Renal transplantation
Disease treated	Renal insufficiency
Quantification of adverse effects	Semen, hormones
No. of patients treated	4
Age group	Young
Treatment period	12 months
Treatment consequences	Sperm parameters, improvement
Efficacy	After transplantation from azoospermia to 20–40 million/ml, sperm motility 40–90%
Randomization of patients	No
Study quality	**3**
Reference	2193: Lim VS, Fang VS. Gonadal dysfunction in uremic men. A study of the hypothalamo-pituitary-testicular axis before and after renal transplantation. Am J Med. 1975 May;58(5):655–62.
Language	English

Compound	Renal Dialysis
Disease treated	Secondary hyperparathyroidism in renal insufficiency
Quantification of adverse effects	Semen
No. of patients treated	19
Age group	29–50 years
Treatment period	3 months
Treatment consequences	Spermatogenesis, impairment
Efficacy	Ten patients improved to normal sperm density ($\geq 20\times10^6$/ml), 9 had oligospermia or remained azoospermic.
Randomization of patients	No
Study quality	**3**
Reference	993: Chou FF, Lee CH, Lee CT, Huang FJ, Hsu KL. Spermatogenesis after parathyroidectomy in patients with symptomatic secondary hyperparathyroidism. J Am Coll Surg. 2003 Jun;196(6):854–8.
Language	English

2.4 Drugs Which Compromise Erectile Function

A02 Drugs for Acid-related Disorders

The prevalence of erectile dysfunction does not appear to be enhanced in patients using these drugs. Cimetidine therapy induced hypoandrogenism leading to erectile dysfunction and breast enlargement as described in numerous case reports and letters. Ranitidine appeared to be less effective in this respect. Results of meaningful prospective clinical studies are not available.

Overall level of evidence of adverse effects : C

Compound	Drugs for acid-related disorders (A02)
Disease treated	Peptic ulcer
Quantification of adverse effects	Interview by GP
No. of patients treated	2010
Age group	>18 years
Treatment period	Various
Dose	Various
Treatment consequences	Incidence of erectile dysfunction
Efficacy	RR not increased
Randomization of patients	No
Study quality	**2–**
Reference	2231: Ricci E, Parazzini F, Mirone V, Imbimbo C, Palmieri A, Bortolotti A, Cintio E di, Landoni M, Lavezzari M. Current drug use as risk factor for erectile dysfunction: results from an Italian epidemiological study. Int J Impot Res. 2003 Jun;15(3):221–4.
Language	English

Compound	Cimetidine (A02BA01), ranitidine
Disease treated	Gastric hypersecretion
Quantification of adverse effects	Sexual function
No. of patients treated	22

Age group	All ages
Treatment period	Continuous
Dose	3.6 g/day
Treatment consequences	Erectile function, impairment; gynaecomastia
Efficacy	60% of patients in cimetidine, disappearance when changing to ranitidine
Randomization of patients	No
Study quality	**2–**
Reference	1463: Jensen RT, Collen MJ, McArthur KE, Howard JM, Maton PN, Cherner JA, Gardner JD. Comparison of the effectiveness of ranitidine and cimetidine in inhibiting acid secretion in patients with gastric hypersecretory states. Am J Med. 1984 Nov 19;77(5B):90–105.
Language	English

Compound	Cimetidine (A02BA01)
Disease treated	Gastric hypersecretion
Quantification of adverse effects	Sexual function, gynaecomastia
No. of patients treated	22
Age group	51 years (mean)
Treatment period	2 years
Dose	Not mentioned
Treatment consequences	Erectile function, impairment, breast enlargement, disappearance 4–8 weeks after discontinuation
Efficacy	11 of 22 patients
Randomization of patients	No
Remarks	Described in numerous case reports and letters
Study quality	**3**
Reference	1464: Jensen RT, Collen MJ, Pandol SJ, Allende HD, Raufman JP, Bissonnette BM, Duncan WC, Durgin PL, Gillin JC, Gardner JD. Cimetidine-induced impotence and breast changes in patients with gastric hypersecretory states. N Engl J Med. 1983 Apr 14;308(15):883–7.
Language	English

Compound	Cimetidine (A02BA01)
Disease treated	Gastric hypersecretion
Quantification of adverse effects	Sexual function, gynaecomastia

No. of patients treated	1
Age group	66 years
Treatment period	Continuous
Dose	3.2 g/day
Treatment consequences	Erectile function, impairment; breast enlargement
Efficacy	Recovery after discontinuation; relapse after reexposition
Randomization of patients	No
Remarks	Described in numerous case reports and letters
Study quality	**3**
Reference	1366: Lardinois CK, Mazzaferri EL. Cimetidine blocks testosterone synthesis. Arch Intern Med. 1985 May;145(5):920–2.
Language	English

Compound	Ranitidine (A02BA02)
Disease treated	Hiatic hernia
Quantification of adverse effects	Erectile function
No. of patients treated	1
Age group	46 years
Treatment period	2 years
Dose	450 mg/day
Treatment consequences	Erectile function, impairment
Efficacy	Improvement after cessation of drug
Study quality	**3**
Reference	1607: Bera F, Jonville-Bera AP, Doustin P, Autret E. Impotence and gynecomastia secondary to hyperprolactinemia induced by ranitidine. Therapie. 1994 Jul–Aug;49(4):361–2.
Language	French

Compound	Cimetidine, ranitidine (A02BA01)
Disease treated	Gastric hypersecretion
Quantification of adverse effects	Sexual function
Age group	All ages
Treatment period	Continuous
Treatment consequences	Erectile function, impairment

Efficacy	Enhanced during cimetidine treatment
Study quality	**4 (review)**
Reference	1462: Biagi P, Milani G. Dysfunction of the hypothalamo–hypophyseal–gonadal axis induced by histamine H2 antagonists. Review of the literature and personal observations. Minerva Med. 1985 Mar 24;76(12):579–86.
Language	Italian

Compound	Omeprazole (A02BC01)
Disease treated	Oesophagitis
Quantification of adverse effects	Erectile function
No. of patients treated	1
Age group	77
Treatment period	6 weeks
Dose	20 mg/day
Treatment consequences	Erection, painful
Efficacy	Development without an increase in libido
Study quality	**3**
Reference	1356: Dutertre JP, Soutif D, Jonville AP, Cadenne M, Valat JP, Autret E. Sexual disturbances during omeprazole therapy. Lancet. 1991 Oct 19;338(8773):1022.
Language	English

A10 Drugs Used in Diabetes

It has been well proven that there is a higher prevalence of erectile dysfunction in diabetic men than in non-diabetic men. The figures of the odds ratio vary between 1.04 and 6.97. In most studies the confidence interval does not include 1.0, i.e. there is a significant difference. Only one study has found no increase of the risk with medication of antidiabetics.

The incidence of erectile dysfunction increases with the duration of the disease: a 10% higher risk was calculated with each year of duration of diabetes, and it was even higher in combination with depression and cardiac disease. In a duration of diabetes >5 years 56% of men had erectile dysfunction, and 72% of men with >20 years of diabetes.

On the other hand, the prevalence of diabetes mellitus in men with erectile dysfunction was significantly higher than in a control group of non-impotent men.

Although there are a number of well-conducted case-control studies, it remains unanswered as to whether the disease itself or the treatment applied impairs erectile function. The increasing incidence of erectile dysfunction with increasing duration of the disease, similar to the diseases in other blood vessels, however, is a strong argument for the association with the disease itself.

Overall level of evidence of adverse effects: B

Compound	Drugs used in diabetes (A10)
Disease treated	Diabetes mellitus
Quantification of adverse effects	Sexual function questionnaire
No. of patients treated	31; 742
Age group	53–90 years
Treatment period	Various
Dose	Various
Treatment consequences	Prevalence of erectile dysfunction as compared with non-diabetic men
Efficacy	OR 1.5 (95% CI 1.2–1.9)
Randomization of patients	No
Study quality	**2++**
Reference	2210: Bacon CG, Mittleman MA, Kawachi I, Giovannucci E, Glasser DB, Rimm EB. Sexual function in men older than 50 years of age: results from the health professionals follow-up study. Ann Intern Med. 2003;139(3):161–8.
Language	English

Compound	Drugs used in diabetes (A10)
Disease treated	Diabetes mellitus
Quantification of adverse effects	Sexual function questionnaire
No. of patients treated	27; 839
Age group	20–75 years
Treatment period	Various
Dose	Various
Treatment consequences	Prevalence of erectile dysfunction as compared with non-diabetic men
Efficacy	4% reporting no erectile dysfunction, 14% reporting erectile dysfunction

2

Randomization of patients	No
Study quality	**2–**
Reference	2208: Rosen RC, Fisher WA, Eardley I, Niederberger C, Nadel A, Sand M. Men's Attitudes to Life Events and Sexuality (MALES) Study. The multinational Men's Attitudes to Life Events and Sexuality (MALES) study: I. Prevalence of erectile dysfunction and related health concerns in the general population. Curr Med Res Opin. 2004 May;20(5):607–17.
Language	English

Compound	Drugs used in diabetes (A10)
Disease treated	Diabetes mellitus
Quantification of adverse effects	IIEF
No. of patients treated	3921
Age group	40–88 years
Treatment period	Various
Dose	Various
Treatment consequences	Prevalence of erectile dysfunction as compared with non-diabetic men
Efficacy	OR 1.45 (95% CI 1.16–1.81)
Randomization of patients	No
Study quality	**2–**
Reference	2206: Grover SA, Lowensteyn I, Kaouache M, Marchand S, Coupal L, DeCarolis E, Zoccoli J, Defoy I. The prevalence of erectile dysfunction in the primary care setting: importance of risk factors for diabetes and vascular disease. Arch Intern Med. 2006 Jan 23;166(2):213–9.
Language	English

Compound	Drugs used in diabetes (A10)
Disease treated	Diabetes mellitus
Quantification of adverse effects	IIEF
No. of patients treated	3566
Age group	>20 years
Treatment period	Various
Dose	Various
Treatment consequences	Prevalence of erectile dysfunction with comorbidities

Efficacy	Diabetes mellitus (OR, 2.69), obesity (OR, 1.60) and hypertension (OR, 1.56)
Randomization of patients	No
Study quality	**2++**
Reference	2223: Saigal CS, Wessells H, Pace J, Schonlau M, Wilt TJ; Urologic Diseases in America Project. Predictors and prevalence of erectile dysfunction in a racially diverse population. Arch Intern Med. 2006 Jan 23;166(2):207–12.
Language	English

Compound	Drugs used in diabetes (A10)
Disease treated	Diabetes mellitus
Quantification of adverse effects	Sexual function questionnaire
No. of patients treated	2674
Age group	20–70 years
Treatment period	Various
Dose	Various
Treatment consequences	Prevalence of erectile dysfunction as compared to non–diabetic men
Efficacy	OR 3.72, (95% CI 2.51–5.71)
Randomization of patients	no
Study quality	**2–**
Reference	2220: Safarinejad MR. Prevalence and risk factors for erectile dysfunction in a population-based study in Iran. Int J Impot Res. 2003 Aug;15(4):246–52.
Language	English

Compound	Drugs used in diabetes (A10)
Disease treated	Diabetes mellitus
Quantification of adverse effects	IIEF
No. of patients treated	2476
Age group	25–70 years
Treatment period	Various
Dose	Various
Treatment consequences	Prevalence of erectile dysfunction as compared with non-diabetic men
Efficacy	OR 4.08 (95% CI 2.57–6.49)

Randomization of patients	No
Study quality	**2++**
Reference	2215: Martin-Morales A, Sanchez-Cruz JJ, Saenz de Tejada I, Rodriguez-Vela L, Jimenez-Cruz JF, Burgos-Rodriguez RJ. Prevalence and independent risk factors for erectile dysfunction in Spain: results of the Epidemiologia de la Disfuncion Erectil Masculina Study. Urol. 2001 Aug;166(2):569–74.
Language	English

Compound	Drugs used in diabetes (A10)
Disease treated	Diabetes mellitus
Quantification of adverse effects	Interview by GP
No. of patients treated	2010
Age group	>18 years
Treatment period	Various
Dose	Various
Treatment consequences	Prevalence of erectile dysfunction as compared with non-diabetic men
Efficacy	RR not increased
Randomization of patients	No
Study quality	**2–**
Reference	2231: Ricci E, Parazzini F, Mirone V, Imbimbo C, Palmieri A, Bortolotti A, Cintio E di, Landoni M, Lavezzari M. Current drug use as risk factor for erectile dysfunction: results from an Italian epidemiological study. Int J Impot Res. 2003 Jun;15(3):221–4.
Language	English

Compound	Drugs used in diabetes (A10)
Disease treated	Diabetes mellitus
Quantification of adverse effects	Single question for erectile function
No. of patients treated	1982
Age group	>40 years
Treatment period	Various
Dose	Various
Treatment consequences	Prevalence of erectile dysfunction as compared with non-diabetic men

Efficacy	OR 2.53 (95% CI 1.77–3.61)
Randomization of patients	No
Study quality	**2++**
Reference	2216: Akkus E, Kadioglu A, Esen A, Doran S, Ergen A, Anafarta K, Hattat H. Turkish Erectile Dysfunction Prevalence Study Group. Prevalence and correlates of erectile dysfunction in Turkey: a population-based study. Eur Urol. 2002 Mar;41(3):298–304.
Language	English

Compound	Drugs used in diabetes (A10)
Disease treated	Diabetes mellitus
Quantification of adverse effects	IIEF
No. of patients treated	1730
Age group	50–80 years
Treatment period	Various
Dose	Various
Treatment consequences	Prevalence of erectile dysfunction as compared with non-diabetic men
Efficacy	OR 2.36 (95% CI 2.02–2.76)
Randomization of patients	No
Study quality	**2+**
Reference	2211: Rosen R, Altwein J, Boyle P, Kirby RS, Lukacs B, Meuleman E, O'Leary MP, Puppo P, Robertson C, Giuliano F. Lower urinary tract symptoms and male sexual dysfunction: the multinational survey of the aging male (MSAM-7). Eur Urol. 2003 Dec;44(6):637–49.
Language	English

Compound	Drugs used in diabetes (A10)
Disease treated	Diabetes mellitus
Quantification of adverse effects	Two questions from the NIH consensus definition
No. of patients treated	1683
Age group	40–69 years
Treatment period	Various
Dose	Various
Treatment consequences	Prevalence of erectile dysfunction as compared with non-diabetic men

Efficacy	RR 2.4 (95% CI 0.9–5.8)
Randomization of patients	No
Study quality	**2+**
Reference	2219: Shiri R, Koskimaki J, Hakama M, Hakkinen J, Tammela TL, Huhtala H, Auvinen A. Effect of chronic diseases on incidence of erectile dysfunction. Urology. 2003 Dec;62(6):1097–102.
Language	English

Compound	**Drugs used in diabetes (A10)**
Disease treated	Diabetes mellitus
Quantification of adverse effects	IIEF
No. of patients treated	729
Age group	30–79 years
Treatment period	Various
Dose	Various
Treatment consequences	Prevalence of erectile dysfunction as compared with non-diabetic men
Efficacy	OR 1.21 (95% CI 0.73–2.02)
Randomization of patients	No
Study quality	**2+**
Reference	2200: Tan JK, Hong CY, Png DJ, Liew LC, Wong ML. Erectile dysfunction in Singapore: prevalence and its associated factors – a population-based study. Singapore Med J. 2003 Jan;44(1):20–6.
Language	English

Compound	**Drugs used in diabetes (A10)**
Disease treated	Diabetes mellitus
Quantification of adverse effects	IIEF
No. of patients treated	518
Age group	58 years (mean)
Treatment period	Various
Dose	Various
Treatment consequences	Prevalence of erectile dysfunction as compared with non-diabetic men
Efficacy	OR 1.04 (95% CI 0.64–1.7)

Randomization of patients	No
Study quality	**2+**
Reference	2201: Roth A, Kalter-Leibovici O, Kerbis Y, Tenenbaum-Koren E, Chen J, Sobol T, Raz I. Prevalence and risk factors for erectile dysfunction in men with diabetes, hypertension, or both diseases: a community survey among 1,412 Israeli men. Clin Cardiol. 2003 Jan;26(1):25–30.
Language	English

Compound	Drugs used in diabetes (A10)
Pharmacological group	Drugs used in diabetes (A10)
Disease treated	Diabetes mellitus
Quantification of adverse effects	IIEF
No. of patients treated	512
Age group	63 years (mean)
Treatment period	Various
Dose	Various
Treatment consequences	Prevalence of erectile dysfunction as compared with non-diabetic men
Efficacy	OR 2.06 (95% CI 1.247–3.406)
Randomization of patients	No
Study quality	**2–**
Reference	2232: Cuellar de Leon AJ, Ruiz Garcia V, Campos Gonzalez JC, Perez Hoyos S, Brotons Multo F. Prevalence erectile dysfunction in patients with hypertension. Med Clin (Barc). 2002 Oct 26;119(14):521–6.
Language	Spanish

Compound	Drugs used in diabetes (A10)
Disease treated	Diabetes mellitus
Quantification of adverse effects	Single question of NIH consensus definition
No. of patients treated	500
Age group	20–80 years
Treatment period	Various
Dose	Various
Treatment consequences	Prevalence of erectile dysfunction as compared with non-diabetic men

2

Efficacy	56% in men with >5 years diabetes, 72% in men with >20 years diabetes
Randomization of patients	No
Study quality	**3**
Reference	2227: Siu SC, Lo SK, Wong KW, Ip KM, Wong YS. Prevalence of and risk factors for erectile dysfunction in Hong Kong diabetic patients. Diabet Med. 2001 Sep;18(9):732–8.
Language	English

Compound	Drugs used in diabetes (A10)
Disease treated	Diabetes mellitus
Quantification of adverse effects	Single question from the NIH consensus definition
No. of patients treated	428
Age group	40–70 years
Treatment period	Various
Dose	Various
Treatment consequences	Incidence of erectile dysfunction within 2 years
Efficacy	RR 2.87 (95% CI 1.21–6.80)
Randomization of patients	No
Study quality	**2+**
Reference	2229: Moreira ED Jr, Abdo CH, Torres EB, Lobo CF, Fittipaldi JA. Prevalence and correlates of erectile dysfunction: results of the Brazilian study of sexual behavior. Urology. 2001 Oct;58(4):583–8.
Language	English

Compound	Drugs used in diabetes (A10)
Disease treated	Diabetes mellitus
Quantification of adverse effects	Single question from the NIH consensus definition
No. of patients treated	428
Age group	40–70 years
Treatment period	Various
Dose	Various
Treatment consequences	Prevalence of erectile dysfunction as compared with non-diabetic men
Efficacy	RR 2.49 (95% CI 1.01–6.14)

Randomization of patients	No
Study quality	**2+**
Reference	2213: Moreira ED Jr, Lobo CF, Diament A, Nicolosi A, Glasser DB. Incidence of erectile dysfunction in men 40 to 69 years old: results from a population-based cohort study in Brazil. Urology. 2003 Feb;61(2):431–6.
Language	English

Compound	Drugs used in diabetes (A10)
Disease treated	Diabetes mellitus
Quantification of adverse effects	IIEF
No. of patients treated	315
Age group	35–75 years
Treatment period	Various
Dose	Various
Treatment consequences	Prevalence of diabetes mellitus in men with erectile dysfunction
Efficacy	20% of patients, 9% of controls, $p<0.05$
Randomization of patients	No
Study quality	**2–**
Reference	2236: Roumeguere T, Wespes E, Carpentier Y, Hoffmann P, Schulman CC. Erectile dysfunction is associated with a high prevalence of hyperlipidemia and coronary heart disease risk. Eur Urol. 2003 Sep;44(3):355–9.
Language	English

Compound	Drugs used in diabetes (A10)
Disease treated	Diabetes mellitus
Quantification of adverse effects	IIEF
No. of patients treated	312
Age group	>20 years
Treatment period	Various
Dose	Various
Treatment consequences	Incidence of erectile dysfunction
Efficacy	10% higher risk with each year duration of diabetes, higher in combination with depression and cardiac disease

Randomization of patients	No
Study quality	**2–**
Reference	2205: Shiri R, Ansari M, Falah Hassani K. Association between comorbidity and erectile dysfunction in patients with diabetes. Int J Impot Res. 2006 Jul–Aug;18(4):348–53.
Language	English

Compound	Drugs used in diabetes (A10)
Disease treated	Diabetes mellitus
Quantification of adverse effects	IIEF
No. of patients treated	239
Age group	40–49 years
Treatment period	Various
Dose	Various
Treatment consequences	Prevalence of erectile dysfunction as compared with non-diabetic men
Efficacy	OR 6.97 (95% CI 0.95–51.3)
Randomization of patients	No
Study quality	**2–**
Reference	2228: Mak R, De Backer G, Kornitzer M, De Meyer JM. Prevalence and correlates of erectile dysfunction in a population-based study in Belgium. Eur Urol. 2002 Feb;41(2):132–8.
Language	English

Compound	Drugs used in diabetes (A10)
Disease treated	Diabetes mellitus
Quantification of adverse effects	Sexual function questionnaire
No. of patients treated	194
Age group	52 years (mean)
Treatment period	Various
Dose	Various
Treatment consequences	Incidence of erectile dysfunction within 8 years
Efficacy	OR 18.83 (95% CI 1.23–2.73)
Randomization of patients	No
Study quality	**2++**

Reference	2204: Johannes CB, Araujo AB, Feldman HA, Derby CA, Kleinman KP, McKinlay JB. Incidence of erectile dysfunction in men 40 to 69 years old: longitudinal results from the Massachusetts male aging study. J Urol. 2000 Feb;163(2):460–3.
Language	English

Compound	Drugs used in diabetes (A10)
Disease treated	Diabetes mellitus
Quantification of adverse effects	Single question
No. of patients treated	88
Age group	40–70 years
Treatment period	Various
Dose	Various
Treatment consequences	Prevalence of erectile dysfunction as compared with non-diabetic men
Efficacy	OR 1.05 (95% CI 1.01–1.10)
Randomization of patients	No
Study quality	**2–**
Reference	2207: Nicolosi A, Moreira ED Jr, Shirai M, Bin Mohd Tambi MI, Glasser DB. Epidemiology of erectile dysfunction in four countries: cross-national study of the prevalence and correlates of erectile dysfunction. Urology. 2003 Jan;61(1):201–6.
Language	English

A14 Anabolic Agents for Systemic Use

Although anabolic steroids influence the hypothalamo-hypophyseal-testicular axis as androgen-like compounds, only case reports on sexual effects are available.

Overall level of evidence of adverse effects: D

Compound	Anabolic steroids (A14A)
Disease treated	Body builders
Quantification of adverse effects	Hamilton rating scale
No. of patients treated	41
Age group	Young

2

Treatment period	Various
Dose	Various
Treatment consequences	Affective syndrome
Efficacy	22 of 41 full syndrome
Randomization of patients	No
Study quality	**3**
Reference	1336: Pope HG Jr, Katz DL. Affective and psychotic symptoms associated with anabolic steroid use. Am J Psychiatry. 1988 Apr;145(4):487–90.
Language	English

Compound	Anabolic steroids (A14A)
Disease treated	Body builder
Quantification of adverse effects	Erectile function
No. of patients treated	1
Age group	Young
Treatment period	Various
Dose	Various
Treatment consequences	Erectile function, impairment
Efficacy	Treatment with hCG successful
Study quality	**3**
Reference	1352: Gill GV. Anabolic steroid induced hypogonadism treated with human chorionic gonadotropin. Postgrad Med J. 1998 Jan;74(867):45–6.
Language	English

C01 Cardiac Therapy

Cardiac Therapy in General

Men with cardiac diseases have a higher prevalence of erectile dysfunction than men without these diseases (significant OR 1.05–3.15). This holds true also for men with poorer health in general, which includes insufficient cardiac capacity. On the other hand, the prevalence of cardiac diseases in men with erectile dysfunction was found to be higher than in men with normal erectile function. In addition, erectile dysfunction preceded cardiac diseases such as myocardial infarction; it may thus be taken as a biomarker of other cardiovascular diseases.

Comparable to the impairment of erectile function in men with diabetes mellitus, in some studies it remained unclear as to whether the erectile dysfunction was associated with the disease itself or with the treatment procedures applied.

Overall level of evidence for adverse effects: B

Compound	Cardiac therapy (C01)
Disease treated	Cardiac disease
Quantification of adverse effects	Sexual function questionnaire
No. of patients treated	27; 839
Age group	20–75 years
Treatment period	Various
Dose	Various
Treatment consequences	Prevalence of erectile dysfunction as compared with men without cardiac diseases
Efficacy	7% reporting no erectile dysfunction, 17% reporting erectile dysfunction
Randomization of patients	No
Study quality	**2–**
Reference	2208: Rosen RC, Fisher WA, Eardley I, Niederberger C, Nadel A, Sand M. Men's Attitudes to Life Events and Sexuality (MALES) Study. The multinational Men's Attitudes to Life Events and Sexuality (MALES) study: I. Prevalence of erectile dysfunction and related health concerns in the general population. Curr Med Res Opin. 2004 May;20(5):607–17.
Language	English

Compound	Cardiac therapy (C01)
Disease treated	Erectile dysfunction
Quantification of adverse effects	Sexual function questionnaire
No. of patients treated	12,825; 12,825
Age group	Old
Treatment period	Various
Dose	Various
Treatment consequences	Prevalence of myocardial infarction
Efficacy	OR 1.99 (95% CI=1.17, 3.38)
Randomization of patients	No

Study quality	**2++**
Reference	2218: Blumentals WA, Gomez-Caminero A, Joo S, Vannappagari V. Should erectile dysfunction be considered as a marker for acute myocardial infarction? Results from a retrospective cohort study. Int J Impot Res. 2004 Aug;16(4):350–3.
Language	English

Compound	Cardiac therapy (C01)
Disease treated	Cardiac disease
Quantification of adverse effects	IIEF
No. of patients treated	3921
Age group	40–88 years
Treatment period	Various
Dose	Various
Treatment consequences	Prevalence of erectile dysfunction as compared with men without cardiac diseases
Efficacy	OR 3.13 (95% CI 2.35–4.16)
Randomization of patients	No
Study quality	**2–**
Reference	2206: Grover SA, Lowensteyn I, Kaouache M, Marchand S, Coupal L, DeCarolis E, Zoccoli J, Defoy I. The prevalence of erectile dysfunction in the primary care setting: importance of risk factors for diabetes and vascular disease. Arch Intern Med. 2006 Jan 23;166(2):213–9.
Language	English

Compound	Cardiac therapy (C01)
Disease treated	Cardiac disease
Quantification of adverse effects	IIEF
No. of patients treated	2476
Age group	25–70 years
Treatment period	Various
Dose	Various
Treatment consequences	Prevalence of erectile dysfunction as compared with men without cardiac diseases
Efficacy	OR 1.79 (95% CI 1.18–2.71)
Randomization of patients	No
Remarks	

Study quality	**2++**
Reference	2215: Martin-Morales A, Sanchez-Cruz JJ, Saenz de Tejada I, Rodriguez-Vela L, Jimenez-Cruz JF, Burgos-Rodriguez RJ. Prevalence and independent risk factors for erectile dysfunction in Spain: results of the Epidemiologia de la Disfuncion Erectil Masculina Study. Urol. 2001 Aug;166(2):569–74.
Language	English

Compound	Cardiac therapy (C01)
Pharmacological group	Cardiac therapy (C01)
Quantification of adverse effects	Single question for erectile function
No. of patients treated	1982
Age group	>40 years
Treatment period	Various
Dose	Various
Treatment consequences	Prevalence of erectile dysfunction as compared with men without cardiac diseases
Efficacy	OR 1.62 (95% CI 1.10–2.38)
Randomization of patients	No
Study quality	**2++**
Reference	2216: Akkus E, Kadioglu A, Esen A, Doran S, Ergen A, Anafarta K, Hattat H; Turkish Erectile Dysfunction Prevalence Study Group. Prevalence and correlates of erectile dysfunction in Turkey: a population-based study. Eur Urol. 2002 Mar;41(3):298–304.
Language	English

Compound	Cardiac therapy (C01)
Disease treated	Cardiac disease
Quantification of adverse effects	Two questions from the NIH consensus definition
No. of patients treated	1683
Age group	40–69 years
Treatment period	Various
Dose	Various
Treatment consequences	Prevalence of erectile dysfunction as compared with men without cardiac diseases
Efficacy	RR 1.3 (95% CI 0.8–2.1)

Randomization of patients	No
Study quality	**2+**
Reference	2219: Shiri R, Koskimaki J, Hakama M, Hakkinen J, Tammela TL, Huhtala H, Auvinen A. Effect of chronic diseases on incidence of erectile dysfunction. Urology. 2003 Dec;62(6):1097–102.
Language	English

Compound	Cardiac therapy (C01)
Disease treated	Cardiac disease
Quantification of adverse effects	IIEF
No. of patients treated	729
Age group	30–79 years
Treatment consequences	Prevalence of erectile dysfunction as compared with men without cardiac diseases
Efficacy	OR 2.84 (95% CI 0.92–8.74)
Randomization of patients	No
Study quality	**2+**
Reference	2200: Tan JK, Hong CY, Png DJ, Liew LC, Wong ML. Erectile dysfunction in Singapore: prevalence and its associated factors – a population-based study. Singapore Med J. 2003 Jan;44(1):20–6.
Language	English

Compound	Cardiac therapy (C01)
Disease treated	Cardiac disease
Quantification of adverse effects	Single question from the NIH consensus definition
No. of patients treated	428
Age group	40–70 years
Treatment period	Various
Dose	Various
Treatment consequences	Prevalence of erectile dysfunction
Efficacy	RR 1.48 (95% CI 0.58–3.77)
Randomization of patients	No
Study quality	**2+**

Reference	2213: Moreira ED Jr, Lobo CF, Diament A, Nicolosi A, Glasser DB. Incidence of erectile dysfunction in men 40 to 69 years old: results from a population-based cohort study in Brazil. Urology. 2003 Feb;61(2):431–6.
Language	English

Compound	Cardiac therapy (C01)
Disease treated	Erectile dysfunction
Quantification of adverse effects	IIEF
No. of patients treated	315
Age group	35–75 years
Treatment period	Various
Dose	Various
Treatment consequences	Prevalence of cardiac diseases in men with erectile dysfunction
Efficacy	13% of patients, 2% of controls, $p<0.05$
Randomization of patients	No
Study quality	**2–**
Reference	2236: Roumeguere T, Wespes E, Carpentier Y, Hoffmann P, Schulman CC. Erectile dysfunction is associated with a high prevalence of hyperlipidemia and coronary heart disease risk. Eur Urol. 2003 Sep;44(3):355–9.
Language	English

Compound	Cardiac therapy (C01)
Disease treated	Myocardial infarction
Quantification of adverse effects	Sexual function questionnaire
No. of patients treated	100; 129
Age group	Middle-aged
Treatment period	Various
Dose	Various
Treatment consequences	Prevalence of erectile dysfunction as compared with men without cardiac diseases
Efficacy	34% of men with myocardial infarction; 18% of men without cardiovascular disease
Randomization of patients	No
Study quality	**2+**

Reference	2239: Stroberg P, Frick E, Hedelin H. Is erectile dysfunction really a clinically useful predictor of cardiovascular disease? Scand J Urol Nephrol. 2005;39(1):62–5.
Language	English

Compound	Cardiac therapy (C01)
Disease treated	Cardiac disease
Quantification of adverse effects	IIEF
No. of patients treated	204
Age group	40–69 years
Treatment period	Various
Dose	Various
Treatment consequences	Prevalence of erectile dysfunction as compared with men without cardiac diseases
Efficacy	OR 0.72 (95% CI 0.24–2.18)
Randomization of patients	No
Study quality	**2–**
Reference	2228: Mak R, De Backer G, Kornitzer M, De Meyer JM. Prevalence and correlates of erectile dysfunction in a population-based study in Belgium. Eur Urol. 2002 Feb;41(2):132–8.
Language	English

Compound	Cardiac therapy (C01)
Disease treated	Cardiac disease
Quantification of adverse effects	Sexual function questionnaire
No. of patients treated	194
Age group	52 years (mean)
Treatment period	Various
Dose	Various
Treatment consequences	Incidence of erectile dysfunction within 8 years of treatment
Efficacy	OR 1.96 (95% CI 1.32–2.91)
Randomization of patients	No
Study quality	**2++**

Reference	2204: Johannes CB, Araujo AB, Feldman HA, Derby CA, Kleinman KP, McKinlay JB. Incidence of erectile dysfunction in men 40 to 69 years old: longitudinal results from the Massachusetts male aging study. J Urol. 2000 Feb;163(2):460–3.
Language	English

Compound	Cardiac therapy (C01)
Disease treated	Cardiac disease
Quantification of adverse effects	Single question
No. of patients treated	178
Age group	40–70 years
Dose	Various
Treatment consequences	Prevalence of erectile dysfunction as compared with men without cardiac diseases
Efficacy	OR 1.05 (95% CI 1.01–1.09) per 1-year duration
Randomization of patients	No
Study quality	**2–**
Reference	2207: Nicolosi A, Moreira ED Jr, Shirai M, Bin Mohd Tambi MI, Glasser DB. Epidemiology of erectile dysfunction in four countries: cross-national study of the prevalence and correlates of erectile dysfunction. Urology. 2003 Jan;61(1):201–6.
Language	English

Compound	Cardiac therapy (C01)
Disease treated	Poor health
Quantification of adverse effects	IIEF
No. of patients treated	28,691
Treatment period	No treatment
Age group	20–75 years
Treatment consequences	Prevalence of erectile dysfunction as compared with men without cardiac diseases
Efficacy	OR 2.0 (95% CI 1.8–2.5)
Randomization of patients	No
Study quality	**2+**

Reference	2217: Shabsigh R, Perelman MA, Lockhart DC, Lue TF, Broderick GA. Health issues of men: prevalence and correlates of erectile dysfunction. J Urol. 2005 Aug;174(2):662–7.
Language	English

Compound	Cardiac therapy (C01)
Disease treated	Poor health
Quantification of adverse effects	IIEF
No. of patients treated	4000
Treatment period	No treatment
Age group	45–75 years
Treatment consequences	Prevalence of erectile dysfunction
Efficacy	Risk factors: age; smoking; diabetes; high cholesterol; hypertension; depression; anxiety disorders
Randomization of patients	No
Study quality	**2+**
Reference	2238: Geirsson G, Thornorgeirsson G, Guethmundsson O, Einarsson G. Risk factors and prevalence of erectile dysfunction amongst Icelandic men aged 45–75. Laeknabladid. 2006 Jul–Aug;92(7–8):533–7.
Language	Icelandian

Compound	Cardiac therapy (C01)
Disease treated	Poor health
Quantification of adverse effects	IIEF
No. of patients treated	832
Treatment period	No treatment
Age group	30–69 years
Treatment consequences	Prevalence of erectile dysfunction
Efficacy	12.5% at 30–39 years; 15.3% at 40–49 years; 27.4% at 50–59 years; 45.2% at 60–69 years
Randomization of patients	No
Study quality	**3**

Reference	2234: Madersbacher S, Temml C, Racz U, Mock K, Ponholzer A, Maier U, Haidinger G. Prevalence and risk factors for erectile dysfunction in Austria: analysis of a health screening project. Wien Klin Wochenschr. 2003 Dec 15;115(23):822–30.
Language	English

Compound	Cardiac therapy (C01)
Disease treated	Poor health
Quantification of adverse effects	Sexual function questionnaire
No. of patients treated	401
Age group	40–70 years
Treatment period	No treatment
Treatment consequences	Progression of severety of erectile dysfunction
Efficacy	Significantly increasing risk with poorer health status
Randomization of patients	No
Study quality	**2++**
Reference	2235: Travison TG, Shabsigh R, Araujo AB, Kupelian V, O'Donnell AB, McKinlay JB. The natural progression and remission of erectile dysfunction: results from the Massachusetts Male Aging Study. J Urol. 2007 Jan;177(1):241–6.
Language	English

C01 Cardiac Therapy

Digoxin and Propaphenon

Digoxin has been suggested to impair sexual functions; however, it remains unanswered as to whether the drug or the disease treated itself causes the effects.

A single case report describes complete impotence in a patient using propaphenon.

Overall level of evidence of adverse effects: D

Compound	Digoxin (C01AA05)
Disease treated	Cardiovascular disease, rheumatic
Quantification of adverse effects	Sexual function scale; hormones

2

No. of patients treated	n.g.
Age group	25–40 years
Treatment period	Continuous
Dose	n.g.
Treatment consequences	Sexual function, depressed; testosterone level, decreased
Efficacy	Significant in digoxin treated group
Randomization of patients	No
Dose arms 1–3	Digoxin; no digoxin
Study quality	**2–**
Reference	1385: Neri A, Zukerman Z, Aygen M, Lidor Y, Kaufman H. The effect of long-term administration of digoxin on plasma androgens and sexual dysfunction. J Sex Marital Ther. 1987 Spring;13(1):58–63.
Language	English

Compound	Digoxin (C01AA05)
Disease treated	Healthy
Quantification of adverse effects	Erectile function
No. of patients treated	6
Age group	Young
Treatment period	4 weeks
Dose	10 nM bis 10 μM per intracavernous injection
Treatment consequences	Erectile rigidity during visual stimulation, decrease
Efficacy	No influence on libido and testosterone
Randomization of patients	Inhibition of corporal smooth muscle sodium pump activity
Study quality	**2–**
Reference	1381: Gupta S, Salimpour P, Saenz de Tejada I, Daley J, Gholami S, Daller M, Krane RJ, Traish AM, Goldstein I. A possible mechanism for alteration of human erectile function by digoxin: inhibition of corpus cavernosum sodium/potassium adenosine triphosphatase activity. J Urol. 1998 May;159(5):1529–36.
Language	English

Compound	Propaphenon (C01BC03)
Disease treated	Cardiac disease
Quantification of adverse effects	Erectile function
No. of patients treated	1
Age group	43
Treatment period	Continuous
Dose	n.g.
Treatment consequences	Erectile function, impairment
Efficacy	No influence on libido and testosterone
Randomization of patients	Complete impotence
Study quality	**3**
Reference	581: Korst HA, Brandes JW, Littmann KP. Disturbances of potency and spermiogenesis due to propafenon. Dtsch Med Wochenschr. 1980 Aug 22;105(34):1187–9.
Language	German

C01C	Cardiac Therapy
	Norepinephrine and Phenylephrine

These two compounds inhibit erectile competence locally in the corpus cavernosum by inhibiting smooth muscle relaxation.

Overall level of evidence of adverse effects: C

Compound	Norepinephrine (C01CA03), phentolamine
Disease treated	Erectile dysfunction
Quantification of dysfunction	Digoxin serum levels after intracavernous injection
No. of patients treated	32
Age group	Old
Treatment period	Single dose
Dose	n.g.
Treatment consequences	Plasma peak of digoxin
Efficacy	40 times higher than after injection of vasodilators

2

Randomization of patients	No
Study quality	**2+**
Reference	1382: de Meyer JM, Oosterlinck W. Pharmacodynamics of intracavernously injected drugs and cavernous wall resistance. Eur Urol. 1997;32(2):184–9.
Language	English

Compound	Phenylephrine (C01CA06)
Disease treated	Cavernous tissue in vitro
Quantification of dysfunction	Smooth muscle contractility
No. of patients treated	38
Age group	Young
Treatment period	Single dose
Dose	n.g.
Treatment consequences	Cavernous tissue, contractility
Efficacy	Antagonists inhibit contractions
Randomization of patients	No
Study quality	**3**
Reference	1594: Christ GJ, Maayani S, Valcic M, Melman A. Pharmacological studies of human erectile tissue: characteristics of spontaneous contractions and alterations in alpha-adrenoceptor responsiveness with age and disease in isolated tissues. Br J Pharmacol. 1990 Oct;101(2):375–81.
Language	English

C01	**Cardiac Therapy**
	Vasodilators Used in Cardiac Therapy (C01D)
	Men being treated with coronary vasodilators have a significantly greater risk to suffer from erectile dysfunction than men without coronary artery disease. The case-control studies, however, do not answer the question about whether the drugs applied or the disease itself are the cause. **Overall level of evidence of adverse effects: B**

Nitroglycerine as a nitrite-releasing compound causes relaxation of cavernous tissue in vitro, thus leading to erection. Controlled clinical studies have revealed disappointing results after primarily positive reports. As a side effect, headache was commonly observed, and it appeared also in the female partner after coitus.

Overall level of evidence of positive effects: C
Overall level of evidence of adverse effects compromising effectiveness: C

Intracavernous injections of the nitric oxide donator linsidomine were tested in erectile dysfunction. It was found to be effective also in controlled studies, but to a lesser extent than alprostadil, the drug most frequently used (see below: G04 Urologicals). No significant adverse effects compromising effectiveness were observed.

Overall level of evidence of positive effects: C
Overall level of evidence of adverse effects compromising effectiveness: C

Compound	Vasodilators used in cardiac therapy (C01D)
Disease treated	Coronary artery disease
Quantification of dysfunction	Sexual function questionnaire
No. of patients treated	2674
Age group	20–70 years
Treatment period	Continuous
Dose	Various
Treatment consequences	Prevalence of erectile dysfunction as compared with men without coronary artery disease
Efficacy	OR 1.61 (95% CI 1.21–2.85)
Randomization of patients	No
Study quality	**2–**
Reference	2220: Safarinejad MR. Prevalence and risk factors for erectile dysfunction in a population-based study in Iran. Int J Impot Res. 2003 Aug;15(4):246–52.
Language	English

Compound	Vasodilators used in cardiac therapy (C01D)
Disease treated	Coronary artery disease
Quantification of dysfunction	Sexual function questionnaire

2

No. of patients treated	512
Age group	63 years (mean)
Treatment period	Continuous
Dose	Various
Treatment consequences	Prevalence of erectile dysfunction as compared with men without coronary artery disease
Efficacy	RR 3.15 (95% CI 1.429–6.947)
Randomization of patients	No
Study quality	**2-**
Reference	2232: Cuellar de Leon AJ, Ruiz Garcia V, Campos Gonzalez JC, Perez Hoyos S, Brotons Multo F. Prevalence erectile dysfunction in patients with hypertension. Med Clin (Barc). 2002 Oct 26;119(14):521–6.
Language	English

Compound	Nitroglycerine (C01DA02)
Disease treated	Erectile dysfunction in various diseases
Quantification of dysfunction	Erectile function
No. of patients treated	33
Age group	Young
Treatment period	Locally applied
Dose	2.5 g of a 10% ointment
Treatment consequences	Erectile function, improvement
Efficacy	Minoxidil better effective than nitroglycerin
Side effects compromising effectiveness	On minoxidil 2 patients with burning pain, on nitroglycerin 8 patients burning pain, 4 headache, 2 hypotension
Randomization of patients	No
Study quality	**3**
Reference	1637: Cavallini G. Minoxidil versus nitroglycerin: a prospective double-blind controlled trial in transcutaneous erection facilitation for organic impotence. J Urol. 1991 Jul;146(1):50–3.
Language	English

Compound	Nitroglycerine (C01DA02)
Disease treated	Erectile dysfunction in spinal cord lesion
Quantification of dysfunction	Penile volume
No. of patients treated	28
Age group	Young
Treatment period	Locally applied
Dose	10% ointment
Treatment consequences	Erectile function, improvement
Efficacy	Less effective than papaverine
Side effects compromising effectiveness	Mild headache in six patients (21%)
Randomization of patients	Cross-over
Dose arms 1–3	Nitroglycerine; papaverine
Study quality	**1–**
Reference	1632: Renganathan R, Suranjan B, Kurien T. Comparison of transdermal nitroglycerin and intracavernous injection of papaverine in the treatment of erectile dysfunction in patients with spinal cord lesions. Spinal Cord. 1997 Feb;35(2):99–103.
Language	English

Compound	Nitroglycerine (C01DA02)
Disease treated	Erectile dysfunction
Quantification of dysfunction	Erectile function
No. of patients treated	26
Age group	Old
Treatment period	Locally applied
Treatment consequences	Erectile function, improvement
Efficacy	Moderate effectivity
Side effects compromising effectiveness	12 patients mild headache, more severe in the youngest patients
Randomization of patients	No
Study quality	**3**

Reference	1639: Claes H, Baert L. Transcutaneous nitroglycerin therapy in the treatment of impotence. Urol Int. 1989;44(5):309–12.
Language	English

Compound	Nitroglycerine (C01DA02)
Disease treated	Erectile dysfunction
Quantification of dysfunction	Erectile function
No. of patients treated	26
Age group	Old
Treatment period	Locally applied
Dose	2% paste
Treatment consequences	Erectile function, improvement
Efficacy	Increase of penile blood flow
Side effects compromising effectiveness	Headache frequent but declining in longer use. Spousal headache possible
Randomization of patients	No
Study quality	**3**
Reference	1638: Owen JA, Saunders F, Harris C, Fenemore J, Reid K, Surridge D, Condra M, Morales A. Topical nitroglycerin: a potential treatment for impotence. J Urol. 1989 Mar;141(3):546–8.
Language	English

Compound	Nitroglycerine (C01DA02)
Disease treated	Erectile dysfunction
Quantification of dysfunction	Relaxation of corporal tissue strips
No. of patients treated	26
Age group	Old
Treatment period	In vitro
Dose	n.g.
Treatment consequences	Cavernous tissue, relaxation
Efficacy	Diminished effectivity in tissue from patients with erectile dysfunction
Randomization of patients	Yes
Dose arms 1–3	Nitroglycerin; placebo

Study quality	**1–**
Reference	1633: Christ GJ, Kim DC, Taub HC, Gondre CM, Melman A. Characterization of nitroglycerine-induced relaxation in human corpus cavernosum smooth muscle: implications to erectile physiology and dysfunction. Can J Physiol Pharmacol. 1995 Dec;73(12):1714–26.
Language	English

Compound	Nitroglycerine (C01DA02)
Disease treated	Erectile dysfunction
Quantification of dysfunction	Erectile function by Rigiscan
No. of patients treated	18
Age group	Old
Treatment period	Locally applied
Dose	10% ointment
Treatment consequences	Erectile function, improvement
Efficacy	No effect
Side effects compromising effectiveness	None
Randomization of patients	Cross-over
Dose arms 1–3	Nitroglycerine; placebo
Study quality	**2–**
Reference	1631: Gramkow J, Lendorf A, Zhu J, Meyhoff HH. Transcutaneous nitroglycerine in the treatment of erectile dysfunction: a placebo controlled clinical trial. Int J Impot Res. 1999 Feb;11(1):35–9.
Language	English

Compound	Nitroglycerine (C01DA02)
Disease treated	Erectile dysfunction in spinal cord lesion
Quantification of dysfunction	Erectile function
No. of patients treated	17
Age group	Young
Treatment period	Locally applied on demand
Dose	10 mg plaster
Treatment consequences	Erectile function, improvement
Efficacy	Positive in 12 men

Side effects compromising effectiveness	6 of 12 headache
Randomization of patients	No
Study quality	**3**
Reference	1635: Sonksen J, Biering-Sorensen F. Transcutaneous nitroglycerin in the treatment of erectile dysfunction in spinal cord injured. Paraplegia. 1992 Aug;30(8):554–7.
Language	English

Compound	Nitroglycerine (C01DA02)
Disease treated	Cavernous tissue in vitro
Quantification of dysfunction	Muscle relaxation
No. of patients treated	16
Age group	42–68 years
Treatment period	In vitro
Dose	5×10^{-4} g
Treatment consequences	Cavernous tissue, relaxation
Efficacy	Poor
Study quality	**2+**
Reference	1438: Barbanti G, Beneforti P, Lapini A, Turini D. Relaxation of isolated corpus cavernosum induced by smooth-muscle relaxant drugs. A comparative study. Urol Res. 1988;16(4):299–302.
Language	English

Compound	Nitroglycerine (C01DA02)
Disease treated	Erectile dysfunction in spinal cord lesion
Quantification of dysfunction	Erectile function
No. of patients treated	10
Age group	Young
Treatment period	Locally applied
Dose	10 mg patch
Treatment consequences	Erectile function, improvement
Efficacy	Positive in all patients

Side effects compromising effectiveness	Headache common
Randomization of patients	No
Study quality	**3**
Reference	1636: Meyhoff HH, Rosenkilde P, Bodker A. Non-invasive management of impotence with transcutaneous nitroglycerin. Br J Urol. 1992 Jan;69(1):88–90.
Language	English

Compound	Nitroglycerine (C01DA02)
Disease treated	Erectile dysfunciton
Quantification of dysfunction	Erectile function
No. of patients treated	3
Age group	Young
Treatment period	Locally applied on demand
Dose	10% ointment
Treatment consequences	Erectile function, improvement
Efficacy	Successful treatment
Side effects compromising effectiveness	Not mentioned
Randomization of patients	No
Study quality	**3**
Reference	1634: Nunez BD, Anderson DC Jr. Nitroglycerin ointment in the treatment of impotence. J Urol. 1993 Oct;150(4):1241–3.
Language	English

Compound	Linsidomine (C01DX18)
Disease treated	Erectile dysfunction
Quantification of dysfunction	Erectile function
No. of patients treated	113
Age group	Old
Treatment period	Single dose intracavernous
Dose	1 mg

Treatment consequences	Erectile rigidity, improvement
Efficacy	69% of patients
Side effects compromising effectiveness	No significant side effects
Randomization of patients	No
Study quality	**3**
Reference	1600: Truss MC, Becker AJ, Djamilian MH, Stief CG, Jonas U. Role of the nitric oxide donor linsidomine chlorhydrate (SIN-1) in the diagnosis and treatment of erectile dysfunction. Urology. 1994 Oct;44(4):553–6.
Language	English

Compound	Linsidomine (C01DX18)
Disease treated	Erectile dysfunction
Quantification of dysfunction	Erectile function
No. of patients treated	113
Age group	Old
Treatment period	Single dose
Dose	1 mg
Treatment consequences	Erectile rigidity, improvement
Efficacy	69% of patients
Side effects compromising effectiveness	No significant side effects
Randomization of patients	No
Study quality	**3**
Reference	1523: Truss MC, Becker AJ, Djamilian MH, Stief CG, Jonas U. Role of the nitric oxide donor linsidomine chlorhydrate (SIN-1) in the diagnosis and treatment of erectile dysfunction. Urology. 1994 Oct;44(4):553–6.
Language	English

Compound	Linsidomine (C01DX18)
Disease treated	Erectile dysfunction
Quantification of dysfunction	Erectile function

No. of patients treated	63
Age group	Old
Treatment period	Single dose
Dose	1 mg
Treatment consequences	Erectile rigidity, improvement
Efficacy	100% comparable to papaverine–phentolamine
Side effects compromising effectiveness	Decreased risk of inducing prolonged erections compared with other papaverine–phentolamine
Randomization of patients	No
Study quality	**3**
Reference	1603: Stief CG, Holmquist F, Djamilian M, Krah H, Andersson KE, Jonas U. Preliminary results with the nitric oxide donor linsidomine chlorhydrate in the treatment of human erectile dysfunction. J Urol. 1992 Nov;148(5):1437–40.
Language	English

Compound	Linsidomine (C01DX18)
Disease treated	Erectile dysfunction
Quantification of dysfunction	Erectile function
No. of patients treated	40
Age group	Old
Treatment period	Decrease of overall functions
Dose	1 mg
Treatment consequences	Erectile rigidity, improvement
Efficacy	92% of linsidomine group, 100% of alprostadile group
Side effects compromising effectiveness	Symptoms of arterial insufficiency after injection
Randomization of patients	Yes
Dose arms 1–3	Linsidomine; alprostadil
Study quality	**1–**
Reference	1602: Porst H. Prostaglandin E1 and the nitric oxide donor linsidomine for erectile failure: a diagnostic comparative study of 40 patients. J Urol. 1993 May;149(5 Pt 2):1280–3.
Language	English

Compound	Linsidomine (C01DX18)
Pharmacological group	Cardiac therapy (C01)
Disease treated	Erectile dysfunction
Quantification of dysfunction	Erection
No. of patients treated	38
Age group	Old
Treatment period	Single dose
Dose	1 mg
Treatment consequences	Erectile function under observation
Efficacy	Alprostadil better than linsidomine
Side effects compromising effectiveness	n.g.
Randomization of patients	No
Study quality	**2–**
Reference	1599: Lemaire A, Buvat J. Erectile response to intracavernous injection of linsidomine in 38 impotent patients. Comparison with prostaglandin E1. Prog Urol. 1998 Jun;8(3):388–91.
Language	French

Compound	Linsidomine (C01DX18)
Disease treated	Erectile dysfunction
Quantification of dysfunction	Erectile function
No. of patients treated	20
Age group	Old
Treatment period	Single dose
Dose	1 mg
Treatment consequences	Erectile rigidity, improvement
Efficacy	Alprostadil better than linsidomine
Side effects compromising effectiveness	No significant side effects
Randomization of patients	Yes

Dose arms 1–3	Linsidomine; alprostadil
Study quality	1+
Reference	1601: Wegner HE, Knispel HH, Klan R, Meier T, Miller K. Prostaglandin E1 versus linsidomine chlorhydrate in erectile dysfunction. Urol Int. 1994;53(4):214–6.
Language	English

C02 Antihypertensives

Erectile dysfunction is claimed to be a frequent side effect of antihypertensive treatment. Also patients themselves are convinced that their impotence is caused by antihypertensive drugs they take, and many physicians support this opinion; however, as early as 1978 Bauer et al. stated that the extent of sexual function impairment is age-related as compared with that observed in men not taking antihypertensives. Ten year later, Bansal (1988) quoted that the reported studies did not clearly indicate whether the impairment is due to the drugs, the influence of the disease, or both. Again 10 years later, other authors concluded: "Scientific evidence that links antihypertensive drugs to sexual dysfunction in placebo-controlled trials is limited" (Grimm et al. 1997).

Nevertheless, patients with hypertension are at greater risk to suffer from erectile dysfunction, irrespective of the treatment, than are healthy men. The OR was found to be significantly greater than 1 in large case-control studies. The erectile dysfunction was frequently associated with intermittent claudication and ischaemic heart disease.

Diuretics, centrally acting sympatholytic drugs, and β-blockers appear to bear a greater impact, while calcium antagonists and ACE inhibitors appear to show a lower impact on erectile function (Fogari et al. 2002; Mikhailidis et al. 2000).

Overall level of evidence of adverse effects: B

Compound	Antihypertensives (C02)
Disease treated	Hypertension
Quantification of adverse effects	Physician's diagnosis
No. of patients treated	285,436
Age group	18–84 years

Treatment period	Various
Treatment consequences	Prevalence of hypertension in men with erectile dysfunction as compared with men without erectile dysfunction
Efficacy	OR 1.38 (p<0.0001)
Randomization of patients	No
Study quality	**2–**
Reference	2226: Sun P, Swindle R. Are men with erectile dysfunction more likely to have hypertension than men without erectile dysfunction? A naturalistic national cohort study. J Urol. 2005 Jul;174(1):244–8.
Language	English

Compound	**Antihypertensives (C02)**
Disease treated	Hypertension
Quantification of adverse effects	Sexual function questionnaire
No. of patients treated	27,839
Age group	20–75 years
Treatment period	Various
Dose	Various
Treatment consequences	Prevalence of erectile dysfunction as compared with normotensive men
Efficacy	19% reporting no erectile dysfunction, 36% reporting erectile dysfunction
Randomization of patients	No
Study quality	**2–**
Reference	2208: Rosen RC, Fisher WA, Eardley I, Niederberger C, Nadel A, Sand M. Men's Attitudes to Life Events and Sexuality (MALES) Study. The multinational Men's Attitudes to Life Events and Sexuality (MALES) study: I. Prevalence of erectile dysfunction and related health concerns in the general population. Curr Med Res Opin. 2004 May;20(5):607–17.
Language	English

Compound	**Antihypertensives (C02)**
Disease treated	Hypertension
Quantification of adverse effects	Sexual function questionnaires
No. of patients treated	2452 patient-years

Age group	35–64 years
Treatment period	24 months
Dose	Various
Treatment consequences	Erectile function, impairment
Efficacy	19.6% of bedrofluamide group, in 5.5% of propranolol group, in 0.9% of placebo group
Randomization of patients	Yes
Dose arms 1-3	Bedrofluazide; propranolol; placebo
Remarks	"Reported incidence figures for suspected adverse reactions are probably lower than the true incidence, since not all reactions will have been mentioned by patients. Side effects such as, for example, impotence, lead less often to withdrawal of drugs than is recorded".
Study quality	**1–**
Reference	1457: Medical Research Council Working Party on mild to moderate hypertension: Adverse reaction to bendrofulazide and propranolog for the treatment of mild hypertension. Lancet 12.9.1981, pp. 539–543.
Language	English

Compound	Antihypertensives (C02)
Disease treated	Hypertension
Quantification of adverse effects	Single question for erectile function
No. of patients treated	1982
Age group	>40 years
Treatment period	Various
Dose	Various
Treatment consequences	Prevalence of erectile dysfunction as compared with normotensive men
Efficacy	OR 2.81 (95% CI 2.16–3.66)
Randomization of patients	No
Study quality	**2++**
Reference	2216: Akkus E, Kadioglu A, Esen A, Doran S, Ergen A, Anafarta K, Hattat H. Turkish Erectile Dysfunction Prevalence Study Group. Prevalence and correlates of erectile dysfunction in Turkey: a population-based study. Eur Urol. 2002 Mar;41(3):298–304.
Language	English

Compound	Antihypertensives (C02)
Disease treated	Hypertension
Quantification of adverse effects	Two questions from the NIH consensus definition
No. of patients treated	1683
Age group	40–69 years
Treatment period	Various
Dose	Various
Treatment consequences	Prevalence of erectile dysfunction as compared with normotensive men
Efficacy	RR 1.1 (95% CI 0.8–1.6)
Randomization of patients	No
Study quality	**2+**
Reference	2219: Shiri R, Koskimaki J, Hakama M, Hakkinen J, Tammela TL, Huhtala H, Auvinen A. Effect of chronic diseases on incidence of erectile dysfunction. Urology. 2003 Dec;62(6):1097–102.
Language	English

Compound	Antihypertensives (C02)
Disease treated	Hypertension
Quantification of adverse effects	Sexual function questionnaires
No. of patients treated	1017
Age group	30–69 years
Treatment period	24 months
Dose	Various
Treatment consequences	Erectile function, alteration
Efficacy	19% in active treatment, 14% in placebo group, 20% in "no tablets" group
Randomization of patients	Yes
Dose arms 1–3	Antihypertensives; placebo; nothing
Remarks	"Failure to sustain erection and failure to ejaculate: both symptoms are age-related in patients taking active drugs or placebo".
Study quality	**1–**
Reference	1456: Bauer GE, Baker J, Hunyour SN, Maarshall P. Side effects of antihypertensive treatment: a placebo controlled study. Clin Sci Mol Med 1978;55: 341s–4s.
Language	English

Compound	Antihypertensives (C02)
Disease treated	Hypertension
Quantification of adverse effects	IIEF
No. of patients treated	729
Age group	30–79 years
Treatment period	Various
Dose	Various
Treatment consequences	Prevalence of erectile dysfunction as compared with normotensive men
Efficacy	OR 2.06 (95% CI 0.96–4.43)
Randomization of patients	No
Study quality	**2+**
Reference	2200: Tan JK, Hong CY, Png DJ, Liew LC, Wong ML. Erectile dysfunction in Singapore: prevalence and its associated factors: a population-based study. Singapore Med J. 2003 Jan;44(1):20–6.
Language	English

Compound	Antihypertensives (C02)
Disease treated	Hypertension
Quantification of adverse effects	Sexual function questionnaires
No. of patients treated	557
Age group	45–69 years
Treatment period	12 months
Dose	Various
Treatment consequences	Sexual dysfunction
Efficacy	Acebutol: no alteration, amlopidine: no alteration, chlorthalidon: E.d. more frequent
Randomization of patients	Yes
Dose arms 1–3	Acebutol; amlopidine; chlorthalidon
Remarks	"Scientific evidence that links antihypertensive drugs to sexual dysfunction in placebo-controlled trials is limited".
Study quality	**1–**
Reference	1450: Grimm RH, Grandits GA, Prineas RJ et al. Long-term effects on sexual function of five antihypertensive drugs and nutritional hygienic treatment in hypertensive men an women. Hypertension 1997;29: 8–14.
Language	English

2

Compound	Antihypertensives (C02)
Disease treated	Hypertension
Quantification of adverse effects	Single question from the NIH consensus definition
No. of patients treated	428
Age group	40–70 years
Dose	Various
Treatment consequences	Incidence of erectile dysfunction within 2 years
Efficacy	RR 2.42 (95% CI 1.42–4.13)
Randomization of patients	No
Study quality	**2+**
Reference	2229: Moreira ED Jr, Abdo CH, Torres EB, Lobo CF, Fittipaldi JA. Prevalence and correlates of erectile dysfunction: results of the Brazilian study of sexual behavior. Urology. 2001 Oct;58(4):583–8.
Language	English

Compound	Antihypertensives (C02)
Disease treated	Hypertension
Quantification of adverse effects	Erection, response to intracavernous papaverine
No. of patients treated	427
Age group	Old
Treatment period	Continuous
Dose	Various
Treatment consequences	Erectile function in response to papaverin, improvement
Efficacy	Better in β-blockers than in thiazides
Randomization of patients	No
Study quality	**2–**
Reference	1562: Muller SC, el-Damanhoury H, Ruth J, Lue TF. Hypertension and impotence. Eur Urol. 1991;19(1):29–34.
Language	English

Compound	Antihypertensives (C02)
Disease treated	Hypertension
Quantification of adverse effects	IIEF
No. of patients treated	315

Age group	35–75 years
Treatment period	No treatment
Treatment consequences	Prevalence of erectile dysfunction as compared with normotensive men
Efficacy	23.2% of patients, 11% of controls, $p<0.05$
Randomization of patients	No
Study quality	**2–**
Reference	2236: Roumeguere T, Wespes E, Carpentier Y, Hoffmann P, Schulman CC. Erectile dysfunction is associated with a high prevalence of hyperlipidemia and coronary heart disease risk. Eur Urol. 2003 Sep;44(3):355–9.
Language	English

Compound	Antihypertensives (C02)
Disease treated	Hypertension
Quantification of adverse effects	Sexual function questionnaire
No. of patients treated	194
Age group	52 years (mean)
Dose	Various
Treatment consequences	Incidence of erectile dysfunction within 8 years in treated hypertension
Efficacy	OR 1.52 (95% CI 1.11–2.07)
Randomization of patients	No
Study quality	**2++**
Reference	2204: Johannes CB, Araujo AB, Feldman HA, Derby CA, Kleinman KP, McKinlay JB. Incidence of erectile dysfunction in men 40 to 69 years old: longitudinal results from the Massachusetts male aging study. J Urol. 2000 Feb;163(2):460–3.
Language	English

Compound	Antihypertensives (C02)
Disease treated	Hypertension
Quantification of adverse effects	Sexual function questionnaire
No. of patients treated	101
Age group	Middle-aged
Treatment period	Various
Dose	Various

2

Treatment consequences	Prevalence of erectile dysfunction as compared with normotensive men
Efficacy	27%, mainly associated with intermittent claudication and ischaemic heart disease
Randomization of patients	No
Study quality	**2–**
Reference	2240: Jensen J, Lendorf A, Stimpel H, Frost J, Ibsen H, Rosenkilde P. The prevalence and etiology of impotence in 101 male hypertensive outpatients. Am J Hypertens. 1999 Mar;12(3):271–5.
Language	English

Compound	Antihypertensives (C02)
Disease treated	Hypertension
Quantification of adverse effects	Erectile function
Age group	Old
Treatment consequences	Erectile function, impairment
Efficacy	Dependent on antihypertensive classes
Remarks	Diuretics, centrally acting sympatholytic drugs, β-blockers have a greater impact ; calcium antagonists and ACE inhibitors lower impact
Study quality	**4 (review)**
Reference	1156: Fogari R, Zoppi A. Effects of antihypertensive therapy on sexual activity in hypertensive men. Curr Hypertens Rep. 2002 Jun;4(3):202–10.
Language	English

Compound	Antihypertensives (C02)
Disease treated	Hypertension
Quantification of adverse effects	Erectile function
Age group	All ages
Treatment consequences	Erectile function, impairment
Efficacy	Dependent on drug type
Remarks	"In general, thiazide diuretics and beta-blockers seem to cause ED more often. In contrast, the alpha-blocker, doxazosin, has not been associated with an increased incidence of ED as a side effect".

Study quality	**4 (review)**
Reference	1195: Mikhailidis DP, Khan MA, Milionis HJ, Morgan RJ. The treatment of hypertension in patients with erectile dysfunction. Curr Med Res Opin. 2000;16 Suppl 1:s31–6.
Language	English

Compound	Antihypertensives (C02)
Disease treated	Coronary artery disease
Quantification of adverse effects	Erectile function assessed by rigiscan
Age group	Old
Treatment consequences	Erectile function, impairment
Efficacy	Dependent on medication
Remarks	Effect of antihypertensive drugs on sleep-related erectile function remains unclear.
Study quality	**4 (review)**
Reference	1284: Rosen RC, Weiner DN. Cardiovascular disease and sleep-related erections. J Psychosom Res. 1997 Jun;42(6):517–30.
Language	English

Compound	Antihypertensives (C02)
Disease treated	Hypertension
Quantification of adverse effects	Sexual function questionnaires
Age group	All ages
Treatment consequences	Erectile function, unaltered
Remarks	"Based on the data reviewed, there is no definite evidence of an increased prevalence of sexual dysfunction in treated hypertensive men. Despite this ... the majority of authors … suggest that hypotensive therapy is an important cause of sexual dysfunction… an area in need of considerable research. It is not clear from the reported studies whether the impairment is due to the drugs, the influence of the disease, or both".
Study quality	**4 (review)**
Reference	1458: Bansal S: Sexual dysfunction in hypertensive men. A critical review of the literature. Hypertension 1988; 12: 1–10.
Language	English

Compound	Antihypertensives (C02)
Disease treated	Hypertension
Quantification of adverse effects	Sexual function questionnaire
No. of patients treated	31,742
Age group	53–90 years
Treatment period	No treatment
Treatment consequences	Prevalence of erectile dysfunction as compared with normotensive men
Efficacy	RR 1.2 (95% CI 1.1–1.3)
Randomization of patients	No
Study quality	**2++**
Reference	2210: Bacon CG, Mittleman MA, Kawachi I, Giovannucci E, Glasser DB, Rimm EB. Sexual function in men older than 50 years of age: results from the health professionals follow-up study. Ann Intern Med. 2003;139(3):161–8.
Language	English

Compound	Antihypertensives (C02)
Disease treated	Hypertension
Quantification of adverse effects	IIEF
No. of patients treated	2476
Age group	25–70 years
Treatment period	No treatment
Treatment consequences	Prevalence of erectile dysfunction as compared with normotensive men
Efficacy	OR 1.58 (95% CI 1.11–2.24)
Randomization of patients	No
Study quality	**2++**
Reference	2215: Martin-Morales A, Sanchez-Cruz JJ, Saenz de Tejada I, Rodriguez-Vela L, Jimenez-Cruz JF, Burgos-Rodriguez RJ. Prevalence and independent risk factors for erectile dysfunction in Spain: results of the Epidemiologia de la Disfuncion Erectil Masculina Study. Urol. 2001 Aug;166(2):569–74.
Language	English

Compound	Antihypertensives (C02)
Disease treated	Hypertension
Quantification of adverse effects	Single question from the NIH consensus definition
No. of patients treated	428
Age group	40–70 years
Treatment period	No treatment
Treatment consequences	Prevalence of erectile dysfunction as compared with normotensive men
Efficacy	RR 1.89 (95% CI 1.07–3.37)
Randomization of patients	No
Study quality	**2+**
Reference	2213: Moreira ED Jr, Lobo CF, Diament A, Nicolosi A, Glasser DB. Incidence of erectile dysfunction in men 40 to 69 years old: results from a population-based cohort study in Brazil. Urology. 2003 Feb;61(2):431–6.
Language	English

Compound	α-adrenoreceptor antagonists (C02CA)
Disease treated	Erectile dysfunction in diabetes mellitus
Quantification of dysfunction	Erectile function
No. of patients treated	3160
Age group	Middle-aged
Treatment period	Continuous
Dose	Various
Treatment consequences	Erectile function, impairment
Efficacy	Increase of risk by alpha blockers (OR=1.54, 95% CI 1.11, 2.12)
Randomization of patients	No
Study quality	**2+**
Reference	1641: Blumentals WA, Brown RR, Gomez-Caminero A. Antihypertensive treatment and erectile dysfunction in a cohort of type II diabetes patients. Int J Impot Res. 2003 Oct;15(5):314–7.
Language	English

Compound	Moxonidine (C02AC05)+metoprolol (C07AB02)
Disease treated	Erectile dysfunction in hypertension
Quantification of dysfunction	Erectile function
No. of patients treated	11
Age group	Middle-aged
Treatment period	8 weeks+8 weeks
Dose	0.4 mg/days
Treatment consequences	Erectile function, improvement
Efficacy	After mononidine; again impairment after metoprolol
Randomization of patients	No
Study quality	**3**
Reference	1596: Piha J, Kaaja R. Effects of moxonidine and metoprolol in penile circulation in hypertensive men with erectile dysfunction: results of a pilot study. Int J Impot Res. 2003 Aug;15(4):287–9.
Language	English

Compound	Monoamine oxidase type-A inhibitors (C02KC)
Disease treated	Depression
Quantification of adverse effects	Erectile function
Age group	Young
Treatment consequences	Erectile function, impairment
Efficacy	Common in depressive patients
Randomization of patients	No
Study quality	**1+ (structured review)**
Reference	1031: Baldwin DS. Sexual dysfunction associated with antidepressant drugs. Expert Opin Drug Saf. 2004 Sep;3(5):457–70.
Language	English

Compound	Yohimbine (not listed)
Disease treated	Erectile dysfunction
Quantification of dysfunction	Erectile function
Age group	Old

Treatment consequences	Erectile function, improvement
Efficacy	Moderate
Randomization of patients	In part
Study quality	**4 (review)**
Reference	1172: Tam SW, Worcel M, Wyllie M. Yohimbine: a clinical review. Pharmacol Ther. 2001 Sep;91(3):215–43.
Language	English

C03 Diuretics

Diuretics used in treatment of hypertension impair sexual function as proved in controlled studies. In case-control studies, the prevalence of erectile dysfunction was found to be significantly enhanced in patients on diuretics. When applied in diabetes mellitus, they may reduce the intrinsic risk of erectile dysfunction (Blumentals et al. 2003).

Overall level of evidence of adverse effects: A

Compound	Diuretics (C03)
Disease treated	Hypertension
Quantification of adverse effects	Erectile function
No. of patients treated	3160
Age group	Middle-aged
Treatment period	Various
Dose	Various
Treatment consequences	Erectile function, impairment
Efficacy	Reduced risk on diuretics (OR=0.73, 95% CI=0.54, 0.99).
Randomization of patients	No
Study quality	**2–**
Reference	1641: Blumentals WA, Brown RR, Gomez-Caminero A. Antihypertensive treatment and erectile dysfunction in a cohort of type II diabetes patients. Int J Impot Res. 2003 Oct;15(5):314–7.
Language	English

Compound	Diuretics (C03)
Disease treated	Hypertension
Quantification of adverse effects	Sexual function questionnaire
No. of patients treated	2837
Age group	55–75 years
Treatment period	5 years
Dose	Various
Treatment consequences	Prevalence of erectile dysfunction as compared with men not using diuretics
Efficacy	RR 1.3 (95% CI 0.7–2.4)
Randomization of patients	No
Study quality	**2+**
Reference	2224: Shiri R, Koskimaki J, Hakkinen J, Auvinen A, Tammela TL, Hakama M. Cardiovascular drug use and the incidence of erectile dysfunction. Int J Impot Res 2007 Mar–Apr;19(2):208–12.
Language	English

Compound	Diuretics (C03)
Disease treated	Hypertension
Quantification of adverse effects	Interview by general practitioner
No. of patients treated	2010
Age group	>18 years
Treatment period	Various
Dose	Various
Treatment consequences	Prevalence of erectile dysfunction as compared with men not using diuretics
Efficacy	RR 3.1 (95% CI 1.4–6.9)
Randomization of patients	No
Study quality	**2–**
Reference	2231: Ricci E, Parazzini F, Mirone V, Imbimbo C, Palmieri A, Bortolotti A, Cintio E di, Landoni M, Lavezzari M. Current drug use as risk factor for erectile dysfunction: results from an Italian epidemiological study. Int J Impot Res. 2003 Jun;15(3):221–4.
Language	English

Compound	Thiazide (C03AA)
Disease treated	Hypertension
Quantification of adverse effects	Sexual function questionnaires
No. of patients treated	697
Age group	21–65 years
Treatment period	6 months
Dose	Various
Treatment consequences	Sexual function, impairment
Efficacy	Sexual satisfaction decreased by 0.27, not in atenolol
Randomization of patients	Yes
Dose arms 1–3	Chlorthalidone; atenolol; placebo
Remarks	Measures of well-being and sexual satisfaction asked on a four-point scale (not a standardized questionnaire).
Study quality	**1+**
Reference	1451: Wassertheil-Smoller S, Blaufox MD, Oberman A, Davis BR, Swencionis C, O'Connell Knerr M, Hawkins CM, Langford HG. Effect of antihypertensives on sexual function and quality of life: The TAIM study. Ann Intern Med 1991;114: 613–620.
Language	English

Compound	Hydrochlorothiazide (C03AA03)
Disease treated	Hypertension
Quantification of adverse effects	Sexual function questionnaires
No. of patients treated	176
Age group	35–70 years
Treatment period	2 months
Dose	50 mg/day
Treatment consequences	Sexual function, impairment
Efficacy	Erection score in hydrochlorothiazide group 1.0; in h+KCl group 0.5; in placebo group 0.0
Randomization of patients	Yes
Dose arms 1–3	Hydrochlorothiazide; h+KCl; placebo

Remarks	"Our analysis found that the relationship between randomised diuretic therapy and increase sexual dysfunction remained significant when controlling for age, diabetes mellitus, and the use of a nondiuretic antihypertensive medication".
Study quality	**1+**
Reference	1452: Chang SW, Fine R, Siegel D et al. The impact of diuretic therapy on reported sexual function. Arch Intern Med 1991;151: 2402–2408.
Language	English

Compound	Hydrochlorothiazide (C03AA03)
Disease treated	Hypertension
Quantification of adverse effects	Nocturnal penile tumescence (NPT)
No. of patients treated	12
Age group	Old
Treatment period	6 months
Dose	Various
Treatment consequences	Erections nocturnal, decrease of duration
Efficacy	No significant difference between groups
Randomization of patients	Yes
Dose arms 1–3	Titrated hydrochlorothiazid; titrated prazosin; placebo
Study quality	**1+**
Reference	1453: Scharf MB, Mayleben DW. Comparative effects of prazosin and hydrochlorothiazide on sexual function in hypertensive men. Am J Med 1989;86: 110–112.
Language	English

Compound	Trichloromethiazide (C03AA06)
Disease treated	Hypertension
Quantification of adverse effects	Erectile function questionnaire, hormones
No. of patients treated	156
Age group	Old
Treatment period	1 year
Dose	4 mg/day
Treatment consequences	Erectile function unaltered, testosterone levels unaltered
Efficacy	Impairment after 4 weeks but unaltered after 1 year

Randomization of patients	No
Dose arms 1–3	Trichloromethiazide; atenolol; captopril
Study quality	**2+**
Reference	1604: Suzuki H, Tominaga T, Kumagai H, Saruta T. Effects of first-line antihypertensive agents on sexual function and sex hormones. J Hypertens Suppl. 1988 Dec;6(4):S649–51.
Language	English

C04 Vasodilators

Drugs acting as vasodilators in the coronary system as well as in peripheral arterial systems showed various side effects on sexual functions. Their use increases the risk of suffering from erectile dysfunction (OR significantly different from 1).

Overall level of evidence for adverse effects: B

On the other hand, the drugs act in the cavernous tissue and may be useful in improving erectile function. They are, however, of limited effectiveness.

Overall level of evidence of positive effects: C
Overall level of evidence of adverse effects compromising effectiveness: C

Compound	Peripheral vasodilators (C04)
Disease treated	Peripheral vascular disorder
Quantification of adverse effects	Physicians diagnosis
No. of patients treated	12,825; 12,825
Age group	43.9 years (mean)
Treatment period	No treatment
Treatment consequences	Prevalence of peripheral vascular disease in erectile dysfunction
Efficacy	OR 1.75 (95% CI 1.06–2.90)
Randomization of patients	No
Study quality	**2–**
Reference	2230: Blumentals WA, Gomez-Caminero A, Joo S, Vannappagari V. Is erectile dysfunction predictive of peripheral vascular disease? Aging Male. 2003 Dec;6(4):217–21.
Language	English

2

Compound	Peripheral vasodilators (C04)
Disease treated	Peripheral vascular disorder
Quantification of adverse effects	Sexual function questionnaire
No. of patients treated	2674
Age group	20–70 years
Treatment period	Various
Dose	Various
Treatment consequences	Prevalence of erectile dysfunction as compared with patients not suffering from peripheral vascular disorders
Efficacy	OR 2.44, 95% CI (1.65–3.74)
Randomization of patients	No
Study quality	**2–**
Reference	2220: Safarinejad MR. Prevalence and risk factors for erectile dysfunction in a population-based study in Iran. Int J Impot Res. 2003 Aug;15(4):246–52.
Language	English

Compound	Topical vasodilators (C04A)
Disease treated	Erectile dysfunction
Quantification of dysfunction	Erectile function
Age group	Old
Treatment consequences	Erectile function, impairment
Efficacy	Various efficacy
Side effects compromising effectiveness	Not mentioned
Randomization of patients	No
Study quality	**4 (review)**
Reference	1225: Floth A. Topical therapy in erectile dysfunction. Wien Med Wochenschr. 2000;150(1–2):14–7.
Language	German

Compound	Tolazoline (C04AB02)
Disease treated	Cavernous tissue in vitro
Quantification of dysfunction	Muscle relaxation
No. of patients treated	16

Age group	42–68 years
Treatment period	In vitro
Dose	5×10^{-4} g
Treatment consequences	Cavernous tissue, relaxation
Efficacy	Poor
Study quality	**2–**
Reference	1438: Barbanti G, Beneforti P, Lapini A, Turini D. Relaxation of isolated corpus cavernosum induced by smooth-muscle relaxant drugs. A comparative study. Urol Res. 1988;16(4):299–302.
Language	English

Compound	Phenoxybenzamine (C04AX02); papaverine–phenotolamine
Disease treated	Erectile dysfunction, vascular
Quantification of dysfunction	Erectile function
No. of patients treated	11
Age group	Old
Treatment period	Single dose
Dose	n.g.
Treatment consequences	Erectile function, tumescence
Efficacy	In all patients to various degree
Side effects compromising effectiveness	Not mentioned
Randomization of patients	Yes
Dose arms 1–3	Phenoxybenzamine; papaverine+phentolamine; placebo
Study quality	**2–**
Reference	1549: Szasz G, Stevenson RW, Lee L, Sanders HD. Induction of penile erection by intracavernosal injection: a double-blind comparison of phenoxybenzamine versus papaverine–phentolamine versus saline. Arch Sex Behav. 1987 Oct;16(5):371–8.
Language	English

Compound	Forskolin (not listed), alprostadil, papaverine, phentolamine
Disease treated	Erectile dysfunction
Quantification of dysfunction	Erectile function

No. of patients treated	31
Age group	Old
Treatment period	n.g.
Dose	n.g.
Treatment consequences	Erectile rigidity, improvement
Efficacy	61% of patients
Side effects compromising effectiveness	None
Randomization of patients	No
Dose arms 1–3	Forskolin; other intracavernous drugs
Study quality	**2–**
Reference	1506: Mulhall JP, Daller M, Traish AM, Gupta S, Park K, Salimpour P, Payton TR, Krane RJ, Goldstein I. Intracavernosal forskolin: role in management of vasculogenic impotence resistant to standard 3-agent pharmacotherapy. J Urol. 1997 Nov;158(5):1752–8; discussion 1758–9.
Language	English

C07 Beta-blocking Agents

When taking history in men who complain of erectile dysfunction, patients and physicians accept the medication of beta-blocking agents as the causal explanation of the disease. This group of drugs is suggested to exert impotence most effectively. The risk of having erectile dysfunction was found to be increased in men using these drugs in large case-controlled studies; however, controlled prospective studies demonstrated a different figure. Only atenolol was shown to impair sexual function after extended use. The incidence of erectile dysfunction during treatment of hypertension with beta-blocking agents appears to be influenced by the expectations of the patient (Silvestri et al. 2003).

Overall level of evidence of adverse effects: B

Compound	Beta-blocking agents (C07A)
Disease treated	Hypertension
Quantification of adverse effects	Sexual function questionnaire

No. of patients treated	31,742
Age group	53–90 years
Treatment period	Various
Dose	Various
Treatment consequences	Prevalence of erectile dysfunction as compared with men not using beta-blocking agents
Efficacy	RR 1.2 (95% CI 1.1–1.5)
Randomization of patients	No
Study quality	**2++**
Reference	2210: Bacon CG, Mittleman MA, Kawachi I, Giovannucci E, Glasser DB, Rimm EB. Sexual function in men older than 50 years of age: results from the health professionals follow-up study. Ann Intern Med. 2003;139(3):161–8.
Language	English

Compound	Beta-blocking agents (C07A)
Disease treated	Hypertension
Quantification of adverse effects	Sexual function questionnaire
No. of patients treated	2837
Age group	55–75 years
Treatment period	Various
Dose	Various
Treatment consequences	Prevalence of erectile dysfunction as compared with men not using beta-blocking agents
Efficacy	RR 1.7 (95% CI 0.9–3.2)
Randomization of patients	No
Study quality	**2+**
Reference	2224: Shiri R, Koskimaki J, Hakkinen J, Auvinen A, Tammela TL, Hakama M. Cardiovascular drug use and the incidence of erectile dysfunction. Int J Impot Res 2007 Mar–Apr;19(2):208–12.
Language	English

Compound	Beta-blocking agents (C07A)
Disease treated	Healthy
Quantification of adverse effects	Erectile function
No. of patients treated	30
Age group	Middle-aged

2

Treatment period	4 weeks
Dose	Various
Treatment consequences	Erectile function, impairment
Efficacy	No conclusive effects
Randomization of patients	Yes
Dose arms 1–3	Atenolol; metoprolol; propranolol
Remarks	Personal vulnerability to propranolol
Study quality	**1+**
Reference	1598: Rosen RC, Kostis JB, Jekelis AW. Beta-blocker effects on sexual function in normal males. Arch Sex Behav. 1988 Jun;17(3):241–55.
Language	English

Compound	Beta-blocking agents (C07A)
Disease treated	Coronary artery disease
Quantification of adverse effects	Erectile function
Age group	Old
Treatment consequences	Erectile function, impairment
Efficacy	Frequent side effect
Study quality	**4 (review)**
Reference	1062: Toda N. Vasodilating beta-adrenoceptor blockers as cardiovascular therapeutics. Pharmacol Ther. 2003 Dec;100(3):215–34.
Language	English

Compound	Metoprolol (C07AB02)
Disease treated	Coronary heart disease
Quantification of adverse effects	Erectile function
No. of patients treated	65
Age group	Middle-aged
Treatment period	4 months
Dose	95mg/day
Treatment consequences	Erectile function according to "Kölner Erhebungsbogen", unaltered
Efficacy	Sex life unaffected
Randomization of patients	Yes

Dose arms 1–3	Metoprolol; placebo
Study quality	**1+**
Reference	1597: Franzen D, Metha A, Seifert N, Braun M, Hopp HW. Effects of beta-blockers on sexual performance in men with coronary heart disease. A prospective, randomized and double blinded study. Int J Impot Res. 2001 Dec;13(6):348–51.
Language	English

Compound	Metoprolol (C07AB02)
Disease treated	Hypertension
Quantification of adverse effects	Erectile function
No. of patients treated	11
Age group	Middle-aged
Treatment period	8 weeks
Dose	100 mg/day
Treatment consequences	Erectile function, impairment
Efficacy	In 9 of 11 patients with metropolol
Randomization of patients	Yes
Dose arms 1–3	Metoprolol; monoxidine
Study quality	**1+**
Reference	1630: Piha J, Kaaja R. Effects of moxonidine and metoprolol in penile circulation in hypertensive men with erectile dysfunction: results of a pilot study. Int J Impot Res. 2003 Aug;15(4):287–9.
Language	English

Compound	Atenolol (C07AB03)
Disease treated	Hypertension
Quantification of adverse effects	Erectile function questionnaire, hormones
No. of patients treated	156
Age group	Old
Treatment period	1 years
Dose	100 mg/day
Treatment consequences	Erectile function, impairment and testosterone level decreased
Efficacy	Mild sexual dysfunction

2

Randomization of patients	No
Study quality	**3**
Reference	1604: Suzuki H, Tominaga T, Kumagai H, Saruta T. Effects of first-line antihypertensive agents on sexual function and sex hormones. J Hypertens Suppl. 1988 Dec;6(4):S649–51.
Language	English

Compound	Atenolol (C07AB03)
Disease treated	Hypertension
Quantification of adverse effects	Sexual function questionnaire
No. of patients treated	110
Age group	40–49 years
Treatment period	16 weeks
Dose	50 mg/day
Treatment consequences	Sexual activity, impairment
Efficacy	Reduced in atenolol, increased in valsartan
Randomization of patients	Yes
Dose arms 1–3	Atenolol; valsartan; placebo
Study quality	**1+**
Reference	1622: Fogari R, Preti P, Derosa G, Marasi G, Zoppi A, Rinaldi A, Mugellini A. Effect of antihypertensive treatment with valsartan or atenolol on sexual activity and plasma testosterone in hypertensive men. Eur J Clin Pharmacol. 2002 Jun;58(3):177–80.
Language	English

Compound	Atenolol (C07AB03)
Disease treated	Cardiovascular disease
Quantification of adverse effects	Sexual function questionnaires
No. of patients treated	96
Age group	52 years (mean)
Treatment period	3 months
Dose	50 mg/day
Treatment consequences	Erectile function, impairment
Efficacy	3.1% of group A, 15.6% of group B, 31.2% of group C

Randomization of patients	Yes
Dose arms 1–3	32 patients blinded to the drug given; 32 informed of the drug given but not its side effects; 32 informed of the side effects on erectile function
Remarks	Knowledge and prejudice about side effects of beta-blockers may contribute to occurrence of erectile function.
Study quality	**2+**
Reference	1560: Silvestri A, Galetta P, Cerquetani E, Marazzi G, Patrizi R, Fini M, Rosano GM. Report of erectile dysfunction after therapy with beta-blockers is related to patient knowledge of side effects and is reversed by placebo. Eur Heart J. 2003 Nov;24(21):1928–32.
Language	English

Compound	Labetalol (C07AG01)
Disease treated	Terminal renal insufficiency
Quantification of adverse effects	Erectile function
No. of patients treated	1
Age group	25
Treatment period	2 months
Dose	800 mg/day
Treatment consequences	Priapism, development
Efficacy	After addition of labetalol
Study quality	**3**
Reference	1383: Law MR, Copland RF, Armitstead JG, Gabriel R. Labetalol and priapism. Br Med J. 1980 Jan 12;280(6207):115.
Language	English

2

C08	Calcium Channel Blockers
	This type of antihypertensive is suggested to exert a limited effect on erectile function. In a large case-control study, a marginal increase of the relative risk in patients on these drugs in comparison with patients not taking calcium channel blockers was found. It remains unclear as to whether the drug or the disease itself is associated with the erectile dysfunction. **Overall level of evidence of adverse effects: D**

Compound	Nifedipine (C08CA05)
Disease treated	Hypertension
Quantification of adverse effects	Erectile function questionnaire, hormones
No. of patients treated	156
Age group	Old
Treatment period	1 year
Dose	80 mg/days
Treatment consequences	Erectile function unaltered, testosterone levels unaltered
Efficacy	In all patients
Randomization of patients	No
Study quality	**3**
Reference	1604: Suzuki H, Tominaga T, Kumagai H, Saruta T. Effects of first-line antihypertensive agents on sexual function and sex hormones. J Hypertens Suppl. 1988 Dec;6(4):S649–51.
Language	English

Compound	Verapamil (C08DA01)
Disease treated	Induratio penis plastica
Quantification of adverse effects	Plaques
No. of patients treated	49
Age group	Old
Treatment period	6 weeks
Dose	Transdermal electromotive
Treatment consequences	Fibrotic plaques
Efficacy	Disappearance in 8%, reduction in 74%, no change in 18% of plaques

Randomization of patients	No
Study quality	**3**
Reference	1619: Stasi SM di, Giannantoni A, Capelli G, Jannini EA, Virgili G, Storti L, Vespasiani G. Transdermal electromotive administration of verapamil and dexamethasone for Peyronie's disease. BJU Int. 2003 Jun;91(9):825–9.
Language	English

Compound	Verapamil (C08DA01)
Disease treated	Cardiac disease
Quantification of adverse effects	Erectile function
No. of patients treated	14
Age group	41–75 years
Treatment period	32 months
Dose	240–480 mg/day
Treatment consequences	Erectile function, impairment
Efficacy	In 3 of 14 patients
Randomization of patients	No
Study quality	**3**
Reference	1387: King BD, Pitchon R, Stern EH, Schweitzer P, Schneider RR, Weiner I. Impotence during therapy with verapamil. Arch Intern Med. 1983 Jun;143(6):1248–9.
Language	English

Compound	Non-selective calcium channel blockers (C08E)
Disease treated	Hypertension
Quantification of adverse effects	Sexual function questionnaire
No. of patients treated	2837
Age group	55–75 years
Treatment period	Various
Dose	Various
Treatment consequences	Prevalence of erectile dysfunction as compared with men not using calcium channel blockers
Efficacy	RR 1.6 (95% CI 1.0–2.4)
Randomization of patients	No

2

Study quality	**2+**
Reference	2224: Shiri R, Koskimaki J, Hakkinen J, Auvinen A, Tammela TL, Hakama M. Cardiovascular drug use and the incidence of erectile dysfunction. Int J Impot Res 2007 Mar–Apr;19(2):208–12.
Language	English

C09	**Agents Acting on the Renin–Angiotensin System**
	There are no reports on sexual side effects. In a large case-control study, however, an increase of the relative risk in patients on these drugs in comparison with patients not taking the drugs was found. Again it remains unclear as to whether the drug or the disease itself is associated with the erectile dysfunction. **Overall level of evidence of adverse effects: C**

Compound	ACE inhibitor (C09A)
Disease treated	Hypertension
Quantification of adverse effects	Erectile function
No. of patients treated	3160
Age group	Middle-aged
Treatment period	Various
Dose	Various
Treatment consequences	Erectile function, impairment
Efficacy	In ACE inhibitors increased risk (OR=1.47, 95% CI=1.21, 1.80)
Randomization of patients	No
Study quality	**3**
Reference	1641: Blumentals WA, Brown RR, Gomez-Caminero A. Antihypertensive treatment and erectile dysfunction in a cohort of type II diabetes patients. Int J Impot Res. 2003 Oct;15(5):314–7.
Language	English

Compound	Agents acting on the renin–angiotensin system (C09)
Disease treated	Hypertension
Quantification of adverse effects	Sexual function questionnaire
No. of patients treated	2837
Age group	55–75 years
Treatment period	Various
Dose	Various
Treatment consequences	Prevalence of of erectile dysfunction as compared with men not using the drugs
Efficacy	RR 2.2 (95% CI 1.0–4.7)
Randomization of patients	No
Study quality	**2+**
Reference	2224: Shiri R, Koskimaki J, Hakkinen J, Auvinen A, Tammela TL, Hakama M. Cardiovascular drug use and the incidence of erectile dysfunction. Int J Impot Res 2007 Mar–Apr;19(2):208–12.
Language	English

Compound	ACE inhibitor (C09A)
Disease treated	Erectile dysfunction, vascular
Quantification of dysfunction	IIEF
No. of patients treated	59
Age group	Old
Treatment period	26 weeks
Dose	n.g.
Treatment consequences	Cavernosal perfusion, improvement
Efficacy	In all patients, no difference between groups
Randomization of patients	Yes
Dose arms 1–3	ACE inhibitor; placebo
Study quality	**1+**
Reference	1640: Speel TG, Kiemeney LA, Thien T, Smits P, Meuleman EJ. Long-term effect of inhibition of the angiotensin-converting enzyme (ACE) on cavernosal perfusion in men with atherosclerotic erectile dysfunction: a pilot study. J Sex Med. 2005 Mar;2(2):207–12.
Language	English

Compound	Captopril (C09AA01)
Disease treated	Hypertension
Quantification of adverse effects	Sexual Symptoms Distress Index
No. of patients treated	213
Age group	35–65 years
Treatment period	6 months
Dose	100 mg/day
Treatment consequences	Sexual function, impairment
Efficacy	No alteration
Randomization of patients	Yes
Dose arms 1–3	Captopril+diuretic; methyldopa; propranolol
Study quality	**1–**
Reference	1354: Croog SH, Levine S, Sudilovsky A, Baume RM, Clive J. Sexual symptoms in hypertensive patients. A clinical trial of antihypertensive medications. Arch Intern Med. 1988 Apr;148(4):788–94.
Language	English

Compound	Captopril (C09AA01)
Disease treated	Hypertension
Quantification of adverse effects	Erectile function questionnaire, hormones
No. of patients treated	156
Age group	Old
Treatment period	1 year
Dose	75 mg/day
Treatment consequences	Erectile function unaltered, testosterone levels unaltered
Randomization of patients	No
Study quality	**3**
Reference	1604: Suzuki H, Tominaga T, Kumagai H, Saruta T. Effects of first-line antihypertensive agents on sexual function and sex hormones. J Hypertens Suppl. 1988 Dec;6(4):S649–51.
Language	English

Compound	Losartan (C09CA01)
Disease treated	Hypertension
Quantification of adverse effects	Erectile function
Age group	Old
Dose	n.g.
Treatment consequences	Erectile function, impairment
Efficacy	No effect
Remarks	Angiotensin II has contractile effects on corporal smooth muscle. Losartian increases relaxation.
Study quality	**4 (review)**
Reference	1119: Ferrario CM, Levy P. Sexual dysfunction in patients with hypertension: implications for therapy. J Clin Hypertens (Greenwich). 2002 Nov–Dec;4(6):424–32.
Language	English

C10 Lipid-modifying Agents

Reviews quote no clear evidence of influences of statins (hydroxymethylglutaryl-CoA reductase inhibitors) or other lipid-modifying agents on erectile function. In case-control studies, there was a significantly increased risk for men suffering from hypercholesterolaemia for having erectile dysfunction. Possibly the disease itself is associated with the erectile dysfunction. No prospective studies are available which correlate lipid lowering and improving of dyslipaemia with erectile function (Schachter 2000).

Overall level of evidence of adverse effects: B

Compound	Lipid-modifying agents (C10)
Disease treated	Hypercholesterolaemia
Quantification of adverse effects	Sexual function questionnaire
No. of patients treated	27,839
Age group	20–75 years
Treatment period	Various
Dose	Various
Treatment consequences	Prevalence of erectile dysfunction as compared with normolipaemic men

Efficacy	16% reporting no erectile dysfunction, 29% reporting erectile dysfunction
Randomization of patients	No
Study quality	**2–**
Reference	2208: Rosen RC, Fisher WA, Eardley I, Niederberger C, Nadel A, Sand M. Men's Attitudes to Life Events and Sexuality (MALES) Study. The multinational Men's Attitudes to Life Events and Sexuality (MALES) study: I. Prevalence of erectile dysfunction and related health concerns in the general population. Curr Med Res Opin. 2004 May;20(5):607–17.
Language	English

Compound	Lipid-modifying agents (C10)
Disease treated	Hypercholesterolaemia
Quantification of adverse effects	IIEF
No. of patients treated	3242
Age group	50–80 years
Treatment period	Various
Dose	Various
Treatment consequences	Prevalence of erectile dysfunction as compared with normolipaemic men
Efficacy	OR 1.19 (95% CI 1.06–1.33)
Randomization of patients	No
Study quality	**2+**
Reference	2211: Rosen R, Altwein J, Boyle P, Kirby RS, Lukacs B, Meuleman E, O'Leary MP, Puppo P, Robertson C, Giuliano F. Lower urinary tract symptoms and male sexual dysfunction: the multinational survey of the aging male (MSAM-7). Eur Urol. 2003 Dec;44(6):637–49.
Language	English

Compound	Lipid-modifying agents (C10)
Disease treated	Hypercholesterolaemia
Quantification of adverse effects	IIEF
No. of patients treated	2476
Age group	25–70 years
Treatment period	Various
Dose	Various

Treatment consequences	Prevalence of erectile dysfunction as compared with men with normolipaemia
Efficacy	OR 1.63 (95% CI 1.07–2.49)
Randomization of patients	No
Study quality	**2++**
Reference	2215: Martin-Morales A, Sanchez-Cruz JJ, Saenz de Tejada I, Rodriguez-Vela L, Jimenez-Cruz JF, Burgos-Rodriguez RJ. Prevalence and independent risk factors for erectile dysfunction in Spain: results of the Epidemiologia de la Disfuncion Erectil Masculina Study. Urol. 2001 Aug;166(2):569–74.
Language	English

Compound	Lipid-modifying agents (C10)
Disease treated	Hypercholesterolaemia
Quantification of adverse effects	Sexual function questionnaire
No. of patients treated	2674
Age group	20–70 years
Treatment period	Various
Dose	Various
Treatment consequences	Prevalence of erectile dysfunction as compared with men with normolipaemia
Efficacy	OR 1.71 (95% CI 1.11–2.65)
Randomization of patients	No
Study quality	**2–**
Reference	2220: Safarinejad MR. Prevalence and risk factors for erectile dysfunction in a population-based study in Iran. Int J Impot Res. 2003 Aug;15(4):246–52.
Language	English

Compound	Atorvastatin (C10AA05)
Disease treated	Erectile dysfunction
Quantification of dysfunction	Erectile function
No. of patients treated	12
Age group	Old
Treatment period	12 weeks
Dose	80 mg/day

2

Treatment consequences	Erectile function, improvement
Efficacy	Increase of domain score of 7.8
Randomization of patients	Yes
Dose arms 1–3	Atorvastatin+sildenafil; atorvastatin+placebo
Study quality	**1+**
Reference	1001: Herrmann HC, Levine LA, Macaluso J, Walsh M, Bradbury D, Schwartz S, Mohler ER, Kimmel SE. Can Atorvastatin improve the response to sildenafil in men with erectile dysfunction not initially responsive to sildenafil? J Sex Med 2006; 3(2): 303–308.
Language	English

Compound	Fibrates (C10AB)
Disease treated	Hyperlipidaemia
Quantification of adverse effects	Erectile function
Age group	Old
Treatment consequences	Erectile function, impairment
Efficacy	No clear evidence of association
Study quality	**4 (review)**
Reference	1165: Rizvi K, Hampson JP, Harvey JN. Do lipid-lowering drugs cause erectile dysfunction? A systematic review. Fam Pract. 2002 Feb;19(1):95–8.
Language	English

Compound	Fibrates (C10AB)
Disease treated	Hyperlipidaemia
Quantification of adverse effects	Erectile function
Age group	All ages
Treatment consequences	Erectile function, impairment
Efficacy	No association
Remarks	No prospective studies are available which correlate lipid lowering and improvment of erectile function
Study quality	**4 (review)**
Reference	1192: Schachter M. Erectile dysfunction and lipid disorders. Curr Med Res Opin. 2000;16 Suppl 1:s9–12.
Language	English

Compound	Gemfibrozil (C10AB04)
Disease treated	Dyslipaemia
Quantification of adverse effects	Erectile function
No. of patients treated	3
Age group	39–56 years
Treatment period	6 weeks
Dose	1200 mg/day
Treatment consequences	Erectile function, impairment
Efficacy	Starting 4 weeks to 7 months after beginning of treatment
Randomization of patients	No
Study quality	**3**
Reference	1365: Figueras A, Castel JM, LaPorte JR, Capella D. Gemfibrozil-induced impotence. Ann Pharmacother. 1993 Jul–Aug;27(7–8):982.
Language	English

Compound	Gemfibrozil (C10AB04)
Disease treated	Coronary artery disease
Quantification of adverse effects	Erectile function
No. of patients treated	1
Age group	53 years
Treatment period	4 weeks
Dose	1200 mg/day
Treatment consequences	Erectile function, impairment
Efficacy	Quick improvement after discontinuation
Study quality	**3**
Reference	1384: Bain SC, Lemon M, Jones AF. Gemfibrozil-induced impotence. Lancet. 1990 Dec 1;336(8727):1389.
Language	English

D04	**Antipruritics**
	There is a single case report on sexual dysfunction caused by methyl bromide in the literature.
	Overall level of evidence of adverse effects: D

Compound	Methyl bromide (D04AA33)
Disease treated	Poisoning
Quantification of adverse effects	Sexual function
No. of patients treated	1
Age group	Old
Treatment period	Continuous
Dose	n.g.
Treatment consequences	Erectile function, impairment
Efficacy	Complete
Remarks	There is only this single report in the literature.
Study quality	**3**
Reference	1571: Park HJ, Lee KM, Nam JK, Park NC. A case of erectile dysfunction associated with chronic methyl bromide intoxication. Int J Impot Res. 2005 Mar–Apr;17(2):207–8.
Language	English

G03	**Sex Hormones and Modulators of the Genital System**
	Testosterone (T)
	Although testosterone, as the male sexual hormone, is essential for growth and differentiation of male sexual function, the association of circulating levels as a result of endogenous production or exogenous supplementation to erectile function is complex. A threshold level seems to be necessary for normal erections. Higher levels do not improve erectile function, but lower levels may induce erectile dysfunction. Treating erectile dysfunction with testosterone supplementation appears to be successful only in hypogonadism. In this stage, the supplementation of testosterone improves the effect of 5-phosphodiesterase inhibitors. It is ineffective when testosterone levels are normal, but the treatment appears to be free of compromising effects.

Overall level of evidence of positive effects: A
Overall level of evidence of adverse effects compromising effectiveness: B

Reports on a stimulation of testosterone production by the anti-oestrogenic compound clomiphene citrate were never confirmed by other groups.

Overall level of positive effects: D

Compound	Testosterone (G03BA03)
Disease treated	Hypogonadism
Quantification of dysfunction	Erectile function
No. of patients treated	656
Treatment consequences	Erectile function, improvement
Efficacy	Effects of T on erectile function inversely related to the mean baseline T concentration
Side effects compromising effectiveness	None
Randomization of patients	Yes
Remarks	T treatment might be useful for improving vasculogenic erectile dysfunction
Study quality	**1++**
Reference	1251: Isidori AM, Giannetta E, Gianfrilli D, Greco EA, Bonifacio V, Aversa A, Isidori A, Fabbri A, Lenzi A. Effects of testosterone on sexual function in men: results of a meta-analysis. Clin Endocrinol (Oxf). 2005 Oct;63(4):381–94.
Language	English

Compound	Testosterone (G03BA03)
Disease treated	Erectile dysfunction in hypogonadism
Quantification of dysfunction	IIEF
No. of patients treated	187
Age group	>45 years
Treatment period	1 year
Dose	250 mg/2 weeks IM
Treatment consequences	PSA level, unaltered

Efficacy	No significant difference between pre- and post-treatment level
Side effects compromising effectiveness	None
Randomization of patients	No
Study quality	**2–**
Reference	1219: El-Sakka AI, Hassoba HM, Elbakry AM, Hassan HA. Prostatic specific antigen in patients with hypogonadism: effect of testosterone replacement. J Sex Med. 2005 Mar;2(2):235–40.
Language	English

Compound	Testosterone (G03BA03)
Disease treated	Erectile dysfunction in diabetes mellitus
Quantification of dysfunction	IIEF
No. of patients treated	120
Age group	43–74 years
Treatment period	2 weeks
Dose	40 mg/day orally
Treatment consequences	Erectile function, improvement
Efficacy	In 84 of 120 sildenafil non-responders, combined therapy with testosterone orally induced a significant increase in IIEF.
Side effects compromising effectiveness	None
Randomization of patients	No
Study quality	**2–**
Reference	1213: Kalinchenko SY, Kozlov GI, Gontcharov NP, Katsiya GV. Oral testosterone undecanoate reverses erectile dysfunction associated with diabetes mellitus in patients failing on sildenafil citrate therapy alone. Aging Male. 2003 Jun;6(2):94–9.
Language	English

Compound	Testosterone (G03BA03)
Disease treated	Cardiac transplants
Quantification of dysfunction	Bone mineral density
No. of patients treated	88
Age group	Old
Treatment period	2 years
Dose	Various
Treatment consequences	Bone mineral density
Efficacy	Decreased in 25% of patients, no increase by T substitution
Study quality	**3**
Reference	1317: Stief J, Sohn HY, Alt A, Uberfuhr P, Theisen K, Stempfle HU. Effect of immunosuppression-induced hypogonadism on bone metabolism after heart transplantation. Dtsch Med Wochenschr. 2004 Jul 30;129(31–32):1674–8.
Language	German

Compound	Testosterone (G03BA03)
Disease treated	Erectile dysfunction in hypogonadism
Quantification of dysfunction	IIEF
No. of patients treated	75
Age group	All ages
Treatment period	12 weeks
Dose	5 mg/day
Treatment consequences	Erectile function, improvement
Efficacy	Better effect of sildenafil when T was added
Side effects compromising effectiveness	None
Randomization of patients	Yes
Dose arms 1–3	T+sildenafil; placebo+sildenafil
Study quality	**1+**
Reference	1202: Shabsigh R, Kaufman JM, Steidle C, Padma-Nathan H. Randomized study of testosterone gel as adjunctive therapy to sildenafil in hypogonadal men with erectile dysfunction who do not respond to sildenafil alone. J Urol. 2004 Aug;172(2):658–63.
Language	English

2

Compound	Testosterone (G03BA03)
Disease treated	Erectile dysfunction in hypogonadism
Quantification of dysfunction	IIEF
No. of patients treated	69
Age group	59 years (mean)
Treatment period	3 months
Dose	5 mg/day
Treatment consequences	Erectile function, improvement
Efficacy	T+tadalafil better than tadalafil alone
Side effects compromising effectiveness	None
Randomization of patients	Yes
Dose arms 1–3	T+tadalafil; tadalafil alone
Study quality	**1+**
Reference	1220: Yassin AA, Saad F, Diede HE. Testosterone and erectile function in hypogonadal men unresponsive to tadalafil: results from an open-label uncontrolled study. Andrologia. 2006 Apr;38(2):61–8.
Language	English

Compound	Testosterone (G03BA03)
Disease treated	Erectile dysfunction in hypogonadism
Quantification of dysfunction	IIEF
No. of patients treated	49
Age group	60.7 years (mean)
Treatment period	20 months
Dose	5 mg/day
Treatment consequences	Erectile function, improvement
Efficacy	31 of 49 patients mean increase from 13.6 to 27
Side effects compromising effectiveness	None
Randomization of patients	No
Study quality	**3**

Reference	1200: Greenstein A, Mabjeesh NJ, Sofer M, Kaver I, Matzkin H, Chen J. Does sildenafil combined with testosterone gel improve erectile dysfunction in hypogonadal men in whom testosterone supplement therapy alone failed? J Urol. 2005 Feb;173(2):530–2.
Language	English

Compound	Testosterone (G03BA03)
Disease treated	Erectile dysfunction not responding to sildenafil
Quantification of dysfunction	IIEF
No. of patients treated	40
Age group	40–70 years
Treatment period	2 months
Dose	1000 mg/12 week
Treatment consequences	Erectile function, improvement
Efficacy	Better effect of sildenafil when T was added
Side effects compromising effectiveness	None
Randomization of patients	No
Study quality	**2–**
Reference	1201: Shamloul R, Ghanem H, Fahmy I, El-Meleigy A, Ashoor S, Elnashaar A, Kamel I. Testosterone therapy can enhance erectile function response to sildenafil in patients with PADAM: a pilot study. J Sex Med. 2005 Jul;2(4):559–64.
Language	English

Compound	Testosterone (G03BA03)
Disease treated	Erectile dysfunction in hypogonadism
Quantification of dysfunction	Measurement of nocturnal penile tumescence (NPT)
No. of patients treated	35
Age group	Old
Treatment period	3 months
Dose	5 mg/day
Treatment consequences	Erectile function, improvement
Efficacy	T treatment for 6 months induced normalization of NPT parameters and restoration of response to sildenafil.

2

Side effects compromising effectiveness	None
Randomization of patients	No
Study quality	**2–**
Reference	1237: Foresta C, Caretta N, Rossato M, Garolla A, Ferlin A. Role of androgens in erectile function. J Urol. 2004 Jun;171(6 Pt 1):2358–62, quiz 2435.
Language	English

Compound	Testosterone (G03BA03)
Disease treated	Erectile dysfunction in hypogonadism
Quantification of dysfunction	IIEF
No. of patients treated	32
Age group	48 years (mean)
Treatment period	1 month
Dose	5 mg/day
Treatment consequences	Erectile function, improvement
Efficacy	Statistical significance was reached for the difference between the baseline and 1 month.
Side effects compromising effectiveness	None
Randomization of patients	No
Study quality	**2–**
Reference	1198: Mulhall JP, Valenzuela R, Aviv N, Parker M. Effect of testosterone supplementation on sexual function in hypogonadal men with erectile dysfunction. Urology. 2004 Feb;63(2):348–52; discussion 352–3.
Language	English

Compound	Testosterone (G03BA03)
Disease treated	Erectile dysfunction in hypogonadism, not responding to sildenafil
Quantification of dysfunction	IIEF
No. of patients treated	32
Age group	All ages

Treatment period	2 months
Dose	40 mg/day orally
Treatment consequences	Erectile function, improvement
Efficacy	In 11 patients with T alone, in 12 patients with T+sildenafil
Side effects compromising effectiveness	None
Randomization of patients	No
Study quality	**2–**
Reference	1203: Hwang TI, Chen HE, Tsai TF, Lin YC. Combined use of androgen and sildenafil for hypogonadal patients unresponsive to sildenafil alone. Int J Impot Res. 2006 Jul–Aug;18(4):400–4. Epub 2006 Jan 5.
Language	English

Compound	Testosterone (G03BA03)
Disease treated	Depression and hypogonadism
Quantification of dysfunction	Erectile function
No. of patients treated	30
Age group	52 years (mean)
Treatment period	6 weeks
Dose	200 mg/week
Treatment consequences	Erectile function, improvement
Efficacy	Self-reported sexual functioning, no between-group difference
Side effects compromising effectiveness	None
Randomization of patients	Yes
Dose arms 1–3	T; placebo
Study quality	**1+**
Reference	1238: Seidman SN, Roose SP. The sexual effects of testosterone replacement in depressed men: randomized, placebo-controlled clinical trial. J Sex Marital Ther. 2006 May–Jun;32(3):267–73.
Language	English

Compound	Testosterone (G03BA03)
Disease treated	Erectile dysfunction in hypogonadism
Quantification of dysfunction	IIEF
No. of patients treated	28
Age group	56 years (mean)
Treatment period	3 months
Dose	80 mg/day orally
Treatment consequences	Erectile function, improvement
Efficacy	Mean IIEF scores from 37.2 to 40.2 after 3 months
Side effects compromising effectiveness	No significant changes in liver function tests, red blood cell count or lipid profiles, no significant adverse reactions leading to cessation
Randomization of patients	No
Study quality	**2–**
Reference	1218: Hong JH, Ahn TY. Oral testosterone replacement in Korean patients with PADAM. Aging Male. 2002 Mar;5(1):52–6.
Language	English

Compound	Testosterone (G03BA03)
Disease treated	Depression and treatment with SSRI
Quantification of adverse effects	Hamilton rating scale
No. of patients treated	26
Age group	46.8 years (mean)
Treatment period	6 weeks
Dose	Escalating doses
Treatment consequences	Hamilton rating scale, improvement
Efficacy	53.8% (7 of 13) in the testosterone group, 23.1% (3 of 13) in the placebo group
Side effects compromising effectiveness	None
Randomization of patients	Yes
Dose arms 1–3	T; placebo
Study quality	**2+**

Reference	1430: Seidman SN, Miyazaki M, Roose SP. Intramuscular testosterone supplementation to selective serotonin reuptake inhibitor in treatment-resistant depressed men: randomized placebo-controlled clinical trial. J Clin Psychopharmacol. 2005 Dec;25(6):584–8.
Language	English

Compound	Testosterone (G03BA03)
Disease treated	Erectile dysfunction in hypogonadism
Quantification of dysfunction	Erectile function
No. of patients treated	23
Age group	Old
Treatment period	60 days
Dose	80 mg/day orally
Treatment consequences	Erectile function, improvement
Efficacy	Restoration of plasma testosterone levels in all patients, but improvement in sexual attitudes and performance in only 61%
Side effects compromising effectiveness	Not mentioned
Randomization of patients	No
Study quality	**2–**
Reference	1234: Morales A, Johnston B, Heaton JP, Lundie M. Testosterone supplementation for hypogonadal impotence: assessment of biochemical measures and therapeutic outcomes. J Urol. 1997 Mar;157(3):849–54.
Language	English

Compound	Testosterone (G03BA03)
Disease treated	Erectile dysfunction, vascular
Quantification of dysfunction	IIEF
No. of patients treated	20
Age group	Old
Treatment period	1 month
Dose	5 mg/day
Treatment consequences	Erectile function, improvement

Efficacy	IIEF score increase in the androgen group increase to 21.8, in the placebo group to 14.4 (p<0.05)
Side effects compromising effectiveness	None
Randomization of patients	Yes
Dose arms 1–3	T; placebo
Study quality	**1+**
Reference	1197: Aversa A, Isidori AM, Spera G, Lenzi A, Fabbri A. Androgens improve cavernous vasodilation and response to sildenafil in patients with erectile dysfunction. Clin Endocrinol (Oxf). 2003 May;58(5):632–8.
Language	English

Compound	Testosterone (G03BA03)
Disease treated	Erectile dysfunction in hypogonadism
Quantification of dysfunction	Erectile function
No. of patients treated	12
Age group	Old
Treatment period	12 months
Dose	1000 mg/12 weeks
Treatment consequences	Erectile function, improvement; occlusion of corporal veins, improvement
Efficacy	5 of 12
Side effects compromising effectiveness	Not mentioned
Randomization of patients	No
Study quality	**3**
Reference	1196: Yassin AA, Saad F, Traish A. Testosterone undecanoate restores erectile function in a subset of patients with venous leakage: a series of case reports. J Sex Med. 2006 Jul;3(4):727–35.
Language	English

Compound	Testosterone (G03BA03)
Disease treated	Erectile dysfunction in hypogonadism after bone marrow transplantation
Quantification of dysfunction	Erectile function

No. of patients treated	8
Age group	22–58 years
Treatment period	6 months
Dose	250 mg/4 weeks
Treatment consequences	Erectile function, improvement
Efficacy	All patients responded favourably.
Side effects compromising effectiveness	None
Randomization of patients	No
Study quality	**3**
Reference	1235: Chatterjee R, Kottaridis PD, McGarrigle HH, Linch DC. Management of erectile dysfunction by combination therapy with testosterone and sildenafil in recipients of high-dose therapy for haematological malignancies. Bone Marrow Transplant. 2002 Apr;29(7):607–10.
Language	English

Compound	Testosterone (G03BA03)
Disease treated	Erectile dysfunction, venous leakage
Quantification of dysfunction	Erectile function
No. of patients treated	1
Age group	56
Treatment period	1 months
Dose	n.g.
Treatment consequences	Erectile function, improvement
Efficacy	Dramatically
Side effects compromising effectiveness	None
Study quality	**3**
Reference	1199: Yassin AA, Saad F. Dramatic improvement of penile venous leakage upon testosterone administration. A case report and review of literature. Andrologia. 2006 Feb;38(1):34–7.
Language	English

Compound	Testosterone (G03BA03)
Disease treated	Hormone deficiency
Quantification of dysfunction	Quality of life (QOL)
Age group	Old
Treatment consequences	QOL, improvement
Efficacy	In most men
Side effects compromising effectiveness	Observation of prostatic side effects necessary
Study quality	**4 (review)**
Reference	1071: Lunenfeld B. Androgen therapy in the aging male. World J Urol. 2003 Nov;21(5):292–305. Epub 2003 Oct 24.
Language	English

Compound	Androgen deprivation (G03BA03)
Disease treated	Prostatic carcinoma
Quantification of dysfunction	Androgen deprivation effects
Age group	Old
Treatment consequences	Androgen deficiency symptoms, sexual dysfunction
Efficacy	Dependent on kind of androgen deprivation
Randomization of patients	No
Study quality	**4 (review)**
Reference	1101: Higano CS. Side effects of androgen deprivation therapy: monitoring and minimizing toxicity. Urology. 2003 Feb;61(2 Suppl 1):32–8.
Language	English

Compound	Clomiphene (not listed)
Pharmacological group	(G03)
Disease treated	Late-onset hypogonadism
Quantification of dysfunction	Hormones; erectile function
No. of patients treated	17
Age group	Middle-aged
Treatment period	2 months
Dose	150 mg/day

Treatment consequences	Hormone levels, alteration; erectile function, alteration
Efficacy	significant increase of LH, FSH, and total and free testosterone levels; no improvement of sexual function
Randomization of patients	Yes
Dose arms 1–3	Clomiphene; placebo
Study quality	**1–**
Reference	1376: Guay AT, Bansal S, Heatley GJ. Effect of raising endogenous testosterone levels in impotent men with secondary hypogonadism: double blind placebo-controlled trial with clomiphene citrate. J Clin Endocrinol Metab. 1995 Dec;80(12):3546–52.
Language	English

G04 Urologicals

G04BE Drugs Used in Erectile Dysfunction

In the past 20 years a number of drugs have been introduced which are able to induce or improve penile erection. There are two main groups of these drugs: the vasoactive drugs applied intracavernously, which cause relaxation of the cavernous smooth muscle and are highly effective in inducing erection, and the 5-phosphodiesterase inhibitors, which may be applied orally. These drugs are designated to treat the disease "erectile dysfunction" and improve sexual health, which is not a severe or life-threatening condition, and treated patients are often otherwise healthy persons; thus, the absence of severe ADEs is essential.

All epidemiological and therapeutic studies agree that the most significant risk factor for the development of erectile dysfunction is age, but also multimorbidity increases the risk.

Overall level of evidence of adverse effects: B

Compound	Drugs used in erectile dysfunction (G04BE)
Disease treated	Erectile dysfunction
Quantification of dysfunction	IIEF
No. of patients treated	2210
Age group	40–79 years
Treatment period	No treatment

2

Treatment consequences	Prevalence of erectile dysfunction
Efficacy	Significantly increasing with age
Randomization of patients	No
Study quality	**2–**
Reference	2221: Lyngdorf P, Hemmingsen L. Epidemiology of erectile dysfunction and its risk factors: a practice-based study in Denmark. Int J Impot Res. 2004 Apr;16(2):105–11.
Language	English

Compound	Drugs used in erectile dysfunction (G04BE)
Disease treated	Erectile dysfunction
Quantification of dysfunction	Standardized sexual function questionnaire
No. of patients treated	655
Age group	>25 years
Treatment period	No treatment
Treatment consequences	Prevalence of erectile dysfunction
Efficacy	Increasing with age; with diabetes mellitus OR 16.7; with hypertension OR 13.5; with cardiac disease OR 16.3
Randomization of patients	No
Study quality	**2–**
Reference	2214: Berrada S, Kadri N, Mechakra-Tahiri S, Nejjari C. Prevalence of erectile dysfunction and its correlates: a population-based study in Morocco. Int J Impot Res. 2003 Apr;15 Suppl 1:S3–7.
Language	English

Compound	Drugs used in erectile dysfunction (G04BE)
Disease treated	Erectile dysfunction
Quantification of dysfunction	Single question from the NIH consensus definition
No. of patients treated	428
Age group	40–70 years
Treatment period	No treatment
Treatment consequences	Prevalence of erectile dysfunction, increment per year of age
Efficacy	RR 1.07 (95% CI 1.04–1.11)

Randomization of patients	No
Study quality	**2+**
Reference	2213: Moreira ED Jr, Lobo CF, Diament A, Nicolosi A, Glasser DB. Incidence of erectile dysfunction in men 40 to 69 years old: results from a population-based cohort study in Brazil. Urology. 2003 Feb;61(2):431–6.
Language	English

Intracavernous Drugs

The injection of alprostadil is followed by penile pain in about 10% or more of patients (up to 29.4%). A study included four men who abstained from sexual activity due to pain after injection (Lee et al. 1989). Prolonged erection is a rare event. Systemic adverse reactions were not described.

Also the injection of papaverine, combined with phentolamine or as a single drug, is followed by discomfort and penile pain. Prolonged erection and priapism was more frequent than after alprostadil; the rate given is up to 18%. Frequent injections may be followed by fibrosis of the corpora cavernosa. Systemic adverse effects were rare.

There are also other studies on both substances which report that there were no significant adverse effects.

Overall level of evidence of positive effects: A

Overall level of evidence of adverse effects compromising effectiveness: B

Compound	Alprostadil (G04BE01)
Disease treated	Erectile dysfunction
Quantification of dysfunction	Erectile function
No. of patients treated	1873
Age group	Old
Treatment consequences	Erectile rigidity, improvement
Efficacy	55% of patients
Side effects compromising effectiveness	Penile pain, urethral trauma

Randomization of patients	No
Study quality	**1+**
Reference	1049: Urciuoli R, Cantisani TA, Carlinil M, Giuglietti M, Botti FM. Prostaglandin E1 for treatment of erectile dysfunction. Cochrane Database Syst Rev. 2004;(2):CD001784.
Language	English

Compound	Alprostadil (G04BE01)
Disease treated	Erectile dysfunction
Quantification of dysfunction	Erectile function
No. of patients treated	1511
Age group	Old
Treatment period	Single dose
Dose	Intraurethrally
Treatment consequences	Erectile rigidity, improvement
Efficacy	58% of patients with "not effective" intracavernous injection
Side effects compromising effectiveness	Penile pain in 7.8% of applications
Randomization of patients	No
Study quality	**2+**
Reference	1503: Engel JD, McVary KT. Transurethral alprostadil as therapy for patients who withdrew from or failed prior intracavernous injection therapy. Urology. 1998 May;51(5):687–92.
Language	English

Compound	Alprostadil (G04BE01), papaverine
Disease treated	Erectile dysfunction
Quantification of dysfunction	Erectile function
No. of patients treated	129
Age group	Old
Treatment period	Single dose
Dose	5 µg, 18 mg
Treatment consequences	Erectile rigidity, improvement
Efficacy	55% alprostadil better than papaverine, 18% papaverine better than alprostadil

Side effects compromising effectiveness	Discomfort during injection in 8.5% on alprostadil, 4.7% on papaverin
Randomization of patients	No
Dose arms 1–3	Alprostadil; papaverine
Study quality	**2–**
Reference	1540: Earle CM, Keogh EJ, Wisniewski ZS, Tulloch AG, Lord DJ, Watters GR, Glatthaar C. Prostaglandin E1 therapy for impotence, comparison with papaverine. J Urol. 1990 Jan;143(1):57–9.
Language	English

Compound	Alprostadil (G04BE01)
Disease treated	Erectile dysfunction
Quantification of dysfunction	Erectile function
No. of patients treated	115
Age group	Old
Treatment period	Test dose
Dose	1000 µg intraurethral
Treatment consequences	Erectile function, improvement
Efficacy	Rigidity score 4 or 5 was achieved in 13.2% after 500µg and 30% after 1000 µg of patients at 30 min.
Side effects compromising effectiveness	47 patients orthostatic hypotension, 21 patients penile pain, penile burning, dizziness, chest pain, 1 patient syncope
Randomization of patients	No
Study quality	**3**
Reference	1243: Fulgham PF, Cochran JS, Denman JL, Feagins BA, Gross MB, Kadesky KT, Kadesky MC, Clark AR, Roehrborn CG. Disappointing initial results with transurethral alprostadil for erectile dysfunction in a urology practice setting. J Urol. 1998 Dec;160(6 Pt 1):2041–6.
Language	English

Compound	Alprostadil (G04BE01)
Disease treated	Erectile dysfunction not responding to sildenafil
Quantification of dysfunction	IIEF
No. of patients treated	67

2

Age group	Old
Treatment period	4 weeks
Dose	40 µg
Treatment consequences	Erectile function, improvement
Efficacy	In questions 3 and 4 in 60 patients, in question 4 in 57 patients
Side effects compromising effectiveness	Penile pain in 25 (29.4%) of 85 patients
Randomization of patients	No
Study quality	**3**
Reference	1236: Shabsigh R, Padma-Nathan H, Gittleman M, McMurray J, Kaufman J, Goldstein I. Intracavernous alprostadil alfadex (EDEX/VIRIDAL) is effective and safe in patients with erectile dysfunction after failing sildenafil (Viagra). Urology. 2000 Apr;55(4):477–80.
Language	English

Compound	Alprostadil (G04BE01), papaverine
Disease treated	Erectile dysfunction, vascular
Quantification of dysfunction	Erectile function
No. of patients treated	54
Age group	Old
Treatment period	Single dose
Dose	20 µg alprostadil, 50 mg papaverine
Treatment consequences	Erectile rigidity, improvement
Efficacy	46% of alprostadil group, 14% of papaverin group
Side effects compromising effectiveness	45% of patients on alprostadil, 44% of patients on papaverine mild pain at the site of injection; in 3 patients dizziness and headache.
Randomization of patients	Yes
Dose arms 1–3	Alprostadil; papaverine
Study quality	**1+**
Reference	1537: Kattan S, Collins JP, Mohr D. Double-blind, cross-over study comparing prostaglandin E1 and papaverine in patients with vasculogenic impotence. Urology. 1991 Jun;37(6):516–8.
Language	English

Compound	Alprostadil (G04BE01), papaverine
Disease treated	Erectile dysfunction
Quantification of dysfunction	Erectile function
No. of patients treated	52
Age group	Old
Treatment period	Single dose
Dose	n.g.
Treatment consequences	Erectile rigidity, improvement
Efficacy	81% of alprostadil group, 89% of papaverine group
Side effects compromising effectiveness	Penile pain in a relevant number of applications
Randomization of patients	Yes
Dose arms 1–3	Alprostadil; papaverine
Study quality	**1+**
Reference	1535: Mahmoud KZ, el Dakhli MR, Fahmi IM, Abdel-Aziz AB. Comparative value of prostaglandin E1 and papaverine in treatment of erectile failure: double-blind crossover study among Egyptian patients. J Urol. 1992 Mar;147(3):623–6.
Language	English

Compound	Alprostadil (G04BE01), papaverine, phentolamine
Disease treated	Erectile dysfunction, vascular
Quantification of dysfunction	Erectile function
No. of patients treated	48
Age group	Old
Treatment period	Single dose
Dose	Various
Treatment consequences	Erectile rigidity, improvement
Efficacy	Two-thirds of patients
Side effects compromising effectiveness	Alprostadil: 20 of 25 pain on injection, 4 men sufficient to preclude sexual activity. Papaverine: 1 of 25 pain on injection
Randomization of patients	No
Study quality	**2–**

Reference	1544: Lee LM, Stevenson RW, Szasz G. Prostaglandin E1 versus phentolamine/papaverine for the treatment of erectile impotence: a double-blind comparison. J Urol. 1989 Mar;141(3):549–50.
Language	English

Compound	Alprostadil (G04BE01), phentolamine
Disease treated	Erectile dysfunction
Quantification of dysfunction	Erectile function
No. of patients treated	42
Age group	Old
Treatment period	14 months
Dose	10 µg+0.5 mg
Treatment consequences	Erectile rigidity, improvement
Efficacy	10 of 42 patients
Side effects compromising effectiveness	5 patients priapism, 4 patients severe pain, 1 patient fibrosis
Study quality	**3**
Reference	1515: Meinhardt W, Fuente RB de la, Lycklama a Nijeholt AA, Vermeij P, Zwartendijk J. Prostaglandin E1 with phentolamine for the treatment of erectile dysfunction. Int J Impot Res. 1996 Mar;8(1):5–7.
Language	English

Compound	Alprostadil (G04BE01)
Disease treated	Erectile dysfunction
Quantification of dysfunction	Erectile function
No. of patients treated	40
Age group	Old
Treatment period	Test dose
Dose	20 µg
Treatment consequences	Erectile function, improvement
Efficacy	Patients with central neurogenic erectile dysfunction required a dose of 5 µg, men with vascular etiologies required 20 µg
Side effects compromising effectiveness	Not mentioned

Randomization of patients	No
Study quality	**3**
Reference	1241: Ismail M, Abbott L, Hirsch IH. Experience with intracavernous PGE-1 in the treatment of erectile dysfunction: dose considerations and efficacy. Int J Impot Res. 1997 Mar;9(1):39–42.
Language	English

Compound	Alprostadil (G04BE01)+calcitonin gene-related peptide (not listed)
Disease treated	Erectile dysfunction
Quantification of dysfunction	Erectile function
No. of patients treated	28
Age group	Old
Treatment period	Single dose
Dose	10 µg
Treatment consequences	Erectile function, improvement
Efficacy	70% of patients
Side effects compromising effectiveness	Not mentioned
Randomization of patients	No
Study quality	**3**
Reference	1527: Truss MC, Becker AJ, Thon WF, Kuczyk M, Djamilian MH, Stief CG, Jonas U. Intracavernous calcitonin gene-related peptide plus prostaglandin E1: possible alternative to penile implants in selected patients. Eur Urol. 1994;26(1):40–5.
Language	English

Compound	Alprostadil (G04BE01), papaverine, sildenafil
Disease treated	Erectile dysfunction
Quantification of dysfunction	Doppler ultrasound, penis
No. of patients treated	20
Age group	Old
Treatment period	Single dose
Dose	10 µg

2

Treatment consequences	Erectile function, duplex sonography, improvement
Efficacy	Identical results with compounds, but sildenafil most convenient
Side effects compromising effectiveness	No patient had side effects or complications from intracavernosal vasoactive agent injection or oral sildenafil citrate.
Randomization of patients	No
Dose arms 1–3	Alprostadil; papaverine; sildenafil
Study quality	**2–**
Reference	1493: Bacar MM, Batislam E, Altinok D, Yilmaz E, Bacar H. Sildenafil citrate for penile hemodynamic determination: an alternative to intracavernosal agents in Doppler ultrasound evaluation of erectile dysfunction. Urology. 2001 Apr;57(4):623–6; discussion 626–7.
Language	English

Compound	Alprostadil (G04BE01), papaverine, phentolamine
Disease treated	Erectile dysfunction
Quantification of dysfunction	Erectile function
No. of patients treated	20
Age group	Old
Treatment period	Two times
Dose	Various
Treatment consequences	Erectile rigidity, improvement
Efficacy	73% of a+p+p group, 28% of p+p group
Side effects compromising effectiveness	Two-drug solution: no pain after injection, one prolonged erection; three-drug solution: three patients pain after injection, two prolonged erections
Randomization of patients	No
Dose arms 1–3	Alprostadil+papaverine+phentolamine; papaverine+phentolamine
Study quality	**2–**
Reference	1518: Shenfeld O, Hanani J, Shalhav A, Vardi Y, Goldwasser B. Papaverine–phentolamine and prostaglandin E1 versus papaverine–phentolamine alone for intracorporeal injection therapy: a clinical double-blind study. J Urol. 1995 Sep;154(3):1017–9.
Language	English

Compound	Alprostadil (G04BE01), papaverine
Disease treated	Erectile dysfunction
Quantification of dysfunction	Erectile function
No. of patients treated	15
Age group	Old
Treatment period	Single dose
Dose	10 µg
Treatment consequences	Erectile rigidity, improvement
Efficacy	9 of 15 patients
Side effects compromising effectiveness	No significant side effects
Randomization of patients	Cross-over
Dose arms 1–3	10 µg alprostadil; 30 mg papaverin
Study quality	**2–**
Reference	1545: Sarosdy MF, Hudnall CH, Erickson DR, Hardin TC, Novicki DE. A prospective double–blind trial of intracorporeal papaverine versus prostaglandin E1 in the treatment of impotence. J Urol. 1989 Mar;141(3):551–3.
Language	English

Compound	Alprostadil (G04BE01), papaverine, phentolamine
Disease treated	Erectile dysfunction
Quantification of dysfunction	Erectile function
No. of patients treated	12
Age group	52 years (mean)
Treatment period	Single dose
Dose	10 µg
Treatment consequences	Erection, rigid; 75% burning sensations
Efficacy	11 of 12 patients
Side effects compromising effectiveness	75% of patients burning sensations during the entire period of erection
Randomization of patients	No
Dose arms 1–3	Alprostadil; papaverine+phentolamine
Study quality	**2–**

Reference	1547: Waldhauser M, Schramek P. Efficiency and side effects of prostaglandin E1 in the treatment of erectile dysfunction. J Urol. 1988 Sep;140(3):525–7.
Language	English

Compound	Alprostadil (G04BE01)
Disease treated	Erectile dysfunction
Quantification of dysfunction	Erectile function
Age group	Old
Treatment period	On demand
Dose	Cream
Treatment consequences	Erectile function, improvement
Efficacy	Good results in patients with mild symptoms
Side effects compromising effectiveness	No significant side effects
Randomization of patients	Yes
Study quality	**4 (review)**
Reference	1052: Becher E. Topical alprostadil cream for the treatment of erectile dysfunction. Expert Opin Pharmacother. 2004 Mar;5(3):623–32.
Language	English

Compound	Papaverine (G04BE02), alprostadil
Disease treated	Erectile dysfunction
Quantification of dysfunction	Erectile function
No. of patients treated	516
Age group	Old
Treatment period	Single dose
Dose	15 mg papaverine, 7–15 μg alprostadil+
Treatment consequences	Erectile rigidity, improvement
Efficacy	60% of alprostadil group, 15% papaverine group
Side effects compromising effectiveness	Not mentioned
Randomization of patients	No

Dose arms 1–3	Papaverine; alprostadil
Study quality	**2–**
Reference	1514: Purvis K, Brekke I, Christiansen E. Determinants of satisfactory rigidity after intracavernosal injection with prostaglandin E1 in men with erectile failure. Int J Impot Res. 1996 Mar;8(1):9–16.
Language	English

Compound	Papaverine (G04BE02), alprostadil, phentolamine, atropine
Disease treated	Erectile dysfunction
Quantification of dysfunction	Erectile function
No. of patients treated	230
Age group	Old
Treatment period	Single dose
Dose	50 mg papaverine+10 µg alprostadil+0.2 mg phentolamine+0.075 mg atropin
Treatment consequences	Erectile rigidity, improvement
Efficacy	45.6% of patients in both groups
Side effects compromising effectiveness	In both groups, about 50% of patients mentioned some painful sensation without significant difference.
Randomization of patients	Yes
Dose arms 1–3	Combination+atropine; combination without atropine
Study quality	**1+**
Reference	1505: Sogari PR, Teloken C, Souto CA. Atropine role in the pharmacological erection test: study of 228 patients. J Urol. 1997 Nov;158(5):1760–3.
Language	English

Compound	Papaverine (G04BE02), phentolamine, alprostadil
Disease treated	Erectile dysfunction
Quantification of dysfunction	Erectile function
No. of patients treated	180
Age group	50.5 years (mean)
Treatment period	1 week
Dose	Papaverine 5–20 mg, phentoalamine 1mg; alprostadil 2.5–10 µg

Treatment consequences	Erectile function, duplex sonography, unaltered
Efficacy	Similar in both treatments
Side effects compromising effectiveness	Priapism in a relevant number
Randomization of patients	Yes
Dose arms 1–3	Nine groups with various doses of papaverine+phentolamine+alprostadil
Study quality	**1–**
Reference	1485: Seyam R, Mohamed K, Akhras AA, Rashwan H. A prospective randomized study to optimize the dosage of trimix ingredients and compare its efficacy and safety with prostaglandin E1. Int J Impot Res. 2005 Jul–Aug;17(4):346–53.
Language	English

Compound	Papaverine (G04BE02), phentolamine
Disease treated	Erectile dysfunction
Quantification of dysfunction	Erectile function
No. of patients treated	172
Age group	Old
Treatment period	12 months
Dose	Various per autoinjection
Treatment consequences	Erectile rigidity, improvement
Efficacy	96% of patients
Side effects compromising effectiveness	3.4% fibrotic plaques, 0.15% prolonged erection
Randomization of patients	No
Study quality	**3**
Reference	1526: Sparwasser C, Drescher P, Pust RA, Madsen PO. Long-term results of therapy with intracavernousal injections and penile venous surgery in chronic erectile dysfunction. Scand J Urol Nephrol Suppl. 1994;157:107–12.
Language	English

Compound	Papaverine (G04BE02), phentolamine, alprostadil
Disease treated	Erectile dysfunction
Quantification of dysfunction	Erectile function
No. of patients treated	168
Age group	Old
Treatment period	6 months self-injection
Dose	Various
Treatment consequences	Cavernous injection, side effects
Efficacy	Highest in papaverine therapy
Side effects compromising effectiveness	No systemic side effects, but mild clinically impalpable fibrosis, 10 patients prolonged erection, 7 patients penile fibrosis, 3 cavernositis, 1 intracavernous needle breakage
Randomization of patients	No
Study quality	**2–**
Reference	1486: Moemen MN, Hamed HA, Kamel II, Shamloul RM, Ghanem HM. Clinical and sonographic assessment of the side effects of intracavernous injection of vasoactive substances. Int J Impot Res. 2004 Apr;16(2):143–5.
Language	English

Compound	Papaverine (G04BE02), alprostadil
Disease treated	Erectile dysfunction
Quantification of dysfunction	Erectile function
No. of patients treated	100
Age group	Old
Treatment period	Three times
Dose	50 mg
Treatment consequences	Erectile rigidity, improvement
Efficacy	60 min duration in 75% of patients
Side effects compromising effectiveness	n.g.
Randomization of patients	No
Dose arms 1–3	Papaverine+alprostadil; alprostadil
Study quality	**2–**

Reference	1504: Zaher TF. Papaverine plus prostaglandin E1 versus prostaglandin E1 alone for intracorporeal injection therapy. Int Urol Nephrol. 1998;30(2):193–6.
Language	English

Compound	Papaverine (G04BE02), phentolamine
Disease treated	Erectile dysfunction
Quantification of dysfunction	Erectile function
No. of patients treated	100
Age group	Old
Treatment period	50 mg
Dose	25mg+0.8 mg
Treatment consequences	Erectile rigidity, improvement
Efficacy	65.7% of vascular erectile dysfunction., 100% of neurogenic erectile dysfunction
Side effects compromising effectiveness	Four of 100 patients with prolonged erection
Randomization of patients	No
Study quality	**2–**
Reference	1554: Sidi AA, Cameron JS, Duffy LM, Lange PH. Intracavernous drug-induced erections in the management of male erectile dysfunction: experience with 100 patients. J Urol. 1986 Apr;135(4):704–6.
Language	English

Compound	Papaverine (G04BE02)+phentolamine; alprostadil
Disease treated	Erectile dysfunction
Quantification of dysfunction	Erectile function
No. of patients treated	60
Age group	58 years (mean)
Treatment period	Single dose
Dose	30, 0.5, 30 mg
Treatment consequences	Erectile rigidity, improvement
Efficacy	54% of patients; 50% with alprostadil

Side effects compromising effectiveness	18% prolonged erections, 15% with alprostadil
Randomization of patients	No
Dose arms 1–3	Papaverine+phentolamine; alprostadil
Study quality	**2–**
Reference	1508: Bechara A, Casabe A, Cheliz G, Romano S, Rey H, Fredotovich N. Comparative study of papaverine plus phentolamine versus prostaglandin E1 in erectile dysfunction. J Urol. 1997 Jun;157(6):2132–4.
Language	English

Compound	Papaverine (G04BE02), phentolamine; apomorphine
Disease treated	Erectile dysfunction
Quantification of dysfunction	Erectile function
No. of patients treated	44
Age group	Old
Treatment period	4 weeks
Treatment consequences	Sexual score, increase
Efficacy	Significant difference to baseline, but no difference between formulations
Side effects compromising effectiveness	With apomorphine nasocongestion, headache frequently
Randomization of patients	Yes
Dose arms 1–3	40 mg phentolamine+6 mg apomorphine; 40 mg phentolamine+150 mg papaverine; 40 mg phentolamine+6 mg apomorphin+150 mg papaverine
Study quality	**1–**
Reference	1489: Lammers PI, Rubio-Aurioles E, Castell R, Castaneda J, Ponce de Leon R, Hurley D, Lipezker M, Loehr LA, Lowrey F. Combination therapy for erectile dysfunction: a randomized, double blind, unblinded active-controlled, cross-over study of the pharmacodynamics and safety of combined oral formulations of apomorphine hydrochloride, phentolamine mesylate and papaverine hydrochloride in men with moderate to severe erectile dysfunction. Int J Impot Res. 2002 Feb;14(1):54–9.
Language	English

Compound	Papaverine (G04BE02), phentolamine, nitroprusside
Disease treated	Erectile dysfunction
Quantification of dysfunction	Erectile function
No. of patients treated	40
Age group	Young
Treatment period	1 weeks
Dose	30, 1, 300 mg
Treatment consequences	Erectile function, improvement
Efficacy	Similar in both treatments
Side effects compromising effectiveness	No side effects with sodium nitroprusside; priapism and local penile pain with papaverin+phentolamine solution
Dose arms 1–3	Papaverine+phentolamine; sodium prusside
Study quality	**2–**
Reference	1483: Shamloul R, Atteya A, Elnashaar A, Gadallah A, Zohdy W, Abdelsalam W. Intracavernous sodium nitroprusside (SNP) versus papaverine/phentolamine in erectile dysfunction: a comparative study of short-term efficacy and side-effects. J Sex Med. 2005 Jan;2(1):117–20.
Language	English

Compound	Papaverine (G04BE02), phentolamine
Disease treated	Erectile dysfunction
Quantification of dysfunction	Erectile function
No. of patients treated	40
Age group	Old
Treatment period	Single dose
Dose	40 mg; 0.5 mg
Treatment consequences	Erectile rigidity, improvement
Efficacy	27% of papaverine group, 48% of papaverine–phentolamine group
Side effects compromising effectiveness	papaverine: 11 men discomfort during injection; combination: 7 men discomfort, 1 patient with prolonged erection
Randomization of patients	Yes
Dose arms 1–3	40 mg papaverine alone; 20 mg papaverine+5 mg phentolamine

Study quality	**1+**
Reference	1541: Keogh EJ, Watters GR, Earle CM, Carati CJ, Wisniewski ZS, Tulloch GS, Lord DJ. Treatment of impotence by intrapenile injections. A comparison of papaverine versus papaverine and phentolamine: a double-blind, crossover trial. J Urol. 1989 Sep;142(3):726–8.
Language	English

Compound	Papaverine (G04BE02), phentolamine, moxisylite
Disease treated	Paraplegics
Quantification of dysfunction	Erectile function
No. of patients treated	36
Age group	31 years (mean)
Treatment period	Single dose
Treatment consequences	Erectile function, improvement
Efficacy	Average dose to obtain grade-4 or grade-5 erection 12.3±4.8 µg alprostadil, 14±5.4 mg moxisylite
Side effects	No significant side effects
Randomization of patients	No
Study quality	**2–**
Reference	1490: Lebib Ben Achour S, Laffont I, Boyer F, Boiteau F, Dizien O. Intracavernous injections in the treatment of erectile dysfunction in spinal cord injured patients: experience with 36 patients. Ann Readapt Med Phys. 2001 Feb;44(1):35–40.
Language	French

Compound	Papaverine (G04BE02), phentolamine
Disease treated	Erectile dysfunction
Quantification of dysfunction	Erectile function
No. of patients treated	30
Age group	Old
Treatment period	4 weeks
Dose	40 mg/0.5 mg
Treatment consequences	Erectile rigidity, improvement
Efficacy	83% of patients

Side effects compromising effectiveness	Penile ecchymosis common, 1 patient prolonged erection
Randomization of patients	Yes
Dose arms 1–3	Papaverine+phentolamine; placebo
Study quality	**1–**
Reference	1552: Gasser TC, Roach RM, Larsen EH, Madsen PO, Bruskewitz RC. Intracavernous self-injection with phentolamine and papaverine for the treatment of impotence. J Urol. 1987 Apr;137(4):678–80.
Language	English

Compound	Papaverine (G04BE02), phentolamine, alprostadil
Disease treated	Erectile dysfunction
Quantification of dysfunction	Priapism
No. of patients treated	29
Age group	Old
Treatment period	Single dose
Dose	40 mg
Treatment consequences	Priapism as a side effect
Efficacy	The disappearance of blood flow in the cavernous artery after 1 h of sustained rigid erection predicts priapism with 100% specificity and sensitivity
Side effects compromising effectiveness	n.g.
Study quality	**3**
Reference	1487: Shamloul R, Ghanem HM, Salem A, Kamel II, Mousa AA. The value of penile duplex in the prediction of intracavernous drug-induced priapism. Int J Impot Res. 2004 Feb;16(1):78–9.
Language	English

Compound	Papaverine intracavernous (G04BE02), nitroglycerin transcutaneously
Disease treated	Erectile dysfunction in spinal cord lesion
Quantification of dysfunction	Erectile function
No. of patients treated	28
Age group	Young

Treatment period	Single dose
Dose	40 mg
Treatment consequences	Erectile rigidity, improvement
Efficacy	93% of papaverin group, 17% of nitroglycerin group
Side effects compromising effectiveness	Mild headache in six (21%) patients
Randomization of patients	No
Dose arms 1–3	Papaverine; nitrogylcerin
Study quality	**2–**
Reference	1509: Renganathan R, Suranjan B, Kurien T. Comparison of transdermal nitroglycerin and intracavernous injection of papaverine in the treatment of erectile dysfunction in patients with spinal cord lesions. Spinal Cord. 1997 Feb;35(2):99–103.
Language	English

Compound	Papaverine (G04BE02), nitroprusside
Disease treated	Erectile dysfunction
Quantification of dysfunction	Electrostimulation of cavernosal nerve
No. of patients treated	22
Age group	Old
Treatment period	Single dose
Dose	60 mg
Treatment consequences	Nerval amplitude, increased
Efficacy	More significant in nitroprusside
Side effects compromising effectiveness	Not mentioned
Randomization of patients	No
Dose arms 1–3	Papaverine; nitroprusside
Study quality	**2–**
Reference	1511: Kayigil O, Atahan O, Metin A. Electromyographic changes of corpus cavernosum due to papaverine and nitroprusside in veno-occlusive dysfunction. J Urol. 1996 Oct;156(4):1316–9.
Language	English

2

Compound	Papaverine transcutaneously (G04BE02)
Disease treated	Erectile dysfunction
Quantification of dysfunction	Erectile function
No. of patients treated	20
Age group	Old
Treatment period	Single dose
Dose	20% gel
Treatment consequences	Peak systolic flow velocity of cavernous artery, increase
Efficacy	26% of tests
Side effects compromising effectiveness	No significant side effects
Randomization of patients	No
Study quality	**3**
Reference	1521: Kim ED, el-Rashidy R, McVary KT. Papaverine topical gel for treatment of erectile dysfunction. J Urol. 1995 Feb;153(2):361–5.
Language	English

Compound	Papaverine (G04BE02), phentolamine
Disease treated	Erectile dysfunction
Quantification of dysfunction	Erectile function
No. of patients treated	18
Age group	25–65 years
Treatment period	Single dose
Dose	30 mg
Treatment consequences	Erectile rigidity, improvement
Efficacy	70% of patients, none in saline group
Side effects compromising effectiveness	No significant side effects
Randomization of patients	No
Dose arms 1–3	Papaverine 30 mg+phentolamine 1 mg; saline solution
Study quality	**2–**

Reference	1551: Kiely EA, Ignotus P, Williams G. Penile function following intracavernosal injection of vasoactive agents or saline. Br J Urol. 1987 May;59(5):473–6.
Language	English

Compound	Papaverine (G04BE02), phentolamine
Disease treated	Cavernous tissue in vitro
Quantification of dysfunction	Muscle relaxation
No. of patients treated	16
Age group	42–68 years
Treatment period	In vitro
Dose	5×10^{-4}g; 5×10^{-4}g
Treatment consequences	Cavernous tissue, relaxation
Efficacy	Good; poor
Study quality	**2–**
Reference	1438: Barbanti G, Beneforti P, Lapini A, Turini D. Relaxation of isolated corpus cavernosum induced by smooth-muscle relaxant drugs. A comparative study. Urol Res. 1988;16(4):299–302.
Language	English

Compound	Papaverine (G04BE02), phentolamine, alprostadil
Disease treated	Erectile dysfunction
Quantification of dysfunction	Erectile function
No. of patients treated	7
Age group	Old
Treatment period	Single dose
Dose	1 mg, 0.5 mg, 5 ug
Treatment consequences	Erectile rigidity, improvement
Efficacy	All patients
Side effects compromising effectiveness	No significant side effects, no penile pain
Randomization of patients	Yes, cross-over
Dose arms 1–3	Papaverine+phentolamine; papaverine+alprostadil

Study quality	**1–**
Reference	1534: Allen RP, Engel RM, Smolev JK, Brendler CB. Objective double-blind evaluation of erectile function with intracorporeal papaverine in combination with phentolamine and/or prostaglandin E1. J Urol. 1992 Oct;148(4):1181–3.
Language	English

Compound	Papaverine (G04BE02)
Disease treated	Erectile dysfunction
Quantification of dysfunction	Erectile function
No. of patients treated	400
Age group	Old
Treatment consequences	Erectile function, improvement
Efficacy	Risk factors for priapism
Side effects compromising effectiveness	Higher in patients with psychogenic or neurogenic impotence than in those with vasculogenic impotence
Study quality	**4 (review)**
Reference	1313: Lomas GM, Jarow JP. Risk factors for papaverine-induced priapism. J Urol. 1992 May;147(5):1280–1.
Language	English

Compound	PNU-83757 (potassium channel opener) (not listed)
Disease treated	Erectile dysfunction, vascular
Quantification of dysfunction	Erectile function
No. of patients treated	66
Age group	Middle-aged
Treatment period	Test dose
Dose	140 µg
Treatment consequences	Erectile function, improvement
Efficacy	Of 25 patients who received 60–140 µg only, 1 had no erectile response, 15 had partial erection and 9 had complete erection.
Side effects compromising effectiveness	No significant side effects

Randomization of patients	No
Study quality	**3**
Reference	1239: Vick RN, Benevides M, Patel M, Parivar K, Linnet O, Carson CC. The efficacy, safety and tolerability of intracavernous PNU-83757 for the treatment of erectile dysfunction. J Urol. 2002 Jun;167(6):2618–23.
Language	English

G04	**Urologicals**
G04BE	*Drugs Used in Erectile Dysfunction*

Phosphodiesterase Inhibitors and Apomorphin

These drugs are designated to be taken orally on demand, each time cohabitation is planned. The easy application permits multiple errors in the dose regimen: healthy men without erectile dysfunction may use it to achieve better sexual performance, patients with insufficient effectiveness may enhance the dose and a combination with other drugs applied for other diseases may induce adverse effects. Risk of all these errors should be excluded for security reasons.

In general, adverse effects of phosphodiesterase inhibitors are mild and self-limited, and withdrawal from clinical studies as a result of drug-related adverse effects was rare. The most frequent side effects are related to their vasodilatory effects, such as headache, flushing, dyspepsia, nasal congestion and rhinitis.

No cardiac side effects were noted in most studies. The synchronous application of antihypertensive medication did not influence the rate of adverse effects. The risk of myocardial infarction was not increased. Absolute contraindication in patients taking nitrate- or molsidomine-containing medications, and an interaction with non-uroselective α-adrenoceptor blockers, was observed.

Overall level of evidence of positive effects: A
Overall level of evidence of adverse effects compromising effectiveness: A

The sequence according to the ATC code has been discarded, in part, in this chapter. The phosphodiesterase-5 inhibitors sildenafil (G04BE03), tadalafil (G08BE03) and vardenafil (G09BE03) are listed consecutively, and apomorphin (G07BE03) thereafter.

2

Sildenafil: A genetic profile may be of relevance for cardiovascular side effects of sildenafil. The rate of myocardial infarction was found to be 0.91 per 100 person-years (PY) in sildernafil, 0.84 per 100 PY in placebo groups and RR 1.08 (95% CI: 0.45–2.77). No significant association with serious cardiovascular events or death was observed. The general risk of sexual intercourse to induce myocardial infarction is 1%. Sildenafil is contraindicated in men who use nitrate medications, because it may cause life-threatening hypotension.

Other adverse effects were mild and self-limited in up to 27% of patients. In all comparative studies the rate was higher than in the placebo groups. Flushing was noted in 10–14%, headache in 3–25%, dyspepsia in 5–14% and visual disturbance in 2–3% of patients. The rate was similar in patients with ischaemic heart disease and patients without ischaemic heart disease. The rate of adverse effects increased to 63% in patients who received doses higher than 100 mg (McMahon et al. 2002). Four of 13 responders in this study refused to continue treatment due to adverse effects.

In patients using intracavernosal injection of alprostadil, the rate of adverse effects is significantly higher than in those taking sildenafil.

Compound	Phosphodiesterase-5 inhibitors (G04BE03)
Disease treated	Coronary artery disease
Quantification of dysfunction	Clinical symptoms
Age group	Old
Treatment consequences	Erectile function, improvement
Efficacy	Various risk groups
Side effects compromising effectiveness	No cardiac side effects
Randomization of patients	No
Remarks	Erectile dysfunction as part of metabolic syndrome
Study quality	**4 (expert opinion)**
Reference	1006: Kostis JB, Jackson G, Rosen R, Barrett-Connor E, Billups K, Burnett AL, Carson C III, Cheitlin M, Debusk R, Fonseca V, Ganz P, Goldstein I, Guay A, Hatzichristou D, Hollander JE, Hutter A, Katz S, Kloner RA, Mittleman M, Montorsi F, Montorsi P, Nehra A, Sadovsky R, Shabsigh R. Sexual dysfunction and cardiac risk (the Second Princeton Consensus Conference). Am J Cardiol. 2005 Jul 15;96(2):313–21. Original 151205

Language	English

Compound	Phosphodiesterase-5 inhibitors (G04BE03)
Disease treated	Diabetes mellitus
Quantification of dysfunction	Erectile function
Age group	Old
Treatment consequences	Erectile function, impairment
Efficacy	Lower than in non-diabetic men
Side effects compromising effectiveness	No cardiac side effects
Study quality	**4 (review)**
Reference	1048: Kloner RA. Assessment of cardiovascular risk in patients with erectile dysfunction: focus on the diabetic patient. Endocrine. 2004 Mar–Apr;23(2–3):125–9.
Language	English

Compound	Phosphodiesterase-5 inhibitors (G04BE03)
Disease treated	Erectile dysfunction
Quantification of dysfunction	Sexual function questionnaire
No. of patients treated	9457
Age group	62 years (mean)
Treatment period	Various
Dose	Various
Treatment consequences	Incidence of myocardial infarction in men complaining of erectile dysfunction as compared with men without erectile dysfunction
Efficacy	OR 1.29 (95% CI 0.96–1.74)
Randomization of patients	No
Study quality	**2++**
Reference	2203: Thompson IM, Tangen CM, Goodman PJ, Probstfield JL, Moinpour CM, Coltman CA. Erectile dysfunction and subsequent cardiovascular disease. J Am Med Assoc. 2005 Dec 21;294(23):2996–3002.
Language	English

Compound	Phosphodiesterase-5 inhibitors (G04BE03)
Disease treated	Erectile dysfunction
Quantification of dysfunction	Erectile function
No. of patients treated	3414
Age group	All ages
Treatment period	Various
Dose	Various
Treatment consequences	Erectile function, impairment
Efficacy	38% patients using antihypertensives, 34% of normal men
Side effects compromising effectiveness	Similar rate for patients taking sildenafil and antihypertensive medication (34%) and those not taking antihypertensive agents (38%)
Randomization of patients	No
Study quality	**2–**
Reference	1556: Kloner RA, Mullin SH, Shook T, Matthews R et al. Erectile dysfunction in the cardiac patient: How common and should we treat? J Urol 2001;170: S46–S50.
Language	English

Compound	Phosphodiesterase-5 inhibitors (G04BE03)
Disease treated	Coronary artery disease
Quantification of dysfunction	Erectile function
Age group	Old
Treatment consequences	Cardiovascular parameters
Efficacy	No influence of phosphodiesterase-5 inhibitors
Side effects compromising effectiveness	No cardiac side effects
Study quality	**4 (review)**
Reference	1066: Brindis RG, Kloner RA. Sildenafil in patients with cardiovascular disease. Am J Cardiol. 2003 Nov 6;92(9A):26M–36M.
Language	English

Compound	Phosphodiesterase-5 inhibitors (G04BE03)
Disease treated	Coronary artery disease
Quantification of dysfunction	Erectile function
Age group	Old
Treatment consequences	Coronary artery disease, improvement with PDE-inhibitors
Efficacy	Good
Side effects compromising effectiveness	No cardiac side effects
Study quality	**4 (review)**
Reference	1016: Kloner R, Padma-Nathan H. Erectile dysfunction in patients with coronary artery disease. Int J Impot Res. 2005 May–Jun;17(3):209–15.
Language	English

Compound	Phosphodiesterase-5 inhibitors (G04BE03)
Disease treated	Erectile dysfunction
Quantification of dysfunction	Erectile function
Age group	Old
Treatment consequences	Erectile function, improvement
Efficacy	Most patients
Side effects compromising effectiveness	Most frequent side effects are related to their vasodilatory effects, such as headache, flushing, dyspepsia, nasal congestion, rhinitis. They are generally reversible.
Remarks	Lower resorption in high-fat food
Study quality	**4 (review)**
Reference	1021: Seftel AD. Phosphodiesterase type 5 inhibitor differentiation based on selectivity, pharmacokinetic, and efficacy profiles. Clin Cardiol. 2004 Apr;27(4 Suppl 1):I14–19.
Language	English

Compound	Phosphodiesterase-5 inhibitors (G04BE03)
Disease treated	Prostatic carcinoma
Quantification of dysfunction	Erectile function
Age group	Old

Treatment consequences	Erectile function, improvement
Efficacy	Sevenfold increase in maintaining erections after nerve-sparing surgery
Side effects compromising effectiveness	Not mentioned
Randomization of patients	No
Study quality	**4 (review)**
Reference	1022: Padma-Nathan H, McCullough A, Forest C. Erectile dysfunction secondary to nerve-sparing radical retropubic prostatectomy: comparative phosphodiesterase-5 inhibitor efficacy for therapy and novel prevention strategies. Curr Urol Rep. 2004 Dec;5(6):467–71.
Language	English

Compound	Phosphodiesterase-5 inhibitors (G04BE03)
Disease treated	Diabetes mellitus
Quantification of dysfunction	Erectile function
Age group	Old
Treatment consequences	Erectile function, improvement
Efficacy	Good
Side effects compromising effectiveness	Headache, nasal congestion and dyspepsia. The drugs are generally well tolerated, and withdrawal from clinical studies as a result of drug-related adverse effects were rare.
Randomization of patients	No
Study quality	**4 (review)**
Reference	1024: Basu A, Ryder RE. New treatment options for erectile dysfunction in patients with diabetes mellitus. Drugs. 2004;64(23):2667–88.
Language	English

Compound	Phosphodiesterase-5 inhibitors (G04BE03)
Disease treated	Prostatic carcinoma
Quantification of dysfunction	Erectile function
Age group	Old
Treatment consequences	Erectile function, improvement

Efficacy	16–82% following radical prostatectomy
Side effects compromising effectiveness	Not mentioned
Study quality	**4 (review)**
Reference	1030: Kendirci M, Hellstrom WJ. Current concepts in the management of erectile dysfunction in men with prostate cancer. Clin Prostate Cancer. 2004 Sep;3(2):87–92.
Language	English

Compound	Phosphodiesterase-5 inhibitors (G04BE03)
Disease treated	Prostatic carcinoma
Quantification of dysfunction	Erectile function
Age group	Old
Treatment consequences	Erectile function, improvement
Efficacy	Phosphodiesterase-5 inhibitors following nerve-sparing operation
Side effects compromising effectiveness	Not mentioned
Study quality	**4 (review)**
Reference	1038: Gontero P, Kirby R. Proerectile pharmacological prophylaxis following nerve-sparing radical prostatectomy (NSRP). Prostate Cancer Prostatic Dis. 2004;7(3):223–6.
Language	English

Compound	Phosphodiesterase-5 inhibitors (G04BE03)
Disease treated	Erectile dysfunction
Quantification of dysfunction	Erectile function
Age group	Old
Treatment consequences	Erectile function, improvement
Efficacy	Highly effective
Side effects compromising effectiveness	Absolute contraindication in patients taking nitrate- or molsidomine-containing medications, interaction with non-uroselective alpha-adrenoceptor blockers
Study quality	**4 (review)**
Reference	1041: Porst H. Erectile dysfunction. New drugs with special consideration of the PDE 5 inhibitors. Urologe A. 2004 Jul;43(7):820–8.

Language	German

Compound	Phosphodiesterase-5 inhibitors (G04BE03)
Disease treated	Erectile dysfunction
Quantification of dysfunction	Erectile function
Age group	Old
Treatment consequences	Erectile function, improvement
Efficacy	43% in radical prostatectomy, 82% in neurological diseases
Side effects compromising effectiveness	Insufficient data on adverse effects of vardenafil and tadalafil, particularly their long-term use and use in high-risk groups
Study quality	**4 (review)**
Reference	1120: Gresser U, Gleiter CH. Erectile dysfunction: comparison of efficacy and side effects of the PDE-5 inhibitors sildenafil, vardenafil and tadalafil: review of the literature. Eur J Med Res. 2002 Oct 29;7(10):435–46.
Language	English

Compound	Sildenafil (G04BE03)
Disease treated	Erectile dysfunction
Quantification of dysfunction	Genotype polymorphism
No. of patients treated	n.g.
Age group	Old
Treatment consequences	Erectile function, improvement
Efficacy	GNB3 825C allele carriers 50%, in genotype TT 90% positive response to sildenafil
Side effects compromising effectiveness	Not mentioned
Randomization of patients	No
Dose arms 1–3	GNB3 825C allele carriers; genotype TT
Remarks	Genetic profile may be of relevance for cardiovascular side effects of sildenafil
Study quality	**2–**
Reference	1087: Eisenhardt A, Siffert W. Genetic risk factors for erectile dysfunction and genetic determinants of drug response: on the way to improve drug safety? Herz. 2003 Jun;28(4):304–13.

Language	English

Compound	Sildenafil (G04BE03)
Disease treated	Erectile dysfunction
Quantification of dysfunction	Erectile function
No. of patients treated	6659
Age group	Old
Treatment period	Various
Dose	Various
Treatment consequences	Erectile function, improvement
Efficacy	83% of sildenafil group, 45% of placebo group
Side effects compromising effectiveness	Flushing (12%), headache (11%), dyspepsia (5%), and visual disturbances (3%). All adverse events were significantly less likely to occur with placebo; no significant association with serious cardiovascular events or death
Randomization of patients	Yes
Dose arms 1–3	Sildenafil; placebo
Study quality	**1+ (meta-analysis)**
Reference	1150: Fink HA, MacDonald R, Rutks IR, Nelson DB, Wilt TJ. Sildenafil for male erectile dysfunction: a systematic review and meta-analysis. Arch Intern Med. 2002 Jun 24;162(12):1349–60.
Language	English

Compound	Sildenafil (G04BE03)
Disease treated	Depression
Quantification of dysfunction	Erectile function
No. of patients treated	500
Age group	Old
Treatment period	12 weeks
Dose	25–100 mg
Treatment consequences	Erectile function, improvement
Efficacy	Various conditions
Side effects compromising effectiveness	Not mentioned

Randomization of patients	Yes
Dose arms 1–3	Untreated minor depression; depression refractory to SSRI; erectile dysfunction after SSRI treatment
Study quality	**1++ (structured review)**
Reference	1121: Nurnberg HG, Seidman SN, Gelenberg AJ, Fava M, Rosen R, Shabsigh R. Depression, antidepressant therapies, and erectile dysfunction: clinical trials of sildenafil citrate (Viagra) in treated and untreated patients with depression. Urology. 2002 Sep;60(2 Suppl 2):58–66.
Language	English

Compound	Sildenafil (G04BE03)
Disease treated	Spinal cord injury
Quantification of dysfunction	Erectile function
No. of patients treated	382
Age group	37 years (mean)
Treatment period	30 days
Dose	50 mg
Treatment consequences	Erectile function, improvement
Efficacy	94%
Side effects compromising effectiveness	Similar rate as in other indications
Randomization of patients	Yes
Dose arms 1–3	Sildenafil; placebo
Remarks	Responder rates higher than in diabetes (65%)
Study quality	**1+ (meta-analysis)**
Reference	1123: Derry F, Hultling C, Seftel AD, Sipski ML. Efficacy and safety of sildenafil citrate (Viagra) in men with erectile dysfunction and spinal cord injury: a review. Urology. 2002 Sep;60(2 Suppl 2):49–57.
Language	English

Compound	Sildenafil (G04BE03)
Disease treated	Erectile dysfunction and ischaemic heart disease
Quantification of dysfunction	IIEF
No. of patients treated	357

Age group	Middle-aged
Treatment period	24 weeks
Dose	200 mg
Treatment consequences	Erectile function, improvement
Efficacy	Mean scores for questions 3 and 4 of the IIEF significantly higher for the sildenafil group than for the placebo group; improved erections in 70% of sildenafil patients and 20% of placebo patients
Side effects compromising effectiveness	Headache 25%, flushing 14% and dyspepsia 12% for patients with ischaemic heart disease; 21, 15 and 10% for patients without ischaemic heart disease
Randomization of patients	Yes
Dose arms 1–3	Sildenafil; placebo
Study quality	**1+**
Reference	1207: Conti CR, Pepine CJ, Sweeney M. Efficacy and safety of sildenafil citrate in the treatment of erectile dysfunction in patients with ischemic heart disease. Am J Cardiol. 1999 Mar 4;83(5A):29C–34C.
Language	English

Compound	Sildenafil (G04BE03)
Disease treated	Erectile dysfunction in various conditions
Quantification of dysfunction	IIEF
No. of patients treated	315
Age group	Middle-aged
Treatment period	26 weeks
Dose	100 mg
Treatment consequences	Erectile function, improvement
Efficacy	Patients' abilities to achieve and maintain an erection in the sildenafil group was significantly improved compared with the placebo group.
Side effects compromising effectiveness	Mild to moderate in 27% of patients in sildenafil group, and in 8% of patients in placebo group
Randomization of patients	Yes
Dose arms 1–3	Sildenafil; placebo
Study quality	**1–**

Reference	1208: Meuleman E, Cuzin B, Opsomer RJ, Hartmann U, Bailey MJ, Maytom MC, Smith MD, Osterloh IH. A dose-escalation study to assess the efficacy and safety of sildenafil citrate in men with erectile dysfunction. BJU Int. 2001 Jan;87(1):75–81.
Language	English

Compound	Sildenafil (G04BE03)
Disease treated	Erectile dysfunction
Quantification of dysfunction	IIEF
No. of patients treated	300
Age group	>18 years
Treatment period	12 weeks
Dose	100 mg
Treatment consequences	Erectile function, improvement
Efficacy	Compared with placebo, sildenafil significantly improved self-esteem, confidence, sexual relationship satisfaction and overall relationship satisfaction.
Side effects compromising effectiveness	Not mentioned
Randomization of patients	Yes
Dose arms 1–3	Sildenafil; placebo
Study quality	**1+**
Reference	1229: Althof SE, O'leary MP, Cappelleri JC, Hvidsten K, Stecher VJ, Glina S, King R, Siegel RL. International SEAR Study Group. Sildenafil citrate improves self-esteem, confidence, and relationships in men with erectile dysfunction: Results from an international, multi-center, double-blind, placebo-controlled trial. J Sex Med. 2006 May;3(3):521–9.
Language	English

Compound	Sildenafil (G04BE03)
Disease treated	Erectile dysfunction, organic
Quantification of adverse effects	IIEF
No. of patients treated	232
Age group	55 years (mean)
Treatment period	2 years

Dose	100 mg
Treatment consequences	Erectile function, improvement
Efficacy	Overall response rate 43%; best response rate in veno-occlusive cases, worst responses from neurogenic causes
Side effects	Not mentioned
Randomization of patients	No
Study quality	**2–**
Reference	1289: Chia SJ, Ramesh K, Earnest A. Clinical application of prognostic factors for patients with organic causes of erectile dysfunction on 100 mg of sildenafil citrate. Int J Urol. 2004 Dec;11(12):1104–9.
Language	English

Compound	Sildenafil (G04BE03)
Disease treated	Erectile dysfunction
Quantification of dysfunction	IIEF
No. of patients treated	141
Age group	27–78 years
Treatment period	6 months
Dose	100 mg
Treatment consequences	Erectile function, improvement
Efficacy	IIEF score increased from 11.80 to 20.70. Positive response in 102 patients, 38 unresponsive
Side effects compromising effectiveness	Not mentioned
Randomization of patients	No
Study quality	**3**
Reference	1224: Basar M, Tekdogan UY, Yilmaz E, Basar H, Atan A, Batislam E. The efficacy of sildenafil in different etiologies of erectile dysfunction. Int Urol Nephrol. 2001;32(3):403–7.
Language	English

Compound	Sildenafil (G04BE03), alprostadil
Disease treated	Erectile dysfunction
Quantification of dysfunction	IIEF

No. of patients treated	93
Age group	56 years (mean)
Treatment period	Long-term
Dose	Various
Treatment consequences	Erectile function, improvement
Efficacy	Good in all drugs
Side effects compromising effectiveness	Twenty-nine of 93 patients treated with intracavernosal injection adverse effects: penile pain in 27; dizziness in 5; headache in 2. Thirty-four of 93 patients treated with sildenafil side effects: headache in 30; facial flushing in 25; dyspepsia in 12; nasal congestion in 9; dizziness in 5; visual disturbances in 1. Twenty of 41 patients on combined therapy side effects: penile pain in 15; headache in 15; facial flushing in 12; dyspepsia in 7; nasal congestion in 3; dizziness in 12; syncope in 1
Randomization of patients	No
Study quality	**2–**
Reference	1499: McMahon CG, Samali R, Johnson H. Treatment of intracorporeal injection nonresponse with sildenafil alone or in combination with triple agent intracorporeal injection therapy. J Urol. 1999 Dec;162(6):1992–7; discussion 1997–8.
Language	English

Compound	Sildenafil (G04BE03)
Disease treated	Erectile dysfunction after brachytherapy of prostate
Quantification of dysfunction	IIEF
No. of patients treated	60
Age group	Old
Treatment period	12 weeks
Dose	100 mg
Treatment consequences	Erectile function, improvement
Efficacy	Significant increase in sildenafil treatment vs placebo
Side effects compromising effectiveness	Mild or moderate
Randomization of patients	Cross-over
Dose arms 1–3	Sildenafil; placebo

Study quality	**2+**
Reference	1246: Incrocci L, Hop WC, Slob AK. Favorable effect of sildenafil on erectile dysfunction in patients after radiotherapy for prostate cancer; randomised, double-blind, placebo-controlled crossover study. Ned Tijdschr Geneeskd. 2003 Aug 30;147(35):1687–90.
Language	Dutch

Compound	Sildenafil (G04BE03)
Disease treated	Prostatic carcinoma
Quantification of dysfunction	Erectile function
No. of patients treated	48
Age group	Old
Treatment period	Various
Dose	Various
Treatment consequences	Erectile function, improvement
Efficacy	71% of patients
Side effects compromising effectiveness	Headache (12%), flushing (10%), blue or blurred vision (2%)
Randomization of patients	No
Dose arms 1–3	Nerve-sparing surgery; unilateral nerve-sparing surgery; no nerve-sparing surgery
Study quality	**2–**
Reference	1085: Raina R, Lakin MM, Agarwal A, Sharma R, Goyal KK, Montague DK, Klein E, Zippe CD. Long-term effect of sildenafil citrate on erectile dysfunction after radical prostatectomy: 3-year follow-up. Urology. 2003 Jul;62(1):110–5.
Language	English

Compound	Sildenafil (G04BE03)
Disease treated	Erectile dysfunction in hypogonadism
Quantification of dysfunction	Nocturnal penile tumescence (NPT) and rigidity monitoring
No. of patients treated	48
Age group	Middle-aged
Treatment period	6 weeks
Dose	50 mg

Treatment consequences	Nocturnal erection, improvement
Efficacy	Significant increase in sildenafil treatment vs placebo
Side effects compromising effectiveness	Not mentioned
Randomization of patients	Yes
Dose arms 1–3	sildenafil; placebo;
Study quality	**1+**
Reference	1245: Rochira V, Balestrieri A, Madeo B, Granata AR, Carani C. Sildenafil improves sleep-related erections in hypogonadal men: evidence from a randomized, placebo-controlled, crossover study of a synergic role for both testosterone and sildenafil on penile erections. J Androl. 2006 Mar–Apr;27(2):165–75. Epub 2005 Nov 8.
Language	English

Compound	Sildenafil (G04BE03)
Disease treated	Erectile dysfunction not responding to sildenafil
Quantification of dysfunction	IIEF
No. of patients treated	45
Age group	60 years (mean)
Treatment period	4 weeks
Dose	200 mg
Treatment consequences	Erectile function, improvement
Efficacy	Treatment was regarded as having improved the erections by 37, 46.3 and 68% of patients with sildenafil 100, 150 and 200 mg, respectively.
Side effects compromising effectiveness	34 of 54: headache (19); facial flushing (32); dyspepsia (14); nasal congestion (11); dizziness (5); visual disturbances (5). Four of 13 responders refused to continue treatment due to adverse effects.
Randomization of patients	No
Remarks	Sildenafil up to 200 mg is an effective salvage therapy for 24.1% of previous sildenafil non-responders: limited by a significantly higher incidence of adverse effects and a 31% treatment discontinuation rate
Study quality	**3**

Reference	1233: McMahon CG. High dose sildenafil citrate as a salvage therapy for severe erectile dysfunction. Int J Impot Res. 2002 Dec;14(6):533–8.
Language	English

Compound	Sildenafil (G04BE03)
Disease treated	Erectile dysfunction in congestive heart failure
Quantification of dysfunction	IIEF
No. of patients treated	35
Age group	Old
Treatment period	12 weeks
Dose	50 mg
Treatment consequences	Erectile function, improvement; depression scores, improvement
Efficacy	Good compared with placebo
Side effects compromising effectiveness	Not mentioned
Randomization of patients	Yes
Dose arms 1–3	Sildenafil; placebo
Study quality	**1+**
Reference	1212: Webster LJ, Michelakis ED, Davis T, Archer SL. Use of sildenafil for safe improvement of erectile function and quality of life in men with New York Heart Association classes II and III congestive heart failure: a prospective, placebo-controlled, double-blind crossover trial. Arch Intern Med. 2004 Mar 8;164(5):514–20.
Language	English

Compound	Sildenafil (G04BE03)
Disease treated	Erectile dysfunction in chronic renal dialysis
Quantification of dysfunction	IIEF
No. of patients treated	35
Age group	48 years (mean)
Treatment period	n.g.
Dose	100 mg/2× per week
Treatment consequences	Erectile function, improvement

Efficacy	IIEF score increased after sildenafil treatment
Side effects compromising effectiveness	Dyspepsia in 2 patients, headache in 1 patient
Randomization of patients	No
Study quality	**2–**
Reference	1231: Turk S, Karalezli G, Tonbul HZ, Yildiz M, Altintepe L, Yildiz A, Yeksan M. Erectile dysfunction and the effects of sildenafil treatment in patients on haemodialysis and continuous ambulatory peritoneal dialysis. Nephrol Dial Transplant. 2001 Sep;16(9):1818–22.
Language	English

Compound	Sildenafil (G04BE03)
Disease treated	Erectile dysfunction after rectal surgery
Quantification of dysfunction	IIEF
No. of patients treated	32
Age group	Middle-aged
Treatment period	n.g.
Dose	50 mg
Treatment consequences	Erectile function, improvement
Efficacy	Erectile function domain scores and total IIEF score: significant improvement in sildenafil, not in placebo
Side effects compromising effectiveness	Seven of 14 patients of sildenafil group, 4 of 18 of placebo group, but mild and well tolerated
Randomization of patients	Yes
Dose arms 1–3	Sildenafil; placebo
Study quality	**1+**
Reference	1247: Lindsey I, George B, Kettlewell M, Mortensen N. Randomized, double-blind, placebo-controlled trial of sildenafil (Viagra) for erectile dysfunction after rectal excision for cancer and inflammatory bowel disease. Dis Colon Rectum. 2002 Jun;45(6):727–32.
Language	English

Compound	Sildenafil (G04BE03)
Disease treated	Erectile dysfunction, sildenafil non-responder
Quantification of dysfunction	IIEF

No. of patients treated	12
Age group	Middle-aged
Treatment period	12 weeks
Dose	n.g.
Treatment consequences	Erectile function, improvement
Efficacy	Co-treatment with atorvastatin resulted in an improvement with sildenafil in IIEF domain score of 7.8
Side effects compromising effectiveness	n.g.
Randomization of patients	Yes
Dose arms 1–3	Sildenafil+atorvastatin; sildenafil+placebo
Study quality	**1+**
Reference	1248: Herrmann HC, Levine LA, Macaluso J Jr, Walsh M, Bradbury D, Schwartz S, Mohler ER III, Kimmel SE. Can atorvastatin improve the response to sildenafil in men with erectile dysfunction not initially responsive to sildenafil? Hypothesis and pilot trial results. J Sex Med. 2006 Mar;3(2):303–8.
Language	English

Compound	Sildenafil (G04BE03)
Disease treated	Erectile dysfunction, fluvoxamine-induced
Quantification of dysfunction	Erectile function
No. of patients treated	1
Age group	Young
Treatment period	n.g.
Dose	n.g.
Treatment consequences	Erectile function, improvement
Efficacy	Mechanism questionable
Side effects compromising effectiveness	n.g.
Study quality	**3**
Reference	1424: Balon R. Fluvoxamine-induced erectile dysfunction responding to sildenafil. J Sex Marital Ther. 1998 Oct–Dec;24(4):313–7.
Language	English

Compound	Sildenafil (G04BE03)
Disease treated	Coronary artery disease
Quantification of dysfunction	Deaths
No. of patients treated	120 clinical trials
Age group	Old
Treatment period	Various
Dose	25–100 mg
Treatment consequences	Cardiovascular death with sildenafil
Efficacy	No difference
Side effects compromising effectiveness	Rate of myocardial infarction: cardiovascular 0.91 per 100 person-years (PY) in sildernafil, 0.84 per 100 PY in placebo groups, RR 1.08 (95% CI: 0.45–2.77).
Randomization of patients	Yes
Dose arms 1–3	Sildenafil; placebo
Study quality	**1+ (meta-analysis)**
Reference	1075: Mittleman MA, Glasser DB, Orazem J. Clinical trials of sildenafil citrate (Viagra) demonstrate no increase in risk of myocardial infarction and cardiovascular death compared with placebo. Int J Clin Pract. 2003 Sep;57(7):597–600.
Language	English

Compound	Sildenafil (G04BE03)
Disease treated	Erectile dysfunction
Quantification of dysfunction	Cardiovascular diseases
Age group	Old
Treatment consequences	Cardiovascular death with sildenafil
Efficacy	No improvement
Side effects compromising effectiveness	Contraindicated in men who use nitrate medications
Randomization of patients	No
Study quality	**4 (review)**
Reference	1105: Herschorn S. Cardiovascular safety of PDE5 inhibitors. Can J Urol. 2003 Feb;10 Suppl 1:23–8.
Language	English

Compound	Sildenafil (G04BE03)
Disease treated	Depression
Quantification of dysfunction	Erectile function
Age group	Old
Treatment consequences	Erectile function, impairment
Efficacy	Effective treatment possible, no impairment of depression
Side effects compromising effectiveness	Not mentioned
Remarks	Be careful with yohimbine
Study quality	**4 (review)**
Reference	1158: Seidman SN. Exploring the relationship between depression and erectile dysfunction in aging men. J Clin Psychiatry. 2002;63 Suppl 5:5–12; discussion 23–5.
Language	English

Compound	Sildenafil (G04BE03)
Disease treated	Hypertension
Quantification of dysfunction	Erectile function
Age group	Old
Treatment consequences	Erectile function, improvement
Efficacy	No hypotension by sildenafil
Side effects compromising effectiveness	Sildenafil+organic nitrates is contraindicated; it may cause life-threatening hypotension. In contrast, sildenafil+antihypertensive agents may lead to additive but not to potentiating blood pressure decreases.
Remarks	Additive effect of sildenafil and antihypertensives
Study quality	**4 (review)**
Reference	1177: Rosenkranz S, Erdmann E. Wechselwirkungen zwischen Sildenafil und Antihypertensiva – was ist gesichert? Dtsch Med Wochenschr. 2001 Oct 12;126(41):1144–9.
Language	German

Compound	Sildenafil (G04BE03)
Disease treated	Coronary artery disease
Quantification of dysfunction	Erectile function

2

Age group	Old
Treatment consequences	Erectile function, impairment
Efficacy	Risk of 1% sexual intercourse to induce myocardial infarction
Side effects compromising effectiveness	Not mentioned
Study quality	**4 (review)**
Reference	1034: Cheitlin MD. Should the patient with coronary artery disease use sildenafil? Prev Cardiol. 2003 Summer;6(3):161–5.
Language	English

Tadalafil: Most common adverse effects were: headache 7–17%; dyspepsia 10%; flushing 5%; back pain 5%. The adverse effects were mild to moderate, and they declined with lower doses. They were rarely the cause for discontinuation of the treatment.

Compound	Tadalafil (G04BE08)
Disease treated	Erectile dysfunction
Quantification of dysfunction	IIEF
No. of patients treated	2501
Age group	Old
Treatment period	Various
Dose	20 mg
Treatment consequences	IIEF score, improvement
Efficacy	Significantly better effect of tadalafil regardless of concomitant thiazide use
Side effects compromising effectiveness	Tadalafil: headache 15%; dyspepsia 8%; back pain 5.3%. Placebo headache 4.0%, dyspepsia 0.7% and back pain 1.2%; no statistically significant difference between thiazide users and non-users.
Randomization of patients	Yes
Dose arms 1–3	Tadalafil; placebo
Study quality	**1– (meta-analysis)**
Reference	1559: Kloner RA, Sadovsky R, Johnson EG, Mo D, Ahuja S. Efficacy of tadalafil in the treatment of erectile dysfunction in hypertensive men on concomitant thiazide diuretic therapy. Int J Impot Res. 2005 Sep–Oct;17(5):450–4.

Language	English

Compound	Tadalafil (G04BE08)
Disease treated	Erectile dysfunction in diabetes mellitus
Quantification of dysfunction	IIEF
No. of patients treated	2318
Age group	56 years (mean)
Treatment period	12 weeks
Dose	20 mg
Treatment consequences	Erectile function, improvement
Efficacy	Diabetes group receiving tadalafil 20 mg; a mean improvement of 7.4 in the IIEF score against baseline versus 0.9 for placebo; 53% of the attempts at intercourse were successful, compared with 22% for placebo
Side effects compromising effectiveness	Not mentioned
Randomization of patients	Yes
Dose arms 1–3	Tadalafil; placebo
Study quality	**1–**
Reference	1216: Fonseca V, Seftel A, Denne J, Fredlund P. Impact of diabetes mellitus on the severity of erectile dysfunction and response to treatment: analysis of data from tadalafil clinical trials. Diabetologia. 2004 Nov;47(11):1914–23. Epub 2004 Nov 25.
Language	English

Compound	Tadalafil (G04BE08)
Disease treated	Erectile dysfunction
Quantification of dysfunction	IIEF
No. of patients treated	2100
Age group	Middle-aged
Treatment period	12 weeks
Dose	20 mg
Treatment consequences	Erectile function, improvement
Efficacy	Satisfactory intercourse almost always (IIEF-Q7) was reported by 59 and 79% of patients with mild ED taking tadalafil 10 mg and 20 mg vs 32% taking placebo

Side effects compromising effectiveness	n.g.
Randomization of patients	Yes
Dose arms 1–3	Tadalafil; placebo
Study quality	**1+**
Reference	1240: Rosen RC, Shabsigh R, Kuritzky L, Wang WC, Sides GD. The efficacy of tadalafil in improving sexual satisfaction and overall satisfaction in men with mild, moderate, and severe erectile dysfunction: a retrospective pooled analysis of data from randomized, placebo-controlled clinical trials. Curr Med Res Opin. 2005 Nov;21(11):1701–9.
Language	English

Compound	Tadalafil (G04BE08)
Disease treated	Erectile dysfunction
Quantification of dysfunction	IIEF
No. of patients treated	443
Age group	Middle-aged
Treatment period	12 weeks
Dose	20 mg
Treatment consequences	Erectile function, improvement
Efficacy	Tadalafil was significant superior to placebo
Side effects compromising effectiveness	Significantly more common with tadalafil than placebo: headache (7.2 vs 1.9%), flushing (4.6 vs 0%). One patient discontinued tadalafil treatment due to back pain.
Randomization of patients	Yes
Dose arms 1–3	Tadalafil; placebo
Study quality	**1+**
Reference	1227: Skoumal R, Chen J, Kula K, Breza J, Calomfirescu N, Basson BR, Kopernicky V. Efficacy and treatment satisfaction with on-demand tadalafil (Cialis) in men with erectile dysfunction. Eur Urol. 2004 Sep;46(3):362–9; discussion 369.
Language	English

Compound	Tadalafil (G04BE08)
Disease treated	Erectile dysfunction
Quantification of dysfunction	IIEF

No. of patients treated	253
Age group	59 years (mean)
Treatment period	12 weeks
Dose	20 mg
Treatment consequences	Erectile function, improvement
Efficacy	Significant improvement, mean IIEF scores were 14.5, 21.2 and 23.3 of 30 for placebo, tadalafil 10 mg and tadalafil 20 mg
Side effects compromising effectiveness	Tadalafil 20 mg: dyspepsia 22%; heache 17%. Tadalafil 10 mg: dyspepsia 9.7%; headache 14.6%. Placebo: dyspepsia 2%; headache 8%
Randomization of patients	Yes
Dose arms 1–3	Tadalafil; placebo
Study quality	**1+**
Reference	1221: Carrier S, Brock GB, Pommerville PJ, Shin J, Anglin G, Whitaker S, Beasley CM Jr. Efficacy and safety of oral tadalafil in the treatment of men in Canada with erectile dysfunction: a randomized, double-blind, parallel, placebo-controlled clinical trial. J Sex Med. 2005 Sep;2(5):685–98.
Language	English

Compound	Tadalafil (G04BE08)
Disease treated	Erectile dysfunction
Quantification of dysfunction	IIEF
No. of patients treated	168; 52
Age group	53 years (mean)
Treatment period	12 weeks
Dose	20 mg
Treatment consequences	Erectile function, improvement
Efficacy	Mean baseline IIIEF domain score 13.5. Tadalafil improved scores by 11.1, vs 0.4 for placebo; 73.9% of sexual intercourse attempts successful in tadalafil group, 29.9% in placebo group.
Side effects compromising effectiveness	Most common (>2%) headache, dyspepsia, flushing, back pain, pain in limb and myalgia, mild to moderate
Randomization of patients	Yes
Dose arms 1–3	Tadalafil; placebo

Study quality	**1–**
Reference	1232: Eardley I, Gentile V, Austoni E, Hackett G, Lembo D, Wang C, Beardsworth A. Efficacy and safety of tadalafil in a Western European population of men with erectile dysfunction. BJU Int. 2004 Oct;94(6):871–7.
Language	English

Compound	Tadalafil (G04BE08)
Disease treated	Erectile dysfunction
Quantification of dysfunction	IIEF
No. of patients treated	195
Age group	Middle-aged
Treatment period	12 weeks
Dose	20 mg
Treatment consequences	Erectile function, improvement
Efficacy	Significantly better in tadalafil group vs placebo
Side effects compromising effectiveness	Mild or moderate headache, dyspepsia, and myalgia most frequent side effects
Randomization of patients	Yes
Dose arms 1–3	Tadalafil; placebo
Study quality	**1–**
Reference	1250: Carson C, Shabsigh R, Segal S, Murphy A, Fredlund P, Kuepfer C. Trial Evaluating the Activity of Tadalafil for Erectile Dysfunction–United States (TREATED-US) Study Group. Efficacy, safety, and treatment satisfaction of tadalafil versus placebo in patients with erectile dysfunction evaluated at tertiary-care academic centers. Urology. 2005 Feb;65(2):353–9.
Language	English

Compound	Tadalafil (G04BE08)
Disease treated	Erectile dysfunction
Quantification of dysfunction	IIEF
No. of patients treated	140
Age group	Middle-aged
Treatment period	6 months
Dose	20 mg

Treatment consequences	Erectile function, improvement
Efficacy	IIEF score 16.2±0.7 at baseline, 24.3±0.8 after 3 months, 24.3±0.9 after 6 months of treatment
Side effects compromising effectiveness	Not mentioned
Randomization of patients	Yes
Dose arms 1–3	Tadalafil; placebo
Study quality	**1–**
Reference	1209: McMahon CG, Carson CC, Fischer CJ, Wang WC, Florio VA, Bradley JD. Tolerance to the therapeutic effect of tadalafil does not occur during 6 months of treatment: a randomized, double-blind, placebo-controlled study in men with erectile dysfunction. J Sex Med. 2006 May;3(3):504–11.
Language	English

Compound	Tadalafil (G04BE08)
Disease treated	Erectile dysfunction
Quantification of dysfunction	Total testosterone (T), free T (f T), oestradiol (E) levels
No. of patients treated	20
Age group	55 years (mean)
Treatment period	12 months
Dose	20 mg
Treatment consequences	Hormone levels, alteration
Efficacy	Significant decrease in E levels, increase in the T:E ratio, no changes in T and f T serum levels
Side effects compromising effectiveness	Not mentioned
Randomization of patients	Yes
Dose arms 1–3	Tadalafil; placebo
Study quality	**1–**
Reference	1226: Greco EA, Pili M, Bruzziches R, Corona G, Spera G, Aversa A. Testosterone:estradiol ratio changes associated with long-term tadalafil administration: a pilot study. J Sex Med. 2006 Jul;3(4):716–22.
Language	English

2

Compound	Tadalafil (G04BE08)
Disease treated	Erectile dysfunction
Quantification of dysfunction	Cardiovascular diseases
Age group	Old
Treatment consequences	Erectile function, improvement
Efficacy	Good
Side effects compromising effectiveness	No significant side effects
Randomization of patients	No
Study quality	**4 (review)**
Reference	1106: Brock GB. Tadalafil: a new agent for erectile dysfunction. Can J Urol. 2003 Feb;10 Suppl 1:17–22.
Language	English

Vardenafil: The most common adverse effects were headache (up to 22%), flushing (up to 13%), rhinitis (up to 17%) and dyspepsia (up to 6%). No reports of abnormal colour vision have been published. Adverse effects were generally mild to moderate and transient in nature. The rates of the adverse events were either constant or declining over time and with lowering of dose.

Compound	Vardenafil (G04BE09)
Disease treated	Erectile dysfunction in different conditions
Quantification of dysfunction	IIEF
No. of patients treated	1385
Age group	Middle-aged
Treatment period	12 weeks
Dose	20 mg
Treatment consequences	Erectile function, improvement
Efficacy	Men treated with 10 or 20 mg showed statistically significant improvements. The greatest improvements relative to placebo were noted in patients with more severe dysfunction.

Side effects compromising effectiveness	Most common: headache; flushing; rhinitis; dyspepsia; dose related, mostly mild to moderate
Randomization of patients	Yes
Dose arms 1–3	Vardenafil; placebo
Study quality	**1+**
Reference	1222: Donatucci C, Eardley I, Buvat J, Gittelman M, Kell P, Segerson T, Homering M, Montorsi F; Vardenafil Study Group. Vardenafil improves erectile function in men with erectile dysfunction irrespective of disease severity and disease classification. J Sex Med. 2004 Nov;1(3):301–9.
Language	English

Compound	Vardenafil (G04BE09)
Disease treated	Erectile dysfunction
Quantification of dysfunction	IIEF
No. of patients treated	580
Age group	Middle-aged
Treatment period	12 weeks
Dose	20 mg
Treatment consequences	Erectile function, improvement
Efficacy	Mean erectile function domain scores of IIEF statistically greater than placebo, irrespective of aetiology, baseline severity or age. Vardenafil significantly improved the IIEF domain scores of erectile function, orgasmic function and intercourse satisfaction.
Side effects compromising effectiveness	Rates of the adverse events (headache, flushing and dyspepsia) either constant or declining over time; generally mild to moderate and transient in nature
Randomization of patients	Yes
Dose arms 1–3	Vardenafil; placebo
Study quality	**1+**
Reference	1223: Porst H, Young JM, Schmidt AC, Buvat J; International Vardenafil Study Group. Efficacy and tolerability of vardenafil for treatment of erectile dysfunction in patient subgroups. Urology. 2003 Sep;62(3):519–23; discussion 523–4.
Language	English

Compound	Vardenafil (G04BE09)
Disease treated	Erectile dysfunction, sildenafil non-responder
Quantification of dysfunction	IIEF
No. of patients treated	463
Age group	>18 years
Treatment period	8 weeks
Dose	20 mg
Treatment consequences	Erectile function, improvement
Efficacy	Significantly better erectile function with vardenafil than with placebo. Normal erectile function was achieved by 30% of patients receiving vardenafil and 6% receiving placebo.
Side effects compromising effectiveness	Infrequent
Randomization of patients	Yes
Dose arms 1–3	Vardenafil; placebo
Study quality	**1+**
Reference	1214: Carson CC, Hatzichristou DG, Carrier S, Lording D, Lyngdorf P, Aliotta P, Auerbach S, Murdock M, Wilkins HJ, McBride TA, Colopy MW; Patient Response with Vardenafil in Slidenafil Non-Responders (PROVEN) Study Group. Erectile response with vardenafil in sildenafil nonresponders: a multicentre, double-blind, 12-week, flexible-dose, placebo-controlled erectile dysfunction clinical trial. BJU Int. 2004 Dec;94(9):1301–9.
Language	English

Compound	Vardenafil (G04BE09)
Disease treated	Erectile dysfunction after nerve-sparing radical prostatectomy
Quantification of dysfunction	IIEF
No. of patients treated	440
Age group	Old
Treatment period	12 weeks
Dose	20 mg
Treatment consequences	Erectile function, improvement

Efficacy	In group with 10 and 20 mg vardenafil doses significantly greater than in placebo group; significant improvement in the satisfaction rate with erection hardness for each vardenafil dose compared with placebo
Side effects compromising effectiveness	Generally well tolerated; common adverse events were headache, vasodilatation and rhinitis
Randomization of patients	Yes
Dose arms 1–3	Vardenafil; placebo
Study quality	**1+**
Reference	1211: Nehra A, Grantmyre J, Nadel A, Thibonnier M, Brock G. Vardenafil improved patient satisfaction with erectile hardness, orgasmic function and sexual experience in men with erectile dysfunction following nerve sparing radical prostatectomy. J Urol. 2005 Jun;173(6):2067–71.
Language	English

Compound	Vardenafil (G04BE09)
Disease treated	Erectile dysfunction
Quantification of dysfunction	IIEF
No. of patients treated	n.g.
Age group	Middle-aged
Treatment period	26
Dose	20 mg
Treatment consequences	Erectile function, improvement
Efficacy	Improvements of IIEF score were significantly greater with vardenafil 10 or 20 mg than with placebo.
Side effects compromising effectiveness	Most common: headache; flushing; rhinitis; dyspepsia; and sinusitis. There were no reports of abnormal colour vision.
Randomization of patients	Yes
Dose arms 1–3	Vardenafil; placebo
Study quality	**1+ (meta-analysis)**
Reference	1210: Keating GM, Scott LJ. Spotlight on vardenafil in erectile dysfunction. Drugs Aging. 2004;21(2):135–40.
Language	English

Compound	Vardenafil (G04BE09)
Disease treated	Erectile dysfunction
Quantification of dysfunction	IIEF
No. of patients treated	n.g.
Age group	Middle-aged
Treatment period	12 weeks
Dose	20 mg
Treatment consequences	Erectile function, improvement
Efficacy	Compared with placebo, patients taking 10 and 20 mg doses of vardenafil showed statistically significantly greater improvement in IIEF domain scores vs placebo.
Side effects compromising effectiveness	Most frequent in the 5, 10 and 20 mg of vardenafil and placebo groups, respectively: headache (10, 22, 21 and 4%); flushing (5, 10, 13 and 0%); dyspepsia (1, 4, 6 and <1%); and rhinitis (9, 14, 17 and 5%); mild or moderate, transient in nature
Randomization of patients	Yes
Dose arms 1–3	Vardenafil; placebo
Study quality	**1+**
Reference	1244: Giuliano F, Donatucci C, Montorsi F, Auerbach S, Karlin G, Norenberg C, Homering M, Segerson T, Eardley I; Vardenafil Study Group. Vardenafil is effective and well-tolerated for treating erectile dysfunction in a broad population of men, irrespective of age. BJU Int. 2005 Jan;95(1):110–6.
Language	English

Apomorphine: The drug appeared to be safe and efficacious in the treatment, irrespective of underlying diseases and concomitant medications, including 5-phosphodiesterase inhibitors. Adverse effects observed were nausea (up to 14%), dizziness (up to 7%), headache (up to 7%) and spontaneous yawning. The effects were mild to moderate and self-limited. In direct comparison with sildenafil, the rate of efficacy and the rate of adverse effects was higher in apomorphine treatment, and 96% of patients expressed a preference for sildenafil as a treatment. Apomorphine is no longer available in Germany.

Overall level of evidence of positive effects: A
Overall level of evidence of adverse effects compromising effectiveness: A

Compound	Apomorphine (G04BE07)
Disease treated	Erectile dysfunction
Quantification of dysfunction	Erectile function
No. of patients treated	5000
Age group	Old
Treatment period	Various
Dose	Various
Treatment consequences	Erectile function, improvement
Efficacy	Good safety profile but syncope at higher doses
Side effects compromising effectiveness	Mild side effects (<7%): nausea; headache; and dizziness
Randomization of patients	In part
Study quality	**1+ (meta-analysis)**
Reference	1184: Bukofzer S, Livesey N. Safety and tolerability of apomorphine SL (Uprima). Int J Impot Res. 2001 Aug;13 Suppl 3:S40–4.
Language	English

Compound	Apomorphine (G04BE07)
Disease treated	Erectile dysfunction
Quantification of dysfunction	Erectile function
No. of patients treated	569
Age group	Old
Treatment period	8 weeks
Dose	2–6 mg
Treatment consequences	Erection sufficient for coitus
Efficacy	Significantly higher in apomorphine group (53%) than in placebo group (35%)
Side effects compromising effectiveness	Nausea was dose related and diminished number of patients on treatment
Randomization of patients	Yes
Dose arms 1–3	Apomorphine; placebo
Study quality	**1+**

Reference	1588: Dula E, Keating W, Siami PF, Edmonds A, O'Neil J, Buttler S. Efficacy and safety of fixed-dose and dose-optimization regimens of sublingual apomorphine versus placebo in men with erectile dysfunction. The Apomorphine Study Group. Urology. 2000 Jul;56(1):130–5.
Language	English

Compound	**Apomorphine (G04BE07)**
Disease treated	Erectile dysfunction
Quantification of dysfunction	Sexual function
No. of patients treated	507
Age group	18–70 years
Treatment period	8 weeks
Dose	2–4 mg
Treatment consequences	Erectile function, improvement
Efficacy	Significantly higher in apomorphine than in placebo
Side effects compromising effectiveness	Greater than 5% of patients in treated group: nausea (9.8%), dizziness (7.1%) and headache (6.7%), compared with 0.4, 2.4 and 4.0%, respectively, in placebo group
Randomization of patients	Yes
Dose arms 1–3	Apomorphine; placebo
Study quality	**1+**
Reference	1584: Keitz AT von, Stroberg P, Bukofzer S, Mallard N, Hibberd M. A European multicentre study to evaluate the tolerability of apomorphine sublingual administered in a forced dose-escalation regimen in patients with erectile dysfunction. BJU Int. 2002 Mar;89(4):409–15.
Language	English

Compound	**Apomorphine (G04BE07)**
Disease treated	Erectile dysfunction
Quantification of dysfunction	Erectile function
No. of patients treated	296
Age group	Old
Treatment period	4 weeks
Dose	4 mg
Treatment consequences	Erection sufficient for coitus
Efficacy	Significantly higher in apomorphine than in placebo

Side effects compromising effectiveness	Nausea in 3.3% of patients on 3 mg, 14.1% on 4 mg and 1.1% of patients on placebo
Randomization of patients	Yes
Dose arms 1–3	Apomorphine; placebo
Study quality	**1+**
Reference	1587: Dula E, Bukofzer S, Perdok R, George M; Apomorphine SL Study Group. Double-blind, crossover comparison of 3 mg apomorphine SL with placebo and with 4 mg apomorphine SL in male erectile dysfunction. Eur Urol. 2001 May;39(5):558–3; discussion 564.
Language	English

Compound	Apomorphine (G04BE07)
Disease treated	Erectile dysfunction
Quantification of dysfunction	IIEF
No. of patients treated	139
Age group	Old
Treatment period	8 weeks
Dose	n.g.
Treatment consequences	Erection sufficient for coitus
Efficacy	35% of apomorphine group, 75% of sildenafil group
Side effects compromising effectiveness	96% expressed a preference for sildenafil as a treatment
Randomization of patients	Yes
Dose arms 1–3	Apomorphine; sildenafil
Study quality	**1+**
Reference	1573: Eardley I, Wright P, MacDonagh R, Hole J, Edwards A. An open-label, randomized, flexible-dose, crossover study to assess the comparative efficacy and safety of sildenafil citrate and apomorphine hydrochloride in men with erectile dysfunction. BJU Int. 2004 Jun;93(9):1271–5.
Language	English

Compound	Apomorphine (G04BE07)
Disease treated	Erectile dysfunction in diabetes mellitus
Quantification of dysfunction	IIEF

No. of patients treated	130
Age group	Old
Treatment period	Four doses
Dose	3 mg
Treatment consequences	Erection sufficient for coitus
Efficacy	22% in apomorphine, 17% in placebo
Side effects compromising effectiveness	Not mentioned
Randomization of patients	Yes
Dose arms 1–3	Apomorphine; placebo
Study quality	**1+**
Reference	1570: Gontero P, D'Antonio R, Pretti G, Fontana F, Panella M, Kocjancic E, Allochis G, Frea B. Clinical efficacy of apomorphine SL in erectile dysfunction of diabetic men. Int J Impot Res. 2005 Jan–Feb;17(1):80–5.
Language	English

Compound	Apomorphine (G04BE07)
Disease treated	Erectile dysfunction
Quantification of dysfunction	IIEF
No. of patients treated	110
Age group	Old
Treatment period	10 weeks
Dose	2–3 mg
Treatment consequences	Erectile function, improvement
Efficacy	15.9–20.4 IIEF score
Side effects compromising effectiveness	The drug is safe and efficacious in the treatment, irrespective of underlying diseases and concomitant medications.
Randomization of patients	No
Study quality	**3**
Reference	1578: Amornvejsukit T. Evaluating dose regimens of apomorphine, an open-label study. Int J Impot Res. 2003 Apr;15 Suppl 2:S10–2.
Language	English

Compound	Apomorphine (G04BE07)
Disease treated	Erectile dysfunction
Quantification of dysfunction	Erectile function
No. of patients treated	77
Age group	Old
Treatment period	4 weeks
Dose	3 mg
Treatment consequences	Erection sufficient for coitus
Efficacy	44% in apomorphine, 85% in sildenafil
Side effects compromising effectiveness	Incidence of adverse events not significantly different for the two drugs
Randomization of patients	Yes
Dose arms 1–3	Apomorphine; sildenafil
Study quality	**1+**
Reference	1569: Pavone C, Curto F, Anello G, Serretta V, Almasio PL, Pavone-Macaluso M. Prospective, randomized, crossover comparison of sublingual apomorphine (3 mg) with oral sildenafil (50 mg) for male erectile dysfunction. J Urol. 2004 Dec;172(6 Pt 1):2347–9.
Language	English

Compound	Apomorphine (G04BE07)
Disease treated	Erectile dysfunction, vascular
Quantification of dysfunction	Sexual function
No. of patients treated	41
Age group	Old
Treatment period	4 weeks
Dose	2–3 mg
Treatment consequences	Erectile function, improvement
Efficacy	32% in apomorphine, 64% in sildenafil
Side effects compromising effectiveness	Higher rate of side effects in apomorphine group than in sildenafil group
Randomization of patients	Yes
Dose arms 1–3	Apomorphine; sildenafil

Study quality	**1+**
Reference	1575: Perimenis P, Gyftopoulos K, Giannitsas K, Markou SA, Tsota I, Chrysanthopoulou A, Athanasopoulos A, Barbalias G. A comparative, crossover study of the efficacy and safety of sildenafil and apomorphine in men with evidence of arteriogenic erectile dysfunction. Int J Impot Res. 2004 Feb;16(1):2–7.
Language	English

Compound	Apomorphine (G04BE07)
Disease treated	Erectile dysfunction
Quantification of dysfunction	Sexual function
No. of patients treated	40
Age group	Old
Treatment period	10 days
Dose	2–3 mg
Treatment consequences	Erectile function, improvement
Efficacy	Statistically better in sildenafil than in apomorphine
Side effects compromising effectiveness	Not mentioned
Randomization of patients	Yes
Dose arms 1–3	Apomorphine; sildenafil
Study quality	**1+**
Reference	1572: Perimenis P, Markou S, Gyftopoulos K, Giannitsas K, Athanasopoulos A, Liatsikos E, Barbalias G. Efficacy of apomorphine and sildenafil in men with nonarteriogenic erectile dysfunction. A comparative crossover study. Andrologia. 2004 Jun;36(3):106–10.
Language	English

Compound	Apomorphine (G04BE07)
Disease treated	Hyperprolactinaemia
Quantification of dysfunction	IIEF
No. of patients treated	34
Age group	Old
Treatment period	4 weeks

Dose	2–3 mg
Treatment consequences	Erectile function, improvement
Efficacy	13 of 20 patients
Side effects compromising effectiveness	Mild or moderate severity in 4 patients taking on-demand and 3 patients taking daily use, nausea, dizziness or headache
Randomization of patients	No
Study quality	**2–**
Reference	1576: Caruso S, Intelisano G, Farina M, DiMari L, Agnello C, Giammusso B. Efficacy and safety of daily intake of apomorphine SL in men affected by erectile dysfunction and mild hyperprolactinemia: a prospective, open-label, pilot study. Urology. 2003 Nov;62(5):922–7.
Language	English

Compound	Apomorphine (G04BE07)
Disease treated	Erectile dysfunction
Quantification of dysfunction	Erectile function assessed by Rigiscan
No. of patients treated	28
Age group	Old
Treatment period	n.g.
Dose	1 mg
Treatment consequences	Erection sufficient for coitus
Efficacy	17 of 28 patients
Side effects compromising effectiveness	Placebo induced spontaneous yawning, antagonized by 3.5 and 5.0 mg/kg apomorphine, but increased by 7.0 mg/kg apomorphine.
Randomization of patients	No
Study quality	**2–**
Reference	1590: Lal S, Tesfaye Y, Thavundayil JX, Thompson TR, Kiely ME, Nair NP, Grassino A, Dubrovsky B. Apomorphine: clinical studies on erectile impotence and yawning. Prog Neuropsychopharmacol Biol Psychiatry. 1989;13(3–4):329–39.
Language	English

Compound	Apomorphine (G04BE07)
Disease treated	Erectile dysfunction
Quantification of dysfunction	Magnetic resonance tomography (MRT), cerebral
No. of patients treated	16
Age group	Young
Treatment period	7 days
Dose	2 mg
Treatment consequences	Activation in thalamus, associtated with erection, during visual stimulation, improvement
Efficacy	Cerebral activation of an area associated with sexual arousal
Side effects compromising effectiveness	Not mentioned
Randomization of patients	No
Dose arms 1–3	Apomorphine; placebo
Study quality	**2–**
Reference	1581: Montorsi F, Perani D, Anchisi D, Salonia A, Scifo P, Rigiroli P, Deho F, Vito ML de, Heaton J, Rigatti P, Fazio F. Brain activation patterns during video sexual stimulation following the administration of apomorphine: results of a placebo-controlled study. Eur Urol. 2003 Apr;43(4):405–11.
Language	English

Compound	Apomorphine (G04BE07)
Disease treated	Erectile dysfunction
Quantification of dysfunction	Cerebral PET scans
No. of patients treated	12
Age group	Young
Treatment period	Single dose
Dose	2 mg
Treatment consequences	Erectile rigidity during visual stimulation
Efficacy	Cerebral activation of an area associated with sexual arousal
Side effects compromising effectiveness	Not mentioned
Randomization of patients	Yes

Dose arms 1–3	Apomorphine; placebo
Study quality	**1–**
Reference	1580: Hagemann JH, Berding G, Bergh S, Sleep DJ, Knapp WH, Jonas U, Stief CG. Effects of visual sexual stimuli and apomorphine SL on cerebral activity in men with erectile dysfunction. Eur Urol. 2003 Apr;43(4):412–20.
Language	English

Compound	Apomorphine (G04BE07)
Disease treated	Erectile dysfunction
Quantification of dysfunction	Erectile function assessed by Rigiscan
No. of patients treated	10
Age group	Middle-aged
Treatment period	Single dose
Dose	5 mg/day
Treatment consequences	Erection sufficient for coitus
Efficacy	67% of patients
Side effects compromising effectiveness	Not mentioned
Randomization of patients	No
Study quality	**3**
Reference	1589: Heaton JP, Morales A, Adams MA, Johnston B, el-Rashidy R. Recovery of erectile function by the oral administration of apomorphine. Urology. 1995 Feb;45(2):200–6.
Language	English

2

G04 Urologicals

G04C Drugs Used in Benign Prostatic Hyperplasia

Patients suffering from lower urinary tract symptoms are at risk of having erectile dysfunction, irrespective of the treatment. In large case-control studies the OR is doubled in comparison with healthy men.

α-adrenoreceptor agonists tend to improve, or at least do not impair, erectile function, owing to the relaxation of smooth muscle. Finasteride impairs erectile function in up to 33%, which may be a consequence of the antiandrogenic effects. This effect is – to a lesser extent – observed also in young men being treated for alopecia androgenetica.

Overall level of evidence of adverse effects: A

Compound	Drugs used in benign prostatic hyperplasia (G04C)
Disease treated	Lower urinary tract symptoms (LUTS)
Quantification of adverse effects	IIEF
No. of patients treated	28,691
Age group	20–75 years
Treatment period	Various
Dose	Various
Treatment consequences	Prevalence of erectile dysfunction as compared with men without LUTS
Efficacy	OR 2.0 (95% CI 1.8–2.5)
Randomization of patients	No
Study quality	**2++**
Reference	2217: Shabsigh R, Perelman MA, Lockhart DC, Lue TF, Broderick GA. Health issues of men: prevalence and correlates of erectile dysfunction. J Urol. 2005 Aug;174(2):662–7.
Language	English

Compound	Drugs used in benign prostatic hyperplasia (G04C)
Disease treated	Lower urinary tract symptoms (LUTS)
Quantification of adverse effects	Kölner Erhebungsbogen
No. of patients treated	4489
Age group	30–80 years

Treatment period	Various
Dose	Various
Treatment consequences	Prevalence of erectile dysfunction as compared with men without LUTS
Efficacy	In men with erectile dysfunction the prevalence of LUTS was 72.2%, in men without erectile dysfunction LUTS were present in 37.7%.
Randomization of patients	No
Study quality	**2–**
Reference	2225: Braun MH, Sommer F, Haupt G, Mathers MJ, Reifenrath B, Engelmann UH. Lower urinary tract symptoms and erectile dysfunction: co-morbidity or typical "Aging Male" symptoms? Results of the "Cologne Male Survey". Eur Urol. 2003 Nov;44(5):588–94.
Language	English

Compound	Drugs used in benign prostatic hyperplasia (G04C)
Disease treated	Lower urinary tract symptoms (LUTS)
Quantification of adverse effects	IIEF, IPSS
No. of patients treated	2858
Age group	20–80 years
Treatment period	Various
Dose	Various
Treatment consequences	Prevalence of erectile dysfunction as compared with men without LUTS
Efficacy	OR 2.2 (95% CI 1.8–2.8) in high IPSS as compared with low IPPS
Randomization of patients	No
Study quality	**2–**
Reference	2222: Ponholzer A, Temml C, Obermayr R, Madersbacher S. Association between lower urinary tract symptoms and erectile dysfunction. Urology. 2004 Oct;64(4):772–6.
Language	English

Compound	Drugs used in benign prostatic hyperplasia (G04C)
Disease treated	Lower urinary tract symptoms (LUTS)
Quantification of adverse effects	Single question for erectile function
No. of patients treated	1982

Age group	>40 years
Treatment period	No treatment
Treatment consequences	Prevalence of erectile dysfunction as compared with men without LUTS
Efficacy	OR 3.03 (95% CI 2.09–4.44)
Randomization of patients	No
Study quality	**2++**
Reference	2216: Akkus E, Kadioglu A, Esen A, Doran S, Ergen A, Anafarta K, Hattat H; Turkish Erectile Dysfunction Prevalence Study Group. Prevalence and correlates of erectile dysfunction in Turkey: a population-based study. Eur Urol. 2002 Mar;41(3):298–304.
Language	English

Compound	Drugs used in benign prostatic hyperplasia (G04C)
Disease treated	Lower urinary tract symptoms (LUTS)
Quantification of adverse effects	IIEF
No. of patients treated	794
Age group	50–80 years
Treatment period	Various
Dose	Various
Treatment consequences	Prevalence of erectile dysfunction with severe LUTS as compared with men without LUTS
Efficacy	OR 7.67 (95% CI 5.87–10.02)
Randomization of patients	No
Study quality	**2+**
Reference	2211: Rosen R, Altwein J, Boyle P, Kirby RS, Lukacs B, Meuleman E, O'Leary MP, Puppo P, Robertson C, Giuliano F. Lower urinary tract symptoms and male sexual dysfunction: the multinational survey of the aging male (MSAM-7). Eur Urol. 2003 Dec;44(6):637–49.
Language	English

Compound	Drugs used in benign prostatic hyperplasia (G04C)
Disease treated	Lower urinary tract symptoms (LUTS)
Quantification of adverse effects	IIEF
No. of patients treated	476
Age group	55 years (mean)

Treatment period	Various
Dose	Various
Treatment consequences	Prevalence of erectile dysfunction
Efficacy	77%; mean age lower than in patients without LUTS
Randomization of patients	No
Study quality	**3**
Reference	2237: El-Sakka AI. Lower urinary tract symptoms in patients with erectile dysfunction: analysis of risk factors. J Sex Med. 2006 Jan;3(1):144–9.
Language	English

Compound	Drugs used in benign prostatic hyperplasia (G04C)
Disease treated	Lower urinary tract symptoms (LUTS)
Quantification of adverse effects	Single question from the NIH consensus definition
No. of patients treated	428
Age group	40–70 years
Treatment period	Various
Dose	Various
Treatment consequences	Prevalence of erectile dysfunction as compared with men without LUTS
Efficacy	RR 3.67 (95% CI 1.17–11.48)
Randomization of patients	No
Study quality	**2+**
Reference	2213: Moreira ED Jr, Lobo CF, Diament A, Nicolosi A, Glasser DB. Incidence of erectile dysfunction in men 40 to 69 years old: results from a population-based cohort study in Brazil. Urology. 2003 Feb;61(2):431–6.
Language	English

Compound	Drugs used in benign prostatic hyperplasia (G04C)
Disease treated	Lower urinary tract symptoms (LUTS)
Quantification of adverse effects	Single question from the NIH consensus definition
No. of patients treated	428
Age group	40–70 years
Dose	Various
Treatment consequences	Incidence of erectile dysfunction within 2 years of duration

Efficacy	RR 1.83 (95% CI 0.65–5.20)
Randomization of patients	No
Study quality	**2+**
Reference	2229: Moreira ED Jr, Abdo CH, Torres EB, Lobo CF, Fittipaldi JA. Prevalence and correlates of erectile dysfunction: results of the Brazilian study of sexual behavior. Urology. 2001 Oct;58(4):583–8.
Language	English

Compound	**Drugs used in benign prostatic hyperplasia (G04C)**
Disease treated	Lower urinary tract symptoms (LUTS)
Quantification of adverse effects	IIEF
No. of patients treated	181
Age group	68.2 years (mean)
Treatment period	Various
Dose	Various
Treatment consequences	Prevalence of erectile dysfunction
Efficacy	Correlation with IIEF-0.12
Randomization of patients	No
Study quality	**3**
Reference	2209: Elliott SP, Gulati M, Pasta DJ, Spitalny GM, Kane CJ, Yee R, Lue TF. Obstructive lower urinary tract symptoms correlate with erectile dysfunction. Urology. 2004 Jun;63(6):1148–52.
Language	English

Compound	**Drugs used in benign prostatic hyperplasia (G04C)**
Disease treated	Infertility
Quantification of adverse effects	Sexual Health Inventory for Men (SHIM)
No. of patients treated	302
Age group	Not mentioned
Treatment period	n.g.
Dose	Various
Treatment consequences	Prevalence of erectile dysfunction
Efficacy	Higher ratio than in healthy controls

Randomization of patients	No
Study quality	**2–**
Reference	2242: O'Brien JH, Lazarou S, Deane L, Jarvi K, Zini A. Erectile dysfunction and andropause symptoms in infertile men. J Urol. 2005 Nov;174(5):1932–4; discussion 1934
Language	English

Compound	Drugs used in benign prostatic hyperplasia (G04C)
Disease treated	Lower urinary tract symptoms (LUTS)
Quantification of adverse effects	IIEF
No. of patients treated	2476
Age group	25–70 years
Treatment period	No treatment
Treatment consequences	Prevalence of erectile dysfunction
Efficacy	OR 2.93 (95% CI 1.86–4.61)
Randomization of patients	No
Study quality	**2++**
Reference	2215: Martin-Morales A, Sanchez-Cruz JJ, Saenz de Tejada I, Rodriguez-Vela L, Jimenez-Cruz JF, Burgos-Rodriguez RJ. Prevalence and independent risk factors for erectile dysfunction in Spain: results of the Epidemiologia de la Disfuncion Erectil Masculina Study. Urol. 2001 Aug;166(2):569–74.
Language	English

Compound	Drugs used in benign prostatic hyperplasia (G04C)
Disease treated	Lower urinary tract symptoms (LUTS)
Quantification of adverse effects	Single question
No. of patients treated	491
Age group	40–70 years
Treatment period	No treatment
Treatment consequences	Prevalence of erectile dysfunction
Efficacy	OR 4.56 (95% CI 2.24–9.27)
Randomization of patients	No
Study quality	**2+**

Reference	2207: Nicolosi A, Moreira ED Jr, Shirai M, Bin Mohd Tambi MI, Glasser DB. Epidemiology of erectile dysfunction in four countries: cross-national study of the prevalence and correlates of erectile dysfunction. Urology. 2003 Jan;61(1):201–6.
Language	English

Compound	Drugs used in benign prostatic hyperplasia (G04C)
Disease treated	Lower urinary tract symptoms (LUTS)
Quantification of adverse effects	Single question from the NIH consensus definition
No. of patients treated	428
Age group	40–70 years
Treatment period	No treatment
Treatment consequences	Prevalence, increment per year of age
Efficacy	RR 1.07 (95% CI 1.04–1.11)
Randomization of patients	No
Study quality	**2+**
Reference	2213: Moreira ED Jr, Lobo CF, Diament A, Nicolosi A, Glasser DB. Incidence of erectile dysfunction in men 40 to 69 years old: results from a population-based cohort study in Brazil. Urology. 2003 Feb;61(2):431–6.
Language	English

Compound	α-adrenoreceptor agonists (G04CA)
Disease treated	Benign prostatic hyperplasia
Quantification of adverse effects	Erectile function
No. of patients treated	1044
Age group	Old
Treatment period	Continuous
Dose	As recommended
Treatment consequences	Erectile function, improvement
Efficacy	Score 35 improves to 50
Randomization of patients	Yes
Dose arms 1–3	Alfuzosin; placebo

Study quality	**1+ (meta-analysis)**
Reference	1100: Larson TR. Current treatment options for benign prostatic hyperplasia and their impact on sexual function. Urology. 2003 Apr;61(4):692–8.
Language	English

Compound	α-adrenoceptor agonists (G04CA)
Disease treated	Benign prostatic hyperplasia
Quantification of adverse effects	Erectile function
No. of patients treated	43
Age group	66 years (mean)
Treatment period	n.g.
Dose	n.g.
Treatment consequences	Sexual function, alteration
Efficacy	84% of patients
Randomization of patients	No
Study quality	**3**
Reference	1116: Leliefeld HH, Stoevelaar HJ, McDonnell J. Sexual function before and after various treatments for symptomatic benign prostatic hyperplasia. BJU Int. 2002 Feb;89(3):208–13.
Language	English

Compound	α-adrenoreceptor agonists (G04CA)
Disease treated	Benign prostatic hyperplasia
Quantification of adverse effects	Sexual function
Age group	Old
Treatment consequences	Sexual function and QOL, improvement
Efficacy	Best improved
Study quality	**4 (review)**
Reference	1012: Martin DJ, Mulhall JP. Enlarging the scope of managing benign prostatic hyperplasia: addressing sexual function and quality of life. Int J Clin Pract. 2005 May;59(5):579–90.
Language	English

2

Compound	α-adrenoreceptor agonists (G04CA)
Disease treated	Lower urinary tract symptoms (LUTS)
Quantification of adverse effects	Sexual function
Age group	Old
Treatment consequences	Erectile function, impairment
Efficacy	Reports on erectile function are inconsistent. Impotence can occur in some patients without clear differences between drugs.
Study quality	**4 (review)**
Reference	1260: van Dijk MM, Rosette JJ de la, Michel MC. Effects of alpha(1)-adrenoceptor antagonists on male sexual function. Drugs. 2006;66(3):287–301.
Language	English

Compound	Alfuzosin (G04CA01)
Disease treated	Lower urinary tract symptoms (LUTS)
Quantification of adverse effects	Sexual function questionnaires
No. of patients treated	2829
Age group	66 years (mean)
Treatment period	12 months
Dose	7.5 mg/day
Treatment consequences	Sexual function rating scale, improvement
Efficacy	191% (correct!)
Side effects compromising effectiveness	13.7% discontinuation
Randomization of patients	No
Study quality	**2–**
Reference	1446: Lukacs B, Grange JC, Comet D and the BPM Group in General Practice: one year follow-up of 2829 patients with moderate to severe lower urinary tract symptoms treated with alfuzosin in genera practice according to IPSS and a health-related quality-of-life questionnaire. Urology 2000;55:540–546.
Language	English

Compound	Alfuzosin (G04CA01)
Disease treated	Lower urinary tract symptoms (LUTS)
Quantification of adverse effects	International Prostate Symptom Score (IPSS)
No. of patients treated	955
Age group	Old
Treatment period	12 weeks
Dose	10 mg/day
Treatment consequences	Erectile function, impairment
Efficacy	None
Randomization of patients	Yes
Dose arms 1–3	Alfuzosin; placebo
Study quality	**1+**
Reference	1261: Roehrborn CG, Van Kerrebroeck P, Nordling J. Safety and efficacy of alfuzosin 10 mg once-daily in the treatment of lower urinary tract symptoms and clinical benign prostatic hyperplasia: a pooled analysis of three double-blind, placebo-controlled studies. BJU Int. 2003 Aug;92(3):257–61.
Language	English

Compound	Alfuzosin (G04CA01)
Disease treated	Lower urinary tract symptoms (LUTS)
Quantification of adverse effects	International Prostatic Symptom score (IPSS), Brief Male Sexual Function Inventory (BSFI)
No. of patients treated	823
Age group	67 years (mean)
Treatment period	2 years
Dose	10 mg/day
Treatment consequences	IPSS, improvement; BSFI, impairment
Efficacy	IPSS by 7 points; BSFI unaltered
Randomization of patients	Real-life practice
Study quality	**3**
Reference	1591: Elhilali M, Emberton M, Matzkin H, van Moorselaar RJ, Hartung R, Harving N, Alcaraz A, Vallancien G; ALF-ONE Study Group. Long-term efficacy and safety of alfuzosin 10 mg once daily: a 2-year experience in "real-life" practice. BJU Int. 2006 Mar;97(3):513–9.
Language	English

Compound	Tamsulosin (G04CA02), alfuzosin
Disease treated	Lower urinary tract symptoms (LUTS)
Quantification of adverse effects	Sexual function questionnaires
No. of patients treated	256
Age group	>45 years
Treatment period	14 weeks
Treatment consequences	Erectile function, impairment
Efficacy	3.1% of tamsulosin group, 2.4% of alfuzosin group
Randomization of patients	Yes
Dose arms 1–3	Tamsulosin 0.4/day; alfuzosin 3×2.5/day; placebo
Remarks	Abnormal ejaculation is related to the pharmacological action.
Study quality	**1–**
Reference	1445: Höfner K, Claes H, De Reijke TM et al. for the European Tamsulosin Study Group: Tamsulosin 0.4 mg once daily: effect on seual function in patients with lower urinary tract symptoms suggestiveof benign prostatic obstruction. Eur Urology 1999;36, 335–341.
Language	English

Compound	Tamsulosin (G04CA02), alfuzosin
Disease treated	Cavernous tissue in vitro
Quantification of adverse effects	Isometric tension
Age group	45–75 years
Treatment consequences	Relaxation, improvement
Efficacy	Tamsulosin and PGE1 strongest effect; relaxation responses to drug mixtures containing tamsulosin significantly better than phentolamine-containing mixtures
Study quality	**1–**
Reference	1262: Kim SC, Seo KK, Lee SK, Song ES, Lee MY. Comparison of the synergistic effects of tamsulosin versus phentolamine on penile erection: in vitro and in vivo studies. Urol Res. 1999 Dec;27(6):437–44. Korea.
Language	English

Compound	Finasteride (G04CB01)
Disease treated	Benign prostatic hyperplasia
Quantification of adverse effects	Sexual dysfunction, self-reported
No. of patients treated	3040
Age group	45–78 years
Treatment period	48 months
Dose	5 mg/day
Treatment consequences	Erectile function, impairment
Efficacy	8.8% of finasterid group, 3.8% of placebo group
Randomization of patients	Yes
Dose arms 1–3	Finasteride 5 mg/day; placebo
Study quality	1++
Reference	1448: Kaplan SA, Holgrevw HL, Buskewitz RC et al. for the PROSCAR Long Term Efficacy, Safety Study group: comparison of the efficacy and safety of finasteride in older versus younger men with benign prostatic hyperlasie. Urology 2001;57:1073–1077.
Language	English

Compound	Finasteride (G04CB01)
Disease treated	Benign prostatic hyperplasia
Quantification of adverse effects	Erectile function
No. of patients treated	3040
Age group	Old
Treatment period	4 years
Dose	5 mg
Treatment consequences	Sexual dysfunction
Efficacy	15% in finasteride group, 7% of placebo group
Randomization of patients	Yes
Dose arms 1–3	Finasteride; placebo
Study quality	1++

Reference	1628: Wessells H, Roy J, Bannow J, Grayhack J, Matsumoto AM, Tenover L, Herlihy R, Fitch W, Labasky R, Auerbach S, Parra R, Rajfer J, Culbertson J, Lee M, Bach MA, Waldstreicher J; PLESS Study Group. Incidence and severity of sexual adverse experiences in finasteride and placebo-treated men with benign prostatic hyperplasia. Urology. 2003 Mar;61(3):579–84.
Language	English

Compound	Finasteride (G04CB01)
Disease treated	Benign prostatic hyperplasia
Quantification of adverse effects	Sexual dysfunction, self-reported
No. of patients treated	472
Age group	45–80 years
Treatment period	24 months
Dose	5 mg/day
Treatment consequences	Sexual dysfunction
Efficacy	15.8% of finasterid group, in 6.3% of placebo group
Randomization of patients	Yes
Dose arms 1–3	Finasteride 5 mg/day; placebo
Study quality	**1++**
Reference	1447: Nickel JC, Fradet Y, Boake RC et al. for the PROSPECT Study Group: Efficacy and safety of finasteride therapy for benign prostatic hyperplasia: results of a 2-year randomized controlled trial. Can Med Assoc J 1996 155, 1251–1259.
Language	English

Compound	Finasteride (G04CB01)
Disease treated	Androgenetic alopecia
Quantification of adverse effects	Sexual dysfunction, self-reported
No. of patients treated	472
Age group	Young
Treatment period	n.g.
Dose	1 mg
Treatment consequences	Sexual dysfunction
Efficacy	No difference between groups

Randomization of patients	No
Dose arms 1–3	Finasteride; untreated age matched
Study quality	**2+**
Reference	1629: Tosti A, Piraccini BM, Soli M. Evaluation of sexual function in subjects taking finasteride for the treatment of androgenetic alopecia. J Eur Acad Dermatol Venereol. 2001 Sep;15(5):418–21.
Language	English

Compound	Finasteride (G04CB01)
Disease treated	Benign prostatic hyperplasia
Quantification of adverse effects	Erectile function
No. of patients treated	48
Age group	Old
Treatment period	6 months
Dose	5 mg
Treatment consequences	Erectile function, impairment
Efficacy	In 33% as compared with baseline
Randomization of patients	No
Study quality	**2–**
Reference	1100: Larson TR. Current treatment options for benign prostatic hyperplasia and their impact on sexual function. Urology. 2003 Apr;61(4):692–8.
Language	English

Compound	Finasteride (G04CB01)
Disease treated	Benign prostatic hyperplasia
Quantification of adverse effects	Erectile function
No. of patients treated	47
Age group	66 years (mean)
Dose	5 mg/day
Treatment consequences	Sexual function, alteration
Efficacy	84% of patients
Randomization of patients	No
Study quality	**2–**

Reference	1116: Leliefeld HH, Stoevelaar HJ, McDonnell J. Sexual function before and after various treatments for symptomatic benign prostatic hyperplasia. BJU Int. 2002 Feb;89(3):208–13.
Language	English

Compound	Finasteride (G04CB01)
Disease treated	Benign prostatic hyperplasia
Quantification of adverse effects	Sexual function
Age group	Old
Treatment consequences	Sexual function and QOL, impairment
Efficacy	Modest
Randomization of patients	No
Study quality	**4 (review)**
Reference	1012: Martin DJ, Mulhall JP. Enlarging the scope of managing benign prostatic hyperplasia: addressing sexual function and quality of life. Int J Clin Pract. 2005 May;59(5):579–90.
Language	English

Compound	Doxazosin (C02CA04)
Disease treated	Lower urinary tract symptoms (LUTS)
Quantification of adverse effects	Erectile function
No. of patients treated	3447
Age group	>40 years
Treatment period	6 months
Dose	4 mg
Treatment consequences	Erectile function, improvement during treatment for 6 months
Efficacy	In 4.5% of patients, 17.5% in the 40–49 years age group and 1.1% in the >70 years age group
Randomization of patients	No
Study quality	**3**
Reference	1265: Hernandez Fernandez C, Moncada Iribarren I, Jara Rascon J, Castano Gonzalez I, Moralejo Garate M. Treatment with Doxazosin in 3347 patients with lower urinary tract symptoms. Impact on sexual function. The impros study. Actas Urol Esp. 2004 Apr;28(4):290–7.

Language	Spanish

Compound	Doxazosin (C02CA04)
Disease treated	Lower urinary tract symptoms (LUTS)
Quantification of adverse effects	IIEF
No. of patients treated	680
Age group	50–80 years
Treatment period	13 weeks
Dose	8 months
Treatment consequences	Erectile function, improvement
Efficacy	Statistically and clinically significant in each dose of doxazosin
Randomization of patients	Yes
Dose arms 1–3	doxazosin; placebo;
Study quality	**1+**
Reference	1264: Kirby RS, O'Leary MP, Carson C. Efficacy of extended-release doxazosin and doxazosin standard in patients with concomitant benign prostatic hyperplasia and sexual dysfunction. BJU Int. 2005 Jan;95(1):103–9.
Language	English

Compound	Doxazosin (C02CA04)
Disease treated	Lower urinary tract symptoms (LUTS)
Quantification of adverse effects	Erectile function
No. of patients treated	305
Age group	Middle-aged
Treatment period	6 months
Dose	4 mg
Treatment consequences	Erectile function, impairment
Efficacy	Transurethral vaporization caused loss of erectile functions in 4 of 14 patients; 1 of 33 patients using doxazosin
Randomization of patients	No
Study quality	**2–**

Reference	1268: Uygur MC, Gur E, Arik AI, Altug U, Erol D. Erectile dysfunction following treatments of benign prostatic hyperplasia: a prospective study. Andrologia. 1998 Feb–Mar;30(1):5–10.
Language	English

Compound	Doxazosin (C02CA04)
Disease treated	Erectile dysfunction
Quantification of adverse effects	IIEF
No. of patients treated	38
Age group	Middle-aged
Treatment period	12 weeks
Dose	4 mg
Treatment consequences	Erectile function, improvement
Efficacy	Intracavernosal therapy: IIEF improved to 36.1±11.4 (17.7%); addition of doxazosin: IIEF improved to 51.5±14.3
Randomization of patients	Yes
Dose arms 1–3	Doxazosin; placebo
Study quality	**1+**
Reference	1267: Kaplan SA, Reis RB, Kohn IJ, Shabsigh R, Te AE. Combination therapy using oral alpha-blockers and intracavernosal injection in men with erectile dysfunction. Urology. 1998 Nov;52(5):739–43.
Language	English

Compound	Doxazosin (C02CA04)
Disease treated	Erectile dysfunction, non-responder to sildenafil
Quantification of adverse effects	IIEF
No. of patients treated	28
Age group	Middle-aged
Treatment period	60 days
Dose	4 mg
Treatment consequences	Erectile function, improvement
Efficacy	11 of 14 patients treated with doxazosin and sildenafil, 1 of 14 patients in the placebo group
Randomization of patients	Yes

Dose arms 1–3	Doxazosin+sildenafil; placebo+sildenafil
Study quality	**1–**
Reference	1266: Rose AF de, Giglio M, Traverso P, Lantieri P, Carmignani G. Combined oral therapy with sildenafil and doxazosin for the treatment of non-organic erectile dysfunction refractory to sildenafil monotherapy. Int J Impot Res. 2002 Feb;14(1):50–3.
Language	English

Compound	Doxazosin (C02CA04)
Disease treated	Cavernous tissue in vitro
Quantification of dysfunction	Relaxation of smooth muscles in vitro
No. of patients treated	n.g.
Age group	Old
Treatment consequences	Cavernous tissue, relaxation
Efficacy	Doxazosin and Y-27632 caused concentration-dependent relaxation
Randomization of patients	Yes
Study quality	**1–**
Reference	1263: Demir O, Murat N, Aslan G, Gidener S, Esen AA. Effect of doxazosin with and without rho-kinase inhibitor on human corpus cavernosum smooth muscle in the presence of bladder outlet obstruction. J Urol. 2006 Jun;175(6):2345–9.
Language	English

Compound	Doxazosin (C02CA04)
Disease treated	Benign prostatic hyperplasia
Quantification of adverse effects	Erectile function
Age group	Old
Treatment consequences	Erectile function, impairment
Efficacy	No effect
Study quality	**4 (review)**
Reference	1126: Flack JM. The effect of doxazosin on sexual function in patients with benign prostatic hyperplasia, hypertension, or both. Int J Clin Pract. 2002 Sep;56(7):527–30.
Language	English

Compound	Endothelin-1 antagonist (not listed)
Disease treated	Erectile dysfunction
Quantification of dysfunction	Erectile function
Age group	Old
Treatment consequences	Erectile function, improvement
Efficacy	Experimental benefit
Study quality	**4 (review)**
Reference	1186: Khan MA, Calvert RC, Sullivan ME, Thompson CS, Mumtaz FH, Morgan RJ, Mikhailidis DP. Normal and pathological erectile function: the potential clinical role of endothelin-1 antagonists. Curr Drug Targets. 2000 Nov;1(3):247–60.
Language	English

H02 Corticosteroids for Systemic Use

There is a single report on severe impairment of sexual function. The design of the trial does not exclude the possibility that the impairment is due to the diseases themselves.

Overall level of evidence of adverse effects: D

Compound	Cortisone (H02AB10)
Disease treated	Various diseases requiring chronic corticoid therapy
Quantification of adverse effects	Hormones; erectile function
No. of patients treated	17
Age group	23–56 years
Treatment period	Continuous
Dose	Various
Treatment consequences	Hormone levels, alteration; erectile function, alteration
Efficacy	58% decreased libido, 52% impotence, 41% lower back pain. T levels significantly lower than in controls, SHBG levels unchanged
Randomization of patients	No
Study quality	**3**

Reference	1375: Contreras LN, Masini AM, Danna MM, Kral M, Bruno OD, Rossi MA, Andrada JA. Glucocorticoids: their role on gonadal function and LH secretion. Minerva Endocrinol. 1996 Jun;21(2):43–6.
Language	English

H03 Thyroid Therapy

Dysfunctions of the thyroid gland, namely hyperthyreosis as well as hypothyreosis, appeared to non-specifically impair male sexual functions. The kind of impairment is unclear. RCTs are not available.

Overall level of evidence of adverse effects: C

Compound	Hyperthyreosis (H03AA)
Disease treated	Thyroid dysregulation
Quantification of adverse effects	Sexual function questionnaire
No. of patients treated	34
Age group	18–70 years
Treatment period	Continuous
Dose	Various
Treatment consequences	Sexual dysfunction
Efficacy	15% of patients
Randomization of patients	No
Remarks	The most frequent disorder was premature ejaculation.
Study quality	**3**
Reference	1002: Carani C, Isidori A, Granata A et al. Multicenter study on the prevalence of sexual symptoms in male hypo- and hyperthyroid patients. J Clin Endocrinol Metab 2005;96:6472–79.
Language	English

Compound	Thyroid hormone (H03AA)
Disease treated	Thyroid dysregulation
Quantification of adverse effects	Sexual function questionnaire
No. of patients treated	14

Age group	18–70 years
Treatment period	Continuous
Dose	Various
Treatment consequences	Sexual dysfunction
Efficacy	64% of patients
Randomization of patients	No
Study quality	**3**
Reference	1002: Carani C, Isidori A, Granata A et al. Multicenter study on the prevalence of sexual symptoms in male hypo- and hyperthyroid patients. J Clin Endocrinol Metab 2005;96: 6472–79.
Language	English

J02 Antimycotics for Systemic Use

Ketokonazol depressed testosterone levels owing to its effect on the enzymes involved in testosterone biosynthesis. The consequence was decrease in libido, erectile dysfunction and gynaecomastia. The effect was also used as androgen deprivation in the treatment of prostatic cancer.

Overall level of evidence of adverse effects: C

Compound	Ketoconazole (J02AB02)
Disease treated	Mycosis
Quantification of adverse effects	Sexual function
No. of patients treated	168
Age group	All ages
Treatment period	3 months
Dose	2000 mg/day
Treatment consequences	Sexual functions, impairment
Efficacy	Gynaecomastia (21%), decreased libido (13%)
Randomization of patients	No
Study quality	**3**
Reference	1277: Sugar AM, Alsip SG, Galgiani JN, Graybill JR, Dismukes WE, Cloud GA, Craven PC, Stevens DA. Pharmacology and toxicity of high-dose ketoconazole. Antimicrob Agents Chemother. 1987 Dec;31(12):1874–8.

Language	English

Compound	Ketoconazole (J02AB02)
Disease treated	Cancer, prostatic
Quantification of adverse effects	Testosterone production
No. of patients treated	138
Age group	All ages
Treatment period	3 months
Dose	3×200 mg/day
Treatment consequences	PSA level, decline
Efficacy	In 39 patients decrease >50%
Randomization of patients	No
Study quality	**2–**
Reference	1274: Nakabayashi M, Xie W, Regan MM, Jackman DM, Kantoff PW, Oh WK. Response to low-dose ketoconazole and subsequent dose escalation to high-dose ketoconazole in patients with androgen-independent prostate cancer. Cancer. 2006 Sep 1;107(5):975–81.
Language	English

Compound	Ketoconazole (J02AB02)
Disease treated	Cancer, prostatic
Quantification of adverse effects	Testosterone production
No. of patients treated	22
Age group	Old
Treatment period	4 weeks
Dose	3×400 mg/day
Treatment consequences	Testosterone levels, decline
Efficacy	Rapidly to castration levels
Randomization of patients	No
Study quality	**3**
Reference	1278: Vanuytsel L, Ang KK, Vantongelen K, Drochmans A, Baert L, van der Schueren E. Ketoconazole therapy for advanced prostatic cancer: feasibility and treatment results. J Urol. 1987 May;137(5):905–8.
Language	English

Compound	Ketoconazole (J02AB02)
Disease treated	Cancer, prostatic
Quantification of adverse effects	Testosterone production
No. of patients treated	19
Age group	Old
Treatment period	7 days
Dose	3×200 mg
Treatment consequences	Testosterone levels, decline
Efficacy	In 33% rapidly to castration levels
Randomization of patients	No
Study quality	**3**
Reference	1282: Nicolle P, Pontin A, Sarembock L. High-dose ketoconazole therapy in prostatic cancer. A pilot study. S Afr Med J. 1985 Jun 1;67(22):888–9.
Language	English

Compound	Ketoconazole (J02AB02)
Disease treated	Cancer, prostatic
Quantification of adverse effects	Testosterone production
No. of patients treated	13
Age group	Old
Treatment period	7 days
Dose	3×400 mg/day
Treatment consequences	Testosterone levels, decline
Efficacy	Rapidly to castration levels within 1 day
Randomization of patients	No
Study quality	**3**
Reference	1283: Trachtenberg J. Ketoconazole therapy in advanced prostatic cancer. J Urol. 1984 Jul;132(1):61–3.
Language	English

Compound	Ketoconazole (J02AB02)
Disease treated	Cancer, prostatic
Quantification of adverse effects	Testosterone production

No. of patients treated	11
Age group	Old
Treatment period	3 days
Dose	3×400 mg/day
Treatment consequences	Testosterone levels, decline
Efficacy	Rapidly to castration levels
Randomization of patients	No
Study quality	**3**
Reference	1279: Aabo K, Kjaer M, Hansen HH. High-dose ketoconazole to untreated stage D prostate cancer. Eur J Cancer Clin Oncol. 1988 Mar;24(3):431–7.
Language	English

Compound	Ketoconazole (J02AB02)
Disease treated	Healthy
Quantification of adverse effects	Testosterone production in response to hCG
No. of patients treated	10
Age group	Young
Treatment period	7 days
Dose	200 mg/day
Treatment consequences	Testosterone levels, decline
Efficacy	Only decline of hCG response
Randomization of patients	No
Study quality	**3**
Reference	1281: Krause W, Effendy I. How does ketoconazole affect testosterone metabolism? Z Hautkr. 1985 Jul 15;60(14):1147–55.
Language	German

Compound	Ketoconazole (J02AB02)
Disease treated	Normal Leydig cells in vitro
Quantification of adverse effects	Testosterone production
No. of patients treated	n.g.
Age group	n.g.
Dose	0.61±0.03 μmol/l

2

Treatment consequences	Testosterone production in vitro, decline
Efficacy	Dose related
Randomization of patients	Yes
Dose arms 1–3	Ketoconazole; placebo
Study quality	**1–**
Reference	1271: Lambert A, Mitchell R, Robertson WR. The effect of ketoconazole on adrenal and testicular steroidogenesis in vitro. Biochem Pharmacol. 1986 Nov 15;35(22):3999–4004.
Language	English

Compound	Ketoconazole (J02AB02)
Disease treated	Mycosis
Quantification of adverse effects	Hormones
Age group	All ages
Treatment period	Continuous
Dose	800–1200 mg/day
Treatment consequences	Erectile function, impairment, libido decreased
Efficacy	Correlated with ketoconazole levels
Randomization of patients	No
Study quality	**4 (review)**
Reference	1475: Pont A, Graybill JR, Craven PC, Galgiani JN, Dismukes WE, Reitz RE, Stevens DA. High-dose ketoconazole therapy and adrenal and testicular function in humans. Arch Intern Med. 1984 Nov;144(11):2150–3.
Language	English

L01	**Antineoplastic Agents and Radiation**
	A number of patients had impairment of sexual functions after radiation for testicular cancer. The figure is of low informational value, because control groups are missing.
	Overall level of evidence of adverse effects: D

Compound	Radiation (not listed)
Disease treated	Cancer, testicular
Quantification of adverse effects	Sexual function by questionnaire
No. of patients treated	84
Age group	Young
Dose	0.61±0.03 μmol/l
Treatment consequences	Sexual functions, impairment
Efficacy	19% low rates of sexual activity, 12% low sexual desire, 15% erectile dysfunction, 10% difficulty reaching orgasm, 14% premature ejaculation; 33% reduced intensity of orgasm, 49% reduced semen volume (49%)
Randomization of patients	No
Study quality	**3**
Reference	2074: Schover LR, Gonzales M, Eschenbach AC von. Sexual and marital relationships after radiotherapy for seminoma. Urology. 1986 Feb;27(2):117–23.
Language	English

Compound	Radiation (not listed)
Disease treated	Lymphoma and leukemia
Quantification of adverse effects	Sexual function by questionnaire
No. of patients treated	66
Age group	Young
Dose	Various
Treatment consequences	Fatigue, mood and sexual function by questionnaire, decrease
Efficacy	No significant differences between men with normal and low T levels
Randomization of patients	No
Study quality	**3**

Reference	2108: Howell SJ, Radford JA, Smets EM, Shalet SM. Fatigue, sexual function and mood following treatment for haematological malignancy: the impact of mild Leydig cell dysfunction. Br J Cancer. 2000 Feb;82(4):789–93.
Language	English

Compound	Radiation (not listed)
Disease treated	Cancer, bladder
Quantification of adverse effects	Sexual function by questionnaire
No. of patients treated	13
Age group	All ages
Dose	Various
Treatment consequences	Erectile functions, impairment
Efficacy	Seven of 13 patients decline in the quality of erections, decreased libido and frequency; 3 of 13 no erections; 4 of 13 reduced intensity of orgasms
Randomization of patients	No
Study quality	**3**
Reference	1320: Little FA, Howard GC. Sexual function following radical radiotherapy for bladder cancer. Radiother Oncol. 1998 Nov;49(2):157–61.
Language	English

L02 Endocrine Therapy

Androgen deprivation therapy for prostatic cancer impairs sexual functions severely. The chance of return to normal sexual functions is limited.

Overall level of evidence of adverse effects: C

Compound	GnRH agonist (L02AE)
Disease treated	Cancer, prostate
Quantification of adverse effects	Health-related quality of life
No. of patients treated	65
Age group	Old
Dose	Various

Treatment consequences	Sexual function, alteration
Efficacy	Reports of impaired sexual function
Randomization of patients	Yes
Dose arms 1–3	GnRH; wait-and-see
Study quality	**1–**
Reference	1372: Green HJ, Pakenham KI, Headley BC, Gardiner RA. Coping and health-related quality of life in men with prostate cancer randomly assigned to hormonal medication or close monitoring. Psychooncology. 2002 Sep–Oct;11(5):401–14.
Language	English

Compound	GnRH agonist (L02AE)
Disease treated	Cancer, prostate
Quantification of adverse effects	Erectile function
No. of patients treated	20
Age group	55–81 years
Dose	Various
Treatment consequences	IIEF, increase
Efficacy	No significant changes after cessation
Randomization of patients	No
Study quality	**3**
Reference	2095: Wilke DR, Parker C, Andonowski A, Tsuji D, Catton C, Gospodarowicz M, Warde P. Testosterone and erectile function recovery after radiotherapy and long-term androgen deprivation with luteinizing hormone-releasing hormone agonists. BJU Int. 2006 May;97(5):963–8.
Language	English

Compound	GnRH pulsatile (L02AE)
Disease treated	Erectile dysfunction
Quantification of dysfunction	Hormones; erectile function
No. of patients treated	20
Age group	Middle-aged
Treatment period	4 weeks
Dose	1 mg/day

Treatment consequences	Hormone levels, alteration; erectile function, alteration
Efficacy	Significant increase in LH levels; no significant increase in erectile function
Randomization of patients	No
Study quality	**3**
Reference	1379: Benkert O, Jordan R, Dahlen HG, Schneider HP, Gammel G. Sexual impotence: a double-blind study of LHRH nasal spray versus placebo. Neuropsychobiology. 1975;1(4):203–10.
Language	English

Compound	GnRH agonist (L02AE)
Disease treated	Cancer, prostate
Quantification of adverse effects	IIEF
No. of patients treated	20
Age group	Old
Treatment period	2 years
Dose	Various
Treatment consequences	Hormone levels, alteration; erectile function, alteration
Efficacy	Median duration of castrate T levels 8 m; no significant changes in the scores of the IIEF
Randomization of patients	No
Study quality	**3**
Reference	1369: Wilke DR, Parker C, Andonowski A, Tsuji D, Catton C, Gospodarowicz M, Warde P. Testosterone and erectile function recovery after radiotherapy and long-term androgen deprivation with luteinizing hormone-releasing hormone agonists. BJU Int. 2006 May;97(5):963–8.
Language	English

Compound	GnRH pulsatile (L02AE)
Disease treated	Diabetes mellitus
Quantification of adverse effects	Hormones; erectile function
No. of patients treated	8
Age group	Middle-aged
Treatment period	4 weeks

Dose	500 µg/8 h
Treatment consequences	Hormone levels, alteration; erectile function, alteration
Efficacy	Significant increase of LH levels; no significant increase in erectile function
Randomization of patients	Yes
Dose arms 1–3	GnRH; placebo
Study quality	**1–**
Reference	1378: Levitt NS, Vinik AI, Sive AA, Klaff LJ, Phillips C. Synthetic luteinizing hormone-releasing hormone in impotent male diabetics. S Afr Med J. 1980 Apr 26;57(17):701–4.
Language	English

Compound	Buserelin (L02AE01)
Disease treated	Cancer, prostate
Quantification of adverse effects	Hormones; erectile function
No. of patients treated	21
Age group	Old
Treatment period	Single dose
Dose	9.45 mg implant
Treatment consequences	Hormone levels, alteration; sexual function, alteration
Efficacy	Testosterone suppression to 0.5 ng/ml, return after 168–344 days; sexual interest present in 52%, erection possible in 60%, hot flushing remained in 24%
Randomization of patients	No
Study quality	**3**
Reference	1368: Pettersson B, Varenhorst E, Petas A, Sandow J. Duration of testosterone suppression after a 9.45 mg implant of the GnRH-analogue buserelin in patients with localised carcinoma of the prostate a 12-month follow-up study. Eur Urol. 2006 Sep;50(3):483–9.
Language	English

Compound	Goserelin (L02AE03)
Disease treated	Cancer, prostate
Quantification of adverse effects	Hormones; erectile function

2

No. of patients treated	818
Age group	Old
Treatment period	6 months
Dose	Various
Treatment consequences	Sexual function, alteration
Efficacy	The majority became sexually inactive during treatment
Randomization of patients	Yes
Dose arms 1–3	Radiation+goserelin; radiation alone
Study quality	**2+**
Reference	1370: Lamb DS, Denham JW, Mameghan H, Joseph D, Turner S, Matthews J, Franklin I, Atkinson C, North J, Poulsen M, Kovacev O, Robertson R, Francis L, Christie D, Spry NA, Tai KH, Wynne C, Duchesne G. Acceptability of short term neo-adjuvant androgen deprivation in patients with locally advanced prostate cancer. Radiother Oncol. 2003 Sep;68(3):255–67.
Language	English

Compound	Triptorelin (L02AE04)
Disease treated	Paraphilia
Quantification of adverse effects	Intensity of Sexual Desire and Symptoms Scale
No. of patients treated	30
Age group	32 years (mean)
Treatment period	Continuous
Dose	3.75 mg/month
Treatment consequences	Sexual fantasies, decrease
Efficacy	From mean (±SD) of 48±10 per week before therapy to zero during therapy
Randomization of patients	No
Study quality	**3**
Reference	1374: Rosler A, Witztum E. Treatment of men with paraphilia with a long-acting analogue of gonadotropin-releasing hormone. N Engl J Med. 1998 Feb 12;338(7):416–22.
Language	English

L03	Immunostimulants
	A study described positive effects of interferon α-2B in induratio penis plastica showing limited effectivity but significant side effects. **Overall level of evidence of positive effects: C** **Overall level of evidence of adverse effects compromising effectivity: C**

Compound	Interferon α-2B
Disease treated	Induratio penis plastica
Quantification of adverse effects	IIEF
No. of patients treated	25
Age group	Old
Treatment period	6 weeks
Dose	2×10^6U/2 weeks
Treatment consequences	Erectile function, improvement
Efficacy	Significantly in 5 of 7 men
Side effects compromising effectivity	Significant improvements in penile pain and curvature
Randomization of patients	No
Study quality	**1–**
Reference	1217: Dang G, Matern R, Bivalacqua TJ, Sikka S, Hellstrom WJ. Intralesional interferon-alpha-2B injections for the treatment of Peyronie's disease. South Med J. 2004 Jan;97(1):42–6.
Language	English

M01 Antiinflammatory and Antirheumatic Products

M03 Muscle Relaxants

An increased prevalence of erectile dysfunction has been described in patients who use these drugs. It remains unanswered as to whether the diseases or the drugs compromise erectile function.

A single report in the literature quoted erectile dysfunction in 8% of patients treated with baclofen.

Overall evidence of adverse effects: B

Compound	Antiinflammatory and antirheumatic products, non-steroids (M01A)
Disease treated	Arthritis
Quantification of adverse effects	Two questions from the NIH consensus definition
No. of patients treated	1683
Age group	40–69 years
Treatment period	Various
Dose	Various
Treatment consequences	Prevalence of erectile dysfunction
Efficacy	RR 1.3 (95% CI 0.9–1.9)
Randomization of patients	No
Study quality	**2+**
Reference	2219: Shiri R, Koskimaki J, Hakama M, Hakkinen J, Tammela TL, Huhtala H, Auvinen A. Effect of chronic diseases on incidence of erectile dysfunction. Urology. 2003 Dec;62(6):1097–102.
Language	English

Compound	Baclofen intrathecal (M03BX01)
Disease treated	Spinal spasticity
Quantification of adverse effects	Erectile function
No. of patients treated	25
Age group	Young
Treatment period	Continuous
Dose	Various
Treatment consequences	Erectile function, impairment

Efficacy	8% of patients
Randomization of patients	No
Study quality	**3**
Reference	1010: Dario A, Scamoni C, Picano M, Casagrande F, Tomei G. Pharmacological complications of the chronic baclofen infusion in the severe spinal spasticity. Personal experience and review of the literature. J Neurosurg Sci. 2004 Dec;48(4):177–81.
Language	English

N01	**Anaesthetics – Cocaine**
	Cocaine was originally introduced as an anaesthetic. The studies quoted here refer to its use as a lifestyle drug. Data on alteration of sexual function is scarce. A severe impairment is not likely, since several studies described unaltered testosterone levels in cocaine users. **Overall level of evidence of adverse effects: C**

Compound	Cocaine (N01BC01)
Disease treated	Cocaine addiction
Quantification of adverse effects	Hormones
No. of patients treated	24
Age group	All ages
Treatment period	Single dose
Dose	0.4 mg/kg
Treatment consequences	Hormone levels, alteration
Efficacy	LH levels increase, T levels unchanged, prolactin levels decrease
Randomization of patients	No
Dose arms 1–3	Cocaine; nicotine
Study quality	**2–**
Reference	1323: Mendelson JH, Sholar MB, Mutschler NH, Jaszyna-Gasior M, Goletiani NV, Siegel AJ, Mello NK. Effects of intravenous cocaine and cigarette smoking on luteinizing hormone, testosterone, and prolactin in men. J Pharmacol Exp Ther. 2003 Oct;307(1):339–48.
Language	English

Compound	Cocaine (N01BC01)
Disease treated	Cocaine addiction
Quantification of adverse effects	Hormones
No. of patients treated	16
Age group	All ages
Treatment period	4 weeks after cessation
Dose	Various
Treatment consequences	Hormone levels, alteration
Efficacy	Prolactin levels increase, LH and T unchanged
Randomization of patients	No
Study quality	**3**
Reference	1326: Mendelson JH, Teoh SK, Lange U, Mello NK, Weiss R, Skupny A, Ellingboe J. Anterior pituitary, adrenal, and gonadal hormones during cocaine withdrawal. Am J Psychiatry. 1988 Sep;145(9):1094–8.
Language	English

Compound	Cocaine (N01BC01)
Disease treated	Cocaine addiction
Quantification of adverse effects	Hormones
No. of patients treated	12
Age group	All ages
Treatment period	Single dose
Dose	2 mg intranasally
Treatment consequences	Hormone levels, alteration
Efficacy	LH levels increase, T levels unchanged, prolactin levels decrease
Randomization of patients	Yes
Dose arms 1–3	Cocaine; placebo
Study quality	**1–**
Reference	1324: Heesch CM, Negus BH, Bost JE, Keffer JH, Snyder RW 2nd, Eichhorn EJ. Effects of cocaine on anterior pituitary and gonadal hormones. J Pharmacol Exp Ther. 1996 Sep;278(3):1195–200.
Language	English

Compound	Cocaine (N01BC01)
Disease treated	Cocaine addiction
Quantification of adverse effects	Hormones
No. of patients treated	8
Age group	All ages
Treatment period	Continuous
Dose	Various
Treatment consequences	Hormone levels, alteration
Efficacy	LH peaks increase
Randomization of patients	No
Study quality	**3**
Reference	1325: Mendelson JH, Mello NK, Teoh SK, Ellingboe J, Cochin J. Cocaine effects on pulsatile secretion of anterior pituitary, gonadal, and adrenal hormones. J Clin Endocrinol Metab. 1989 Dec;69(6):1256–60.
Language	English

N02 Analgesics

There are few reports on limited adverse effects of analgesics on erectile function. Ergotamine induced relaxation of cavernosal smooth muscles, but clinical studies are not available.

Overall level of evidence of adverse effects: C

Compound	Buprenorphine (N02AE01)
Disease treated	Opiate addiction
Quantification of adverse effects	Sexual function scale; hormones
No. of patients treated	105
Age group	Young
Treatment period	Continuous
Dose	Various
Treatment consequences	Sexual function, impairment; testosterone level, increased
Efficacy	Significantly higher in buprenorphine group than in methadone group

2

Randomization of patients	No
Dose arms 1–3	Methadone; buprenorphine; healthy blood donors
Study quality	**2–**
Reference	1398: Bliesener N, Albrecht S, Schwager A, Weckbecker K, Lichtermann D, Klingmuller D. Plasma testosterone and sexual function in men receiving buprenorphine maintenance for opioid dependence. J Clin Endocrinol Metab. 2005 Jan;90(1):203–6. Epub 2004 Oct 13.
Language	English

Compound	Dihydergotamine (N02CA01)
Disease treated	Erectile dysfunction
Quantification of adverse effects	Erectile function
No. of patients treated	n.g.
Age group	Old
Treatment period	On demand
Dose	5 mg
Treatment consequences	Erectile function, duplex sonography, improvement
Efficacy	In non-responders to sildenafil
Randomization of patients	No
Study quality	**3**
Reference	1625: Dunzendorfer U, Behm A, Dunzendorfer E, Dunzendorfer A. Drug combinations in the therapy of low response to phosphodiesterase 5 inhibitors in patients with erectile dysfunction. In Vivo. 2002 Sep–Oct;16(5):345–8.
Language	English

Compound	Ergotamine (N02CA02)
Disease treated	Cavernous tissue in vitro
Quantification of adverse effects	Muscle relaxation
No. of patients treated	16
Age group	42–68 years
Treatment period	In vitro
Dose	5×10^{-4}g
Treatment consequences	Cavernous tissue, relaxation

Efficacy	Poor
Study quality	**2–**
Reference	1438: Barbanti G, Beneforti P, Lapini A, Turini D. Relaxation of isolated corpus cavernosum induced by smooth-muscle relaxant drugs. A comparative study. Urol Res. 1988;16(4):299–302.
Language	English

N03 Antiepileptics

This class of drugs generally impairs sexual function, in particular erectile function, although no depression, but even an *increase* of testosterone levels, was observed; however, also untreated patients with epilepsy suffer from impaired sexual functions, so the attribution to antiepileptics is questionable.

Overall level of evidence of adverse effects: C

Compound	Antiepileptics (N03A)
Disease treated	Epilepsy
Quantification of adverse effects	Sexual function scale; hormones
No. of patients treated	85
Age group	Young
Treatment period	6 months
Dose	Various
Treatment consequences	Sexual function, impairment; testosterone level, increased
Efficacy	Various
Randomization of patients	No
Dose arms 1–3	Carbamazepine; phenytoin; untreated epilepsy
Study quality	**2–**
Reference	1364: Herzog AG, Drislane FW, Schomer DL, Pennell PB, Bromfield EB, Dworetzky BA, Farina EL, Frye CA. Differential effects of antiepileptic drugs on sexual function and hormones in men with epilepsy. Neurology. 2005 Oct 11;65(7):1016–20.
Language	English

Compound	Antiepileptics (N03A)
Disease treated	Epilepsy
Quantification of adverse effects	Erectile function
Age group	Young
Treatment consequences	Erectile function, impairment
Efficacy	Dependent on medication
Study quality	**4 (review)**
Reference	1357: Mattson RH, Cramer JA. Epilepsy, sex hormones, and antiepileptic drugs. Epilepsia. 1985;26 Suppl 1:S40–51.
Language	English

Compound	Antiepileptics (N03A)
Disease treated	Epilepsy
Quantification of adverse effects	Hormones
No. of patients treated	54
Treatment period	No treatment
Age group	Young
Treatment consequences	Sexual activity decreased; LH, FSH, prolactin, and sex-hormone binding globulin (SHBG) levels increased
Efficacy	Significant
Study quality	**2–**
Reference	1412: Toone BK, Wheeler M, Fenwick PB. Sex hormone changes in male epileptics. Clin Endocrinol (Oxf). 1980 Apr;12(4):391–5.
Language	English

Compound	Antiepileptics (N03A)
Disease treated	Epilepsy
Quantification of adverse effects	Hormones
No. of patients treated	20
Age group	Young
Treatment period	No treatment
Treatment consequences	Sexual libido decrease, gonadotropin levels decreased
Efficacy	11 of 20 patients
Study quality	**3**

Reference	1410: Herzog AG, Seibel MM, Schomer DL, Vaitukaitis JL, Geschwind N. Reproductive endocrine disorders in men with partial seizures of temporal lobe origin. Arch Neurol. 1986 Apr;43(4):347–50.
Language	English

Compound	Antiepileptics (N03A)
Disease treated	Epilepsy
Quantification of adverse effects	Sexual function
Age group	All ages
Treatment period	No treatment
Treatment consequences	Sexual functions, impaired
Efficacy	In 30–66% of men
Remarks	Epileptic discharges in limbic structures may contribute to sexual dysfunction.
Study quality	**4 (review)**
Reference	1355: Morrell MJ. Sexual dysfunction in epilepsy. Epilepsia. 1991;32 Suppl 6:S38–45.
Language	English

Compound	Phenytoin (N03AB02)
Disease treated	Epilepsy
Quantification of adverse effects	Sexual function scale; hormones
No. of patients treated	152
Age group	Young
Treatment period	Continuous
Dose	Various
Treatment consequences	Sexual function, impairment; testosterone level increased, SHBG level increased, DHEA level unaltered
Efficacy	Significant
Randomization of patients	No
Study quality	**3**
Reference	1371: Duncan S, Blacklaw J, Beastall GH, Brodie MJ. Antiepileptic drug therapy and sexual function in men with epilepsy. Epilepsia. 1999 Feb;40(2):197–204.
Language	English

Compound	Clonazepam (N03AE01)
Disease treated	Post-traumatic stress disorder (PTSD)
Quantification of adverse effects	Sexual function questionnaire
No. of patients treated	100
Age group	Middle-aged
Treatment period	Continuous
Dose	3.4 mg/day
Treatment consequences	Sexual dysfunction
Efficacy	43% of patients
Randomization of patients	No
Study quality	**3**
Reference	1624: Fossey MD, Hamner MB. Clonazepam-related sexual dysfunction in male veterans with PTSD. Anxiety. 1994–95;1(5):233–6.
Language	English

Compound	Carbamazepine (N03AF01)
Disease treated	Epilepsy
Quantification of adverse effects	Sexual function scale; hormones
No. of patients treated	184
Age group	18–65 years
Treatment period	Continuous
Dose	Various
Treatment consequences	Sexual function, depressed; testosterone level unaltered, SHBG level increase, DHEA level decreased
Efficacy	Men receiving antiepileptic drugs embraced a stricter sexual morality than the controls and untreated, and expressed greater satisfaction with their marriages than the control and untreated groups.
Randomization of patients	No
Study quality	**3**
Reference	1371: Duncan S, Blacklaw J, Beastall GH, Brodie MJ. Antiepileptic drug therapy and sexual function in men with epilepsy. Epilepsia. 1999 Feb;40(2):197–204.
Language	English

Compound	Valproate (N03AG01)
Disease treated	Epilepsy
Quantification of adverse effects	Sexual function scale; hormones
No. of patients treated	152
Age group	Young
Treatment period	Continuous
Dose	Various
Treatment consequences	Sexual function, depressed; testosterone level unaltered, SHBG level unaltered, DHEA level unaltered
Efficacy	On average
Randomization of patients	No
Study quality	**3**
Reference	1371: Duncan S, Blacklaw J, Beastall GH, Brodie MJ. Antiepileptic drug therapy and sexual function in men with epilepsy. Epilepsia. 1999 Feb;40(2):197–204.
Language	English

Compound	Lamotrigine (N03AX09)
Disease treated	Epilepsy
Quantification of adverse effects	Erectile function
No. of patients treated	3
Age group	Young
Treatment period	8 months
Dose	Various
Treatment consequences	Sexual function, improvement
Efficacy	After cessation of other antileptics
Randomization of patients	No
Study quality	**3**
Reference	1592: Husain AM, Carwile ST, Miller PP, Radtke RA. Improved sexual function in three men taking lamotrigine for epilepsy. South Med J. 2000 Mar;93(3):335–6.
Language	English

2

N04	Anti-Parkinson Drugs

A higher prevalence of erectile dysfunction in patients using anticholinergics than in healthy men has been described. Again, it is not possible to decide whether the disease itself or the drugs used are causative.

The development of hypersexuality during application of anti-Parkinson drugs is rare.

Overall level of evidence of adverse effects: C

Compound	Anticholinergic agents (N04A)
Disease treated	Parkinson's disease
Quantification of adverse effects	Interview by general practitioner
No. of patients treated	2010
Age group	>18 years
Treatment period	Various
Dose	Various
Treatment consequences	Incidence of erectile dysfunction
Efficacy	RR 12.8 (95% CI 2.7–60.1)
Randomization of patients	No
Study quality	**2–**
Reference	2231: Ricci E, Parazzini F, Mirone V, Imbimbo C, Palmieri A, Bortolotti A, Cintio E di, Landoni M, Lavezzari M. Current drug use as risk factor for erectile dysfunction: results from an Italian epidemiological study. Int J Impot Res. 2003 Jun;15(3):221–4.
Language	English

Compound	Anti-Parkinson drugs (N04A)
Disease treated	Parkinson's disease
Quantification of adverse effects	Questionnaires
No. of patients treated	297
Age group	Old
Treatment period	Various
Dose	Various
Treatment consequences	Hypersexuality in Parkinson's disease

Efficacy	2.4%
Randomization of patients	No
Study quality	**2–**
Reference	2168: Voon V, Hassan K, Zurowski M, de Souza M, Thomsen T, Fox S, Lang AE, Miyasaki J. Prevalence of repetitive and reward-seeking behaviors in Parkinson disease. Neurology. 2006 Oct 10;67(7):1254–7.
Language	English

N05 Psycholeptics

Impairment of sexual functions is common in patients treated with psycholeptics, but also in patients suffering from the treated diseases alone. In most cases, it was associated with decreased testosterone levels. Phosphodiesterase-5 inhibitors were of benefit.

Overall level of evidence of adverse effects: C

Compound	Antipsychotics (N05A)
Disease treated	Psychosis
Quantification of adverse effects	Interview by general practitioner
No. of patients treated	2010
Age group	>18 years
Treatment period	Various
Dose	Various
Treatment consequences	Incidence of erectile dysfunction
Efficacy	RR 9.0 (95% CI 1.8–44.4)
Randomization of patients	No
Study quality	**2–**
Reference	2231: Ricci E, Parazzini F, Mirone V, Imbimbo C, Palmieri A, Bortolotti A, Cintio E di, Landoni M, Lavezzari M. Current drug use as risk factor for erectile dysfunction: results from an Italian epidemiological study. Int J Impot Res. 2003 Jun;15(3):221–4.
Language	English

2

Antipsychotic drugs	Antipsychotics (N05A)
Disease treated	Schizophrenia
Quantification of adverse effects	Erectile function
No. of patients treated	139
Age group	Young
Treatment period	Continuous
Dose	Various
Treatment consequences	Sexual function, impairment
Efficacy	45.3%
Randomization of patients	No
Study quality	**2–**
Reference	1314: Olfson M, Uttaro T, Carson WH, Tafesse E. Male sexual dysfunction and quality of life in schizophrenia. J Clin Psychiatry. 2005 Mar;66(3):331–8
Language	English

Compound	Antipsychotics (N05A)
Disease treated	Schizophrenia
Quantification of adverse effects	Erectile function
No. of patients treated	25
Age group	Young
Treatment period	Continuous
Dose	Various
Treatment consequences	Sexual function, impairment of overall functions
Efficacy	40–71%
Randomization of patients	No
Study quality	**3**
Reference	1593: Wirshing DA, Pierre JM, Marder SR, Saunders CS, Wirshing WC. Sexual side effects of novel antipsychotic medications. Schizophr Res. 2002 Jul 1;56(1–2):25–30.
Language	English

Compound	Antipsychotics (N05A)
Disease treated	Schizophrenia
Quantification of adverse effects	Erectile function

No. of patients treated	122
Age group	Young
Treatment period	No treatment
Treatment consequences	Sexual function, impairment
Efficacy	High frequency
Randomization of patients	No
Study quality	**3**
Reference	1316: Aizenberg D, Zemishlany Z, Dorfman-Etrog P, Weizman A. Sexual dysfunction in male schizophrenic patients. J Clin Psychiatry. 1995 Apr;56(4):137–41.
Language	English

Compound	Haloperidol (N05AD01)
Disease treated	Schizophrenia
Quantification of adverse effects	Hormones
No. of patients treated	30
Age group	Young
Treatment period	4 weeks
Treatment consequences	Prolactin levels increased, testosterone levels decreased
Efficacy	In higher dose
Randomization of patients	No
Dose arms 1–3	7.5 mg and 15 mg haloperidol; 30 mg and 60 mg haloperidol
Study quality	**2–**
Reference	1388: Rinieris P, Hatzimanolis J, Markianos M, Stefanis C. Effects of treatment with various doses of haloperidol on the pituitary–gonadal axis in male schizophrenic patients. Neuropsychobiology. 1989;22(3):146–9.
Language	English

Compound	Olanzapine (N05AH03)
Disease treated	Psychosis
Quantification of adverse effects	Erectile function
No. of patients treated	10
Age group	Middle-aged
Treatment period	Continuous

Dose	Various
Treatment consequences	Erectile function, impairment
Efficacy	Improved with sildenafil
Randomization of patients	No
Study quality	**3**
Reference	1605: Atmaca M, Kuloglu M, Tezcan E. Sildenafil use in patients with olanzapine-induced erectile dysfunction. Int J Impot Res. 2002 Dec;14(6):547–9.
Language	English

Compound	Sulpiride (N05AL01)
Disease treated	Psychosis
Quantification of adverse effects	Erectile function
No. of patients treated	13
Age group	Middle-aged
Treatment period	3 weeks
Dose	600 mg
Treatment consequences	Erectile function, improvement
Efficacy	After reduction or discontinuation of sulpiride
Randomization of patients	No
Study quality	**3**
Reference	1626: Weizman A, Maoz B, Treves I, Asher I, Ben-David M. Sulpiride-induced hyperprolactinemia and impotence in male psychiatric outpatients. Prog Neuropsychopharmacol Biol Psychiatry. 1985;9(2):193–8.
Language	English

Compound	Lithium (N05AN01), benzodiazepines
Disease treated	Bipolar psychosis
Quantification of adverse effects	Sexual function score
No. of patients treated	45
Age group	Young
Treatment period	Continuous
Dose	Various
Treatment consequences	Sexual function, alteration

Efficacy	49% of patients difficulties in combined treatment with lithium+benzodiazepines
Randomization of patients	No
Study quality	**2–**
Reference	1392: Ghadirian AM, Annable L, Belanger MC. Lithium, benzodiazepines, and sexual function in bipolar patients. Am J Psychiatry. 1992 Jun;149(6):801–5.
Language	English

Compound	Risperidone (N05AX08)
Disease treated	Schizophrenia
Quantification of adverse effects	Erectile function
No. of patients treated	25
Age group	Young
Treatment period	6 weeks
Dose	3 mg/day
Treatment consequences	Erectile function, impairment
Efficacy	Less impaired in patients treated with quetiapine than with risperidone
Randomization of patients	No
Study quality	**2–**
Reference	1414: Knegtering R, Castelein S, Bous H, Van Der Linde J, Bruggeman R, Kluiter H, van den Bosch RJ. A randomized open-label study of the impact of quetiapine versus risperidone on sexual functioning. J Clin Psychopharmacol. 2004 Feb;24(1):56–61.
Language	English

Compound	Risperidone (N05AX08)
Disease treated	Schizophrenia
Quantification of adverse effects	Erectile function
No. of patients treated	14
Age group	18–65 years
Treatment period	3 months
Dose	3 mg/day
Treatment consequences	Erectile function, improvement

Efficacy	Associated with prolactin rise, contrary to expectation
Randomization of patients	No
Study quality	**2–**
Reference	1413: Spollen JJ III, Wooten RG, Cargile C, Bartztokis G. Prolactin levels and erectile function in patients treated with risperidone. J Clin Psychopharmacol. 2004 Apr;24(2):161–6.
Language	English

N06	**Psychoanaleptics**

Antidepressants hold a high risk of induction of sexual dysfunction. Large case-control studies report an OR of up to 2.0, but not in all studies does the 95% CI exclude 1. In particular, the selective serotonin reuptake inhibitors (SSRI) exert sexual side effects due to overlapping neuroregulatory mechanims. Up to half of patients complain of various dysfunctions. In comparison studies (RCTs are not available) the rate in treated patients was significantly higher than in the placebo groups; however, there are also studies which describe no alteration of sexual functions. Erectile dysfunction in the patients treated with psychoanaleptics may be treated with drugs which improve erection. The association of various symptoms with definite drugs is questionable. Priapism has been recorded to be a consequence of therapy with tradozone.

Overall level of evidence of adverse effects: B

Sexual dysfunction has a high prevalence also in depressed men without treatment. An OR of about 2 is reported for depressed men in comparison with healthy men.

Overall level of evidence of adverse effects: A

Compound	Antidepressants (N06A)
Disease treated	Depression
Quantification of adverse effects	Sexual function
No. of patients treated	11 RCT studies quoted (25–189 patients)
Age group	All ages
Treatment consequences	Sexual dysfunction (loss of libido, orgasmic dysfunction)

Efficacy	Up to 61% varying for various drugs
Randomization	Yes
Study quality	**1++– (structured review)**
Reference	1031: Baldwin DS. Sexual dysfunction associated with antidepressant drugs. Expert Opin Drug Saf. 2004 Sep;3(5):457–70.
Language	English

Compound	Antidepressants (N06A)
Disease treated	Depression
Quantification of adverse effects	Sexual function questionnaire
No. of patients treated	31,742
Age group	53–90 years
Treatment period	Various
Dose	Various
Treatment consequences	Incidence of erectile dysfunction
Efficacy	RR 1.7 (95% CI 1.2–2.2)
Randomization of patients	No
Study quality	**2++**
Reference	2210: Bacon CG, Mittleman MA, Kawachi I, Giovannucci E, Glasser DB, Rimm EB. Sexual function in men older than 50 years of age: results from the health professionals follow-up study. Ann Intern Med. 2003;139(3):161–8.
Language	English

Compound	Antidepressants (N06A)
Disease treated	Depression
Quantification of adverse effects	Sexual function questionnaire
No. of patients treated	27,839
Age group	20–75 years
Treatment period	Various
Dose	Various
Treatment consequences	Prevalence of erectile dysfunction
Efficacy	13% reporting no erectile dysfunction, 25% reporting erectile dysfunction
Randomization of patients	No

Study quality	**2–**
Reference	2208: Rosen RC, Fisher WA, Eardley I, Niederberger C, Nadel A, Sand M; Men's Attitudes to Life Events and Sexuality (MALES) Study. The multinational Men's Attitudes to Life Events and Sexuality (MALES) study: I. Prevalence of erectile dysfunction and related health concerns in the general population. Curr Med Res Opin. 2004 May;20(5):607–17.
Language	English

Compound	Antidepressants (N06A)
Disease treated	Depression
Quantification of adverse effects	Single question from the NIH consensus definition
No. of patients treated	428
Age group	40–70 years
Treatment period	Various
Dose	Various
Treatment consequences	Incidence of erectile dysfunction within 2 years
Efficacy	RR 1.94 (95% CI 0.60–6.26)
Randomization of patients	No
Study quality	**2+**
Reference	2229: Moreira ED Jr, Abdo CH, Torres EB, Lobo CF, Fittipaldi JA. Prevalence and correlates of erectile dysfunction: results of the Brazilian study of sexual behavior. Urology. 2001 Oct;58(4):583–8.
Language	English

Compound	Antidepressants (N06A)
Disease treated	Depression
Quantification of adverse effects	Sexual function
No. of patients treated	412
Age group	Young
Treatment period	Various
Dose	Various
Treatment consequences	Sexual dysfunction
Efficacy	Up to 59.1% varying for various drugs
Study quality	**2–**

Reference	1558: Montejo AL, Llorca G, Izquierdo JA, Rico-Villademoros F. Incidence of sexual dysfunction associated with antidepressant agents: a prospective multicenter study of 1022 outpatients. Spanish Working Group for the Study of Psychotropic-Related Sexual Dysfunction. J Clin Psychiatry. 2001;62 Suppl 3:10–21.
Language	English

Compound	Antidepressants (N06A)
Disease treated	Depression
Quantification of adverse effects	IIEF
No. of patients treated	242
Age group	40–69 years
Treatment period	Various
Dose	Various
Treatment consequences	Prevalence of erectile dysfunction in patients 40–49 years old
Efficacy	OR 1.14 (95% CI 0.51–2.54)
Randomization of patients	No
Study quality	**2–**
Reference	2228: Mak R, De Backer G, Kornitzer M, De Meyer JM. Prevalence and correlates of erectile dysfunction in a population-based study in Belgium. Eur Urol. 2002 Feb;41(2):132–8.
Language	English

Compound	Antidepressants (N06A)
Disease treated	Depression
Quantification of adverse effects	Single question
No. of patients treated	81
Age group	40–70 years
Treatment period	Various
Dose	Various
Treatment consequences	Prevalence of erectile dysfunction
Efficacy	OR 2.09 (95% CI 1.60– 2.74)
Randomization of patients	No

Study quality	**2–**
Reference	2207: Nicolosi A, Moreira ED Jr, Shirai M, Bin Mohd Tambi MI, Glasser DB. Epidemiology of erectile dysfunction in four countries: cross-national study of the prevalence and correlates of erectile dysfunction. Urology. 2003 Jan;61(1):201–6.
Language	English

Compound	Antidepressants (N06A)
Disease treated	Lower urinary tract symptoms (LUTS)
Quantification of adverse effects	IIEF
No. of patients treated	24
Age group	68.2 years (mean)
Treatment period	Various
Dose	Various
Treatment consequences	Prevalence of erectile dysfunction
Efficacy	Correlation with IIEF-0.12
Randomization of patients	No
Study quality	**2–**
Reference	2209: Elliott SP, Gulati M, Pasta DJ, Spitalny GM, Kane CJ, Yee R, Lue TF. Obstructive lower urinary tract symptoms correlate with erectile dysfunction. Urology. 2004 Jun;63(6):1148–52.
Language	English

Compound	Antidepressants (N06A)
Disease treated	Depression
Quantification of adverse effects	Sexual function
No. of patients treated	24
Age group	Young
Treatment period	Various
Dose	Various
Treatment consequences	Sexual dysfunction
Efficacy	43%, not associated with diagnosis or antidepressant
Randomization of patients	No

Study quality	**2–**
Reference	1557: Balon R, Yeragani VK, Pohl R, Ramesh C. Sexual dysfunction during antidepressant treatment. J Clin Psychiatry. 1993 Jun;54(6):209–12.
Language	English

Compound	Antidepressants (N06A)
Disease treated	Epilepsy
Quantification of adverse effects	Erectile function
No. of patients treated	1
Age group	Young
Treatment period	Various
Dose	Various
Treatment consequences	Erectile function, impairment
Side effects	Increased synthesis of SHBG
Randomization of patients	No
Dose arms 1–3	Carbamazepine; oxycarbazepine fewer side effects
Study quality	**3**
Reference	1363: Sachdeo R, Sathyan RR. Amelioration of erectile dysfunction following a switch from carbamazepine to oxcarbazepine: recent clinical experience. Curr Med Res Opin. 2005 Jul;21(7):1065–8.
Language	English

Compound	Antidepressants (N06A)
Disease treated	Depression
Quantification of adverse effects	Erectile function
Age group	Old
Treatment consequences	Erectile function, improvement
Efficacy	Treatment of erectile dysfunction increases compliance
Study quality	**4 (review)**
Reference	1080: Rosen RC, Marin H. Prevalence of antidepressant-associated erectile dysfunction. J Clin Psychiatry. 2003;64 Suppl 10:5–10.
Language	English

2

Compound	Antidepressants (N06A)
Disease treated	Psychosis
Quantification of adverse effects	Priapism
Age group	Old
Treatment consequences	Priapism as a side effect
Efficacy	Frequency below 1:1000, but considerable risk
Remarks	Presumably related to an adrenergic antagonism
Study quality	**4 (review)**
Reference	1188: Compton MT, Miller AH. Priapism associated with conventional and atypical antipsychotic medications: a review. J Clin Psychiatry. 2001 May;62(5):362–6.
Language	English

Compound	Antidepressants (N06A)
Disease treated	Depression
Quantification of adverse effects	Erectile function
Age group	Old
Treatment consequences	Erectile function, improvement
Efficacy	Reliable effect not shown in comparing studies
Remarks	Sexual side effects of SSRI are due to overlapping neuroregulatory mechanisms
Study quality	**4 (review)**
Reference	1079: Labbate LA, Croft HA, Oleshansky MA. Antidepressant-related erectile dysfunction: management via avoidance, switching antidepressants, antidotes, and adaptation. J Clin Psychiatry. 2003;64 Suppl 10:11–19.
Language	English

Compound	Antidepressants (N06A)
Disease treated	Depression
Quantification of adverse effects	Erectile function
Age group	Young
Treatment consequences	Erectile function, impairment
Efficacy	Dependent on medication

Study quality	**4 (review)**
Reference	1362: Mitchell JE, Popkin MK. Antidepressant drug therapy and sexual dysfunction in men: a review. J Clin Psychopharmacol. 1983 Apr;3(2):76–9.
Language	English

Compound	Antidepressants (N06A)
Disease treated	Depression
Quantification of adverse effects	Sexual functions
Age group	Young
Treatment consequences	Sexual dysfunction
Efficacy	Painful ejaculation in imipramine, priapism in tradozone
Study quality	**4 (review)**
Reference	1428: Margolese HC, Assalian P. Sexual side effects of antidepressants: a review. J Sex Marital Ther. 1996 Fall;22(3):209–17. McGill University, Canada.
Language	English

Compound	Antidepressants (N06A)
Disease treated	Depression
Quantification of adverse effects	Single question for erectile function
No. of patients treated	1982
Age group	>40 years
Treatment period	No treatment
Treatment consequences	Prevalence of erectile dysfunction as compared with non-depressed men
Efficacy	OR 1.18 (95% CI 1.11–1.26)
Randomization of patients	No
Study quality	**2++**
Reference	2216: Akkus E, Kadioglu A, Esen A, Doran S, Ergen A, Anafarta K, Hattat H; Turkish Erectile Dysfunction Prevalence Study Group. Prevalence and correlates of erectile dysfunction in Turkey: a population-based study. Eur Urol. 2002 Mar;41(3):298–304.
Language	English

Compound	Antidepressant (N06A)
Disease treated	Depression
Quantification of adverse effects	AUA criteria
No. of patients treated	1709
Age group	40–70 years
Treatment period	No treatment
Treatment consequences	Prevalence of erectile dysfunction as compared with non-depressed men
Efficacy	OR 1.81 (95% CI 1.28– 2.55)
Randomization of patients	No
Study quality	**2+**
Reference	2212: Nicolosi A, Moreira ED Jr, Villa M, Glasser DB. A population study of the association between sexual function, sexual satisfaction and depressive symptoms in men. J Affect Disord. 2004 Oct 15;82(2):235–43.
Language	English

Compound	Antidepressants (N06A)
Disease treated	Depression
Quantification of adverse effects	Single question from the NIH consensus definition
No. of patients treated	428
Age group	40–70 years
Treatment period	No treatment
Treatment consequences	Prevalence of erectile dysfunction as compared with non-depressed men
Efficacy	RR 1.16 (95% CI 0.33–4.07)
Randomization of patients	No
Study quality	**2+**
Reference	2213: Moreira ED Jr, Lobo CF, Diament A, Nicolosi A, Glasser DB. Incidence of erectile dysfunction in men 40 to 69 years old: results from a population-based cohort study in Brazil. Urology. 2003 Feb;61(2):431–6.
Language	English

Compound	Antidepressants (N06A)
Disease treated	Depression
Quantification of adverse effects	IIEF

No. of patients treated	334
Age group	>18 years
Treatment period	No treatment
Treatment consequences	Prevalence of erectile dysfunction as compared with non-depressed men
Efficacy	6.3%, no statistical significant association
Randomization of patients	No
Study quality	**2–**
Reference	2233: Kantor J, Bilker WB, Glasser DB, Margolis DJ. Prevalence of erectile dysfunction and active depression: an analytic cross-sectional study of general medical patients. Am J Epidemiol. 2002 Dec 1;156(11):1035–42.
Language	English

Compound	Antidepressants (N06A)
Disease treated	Depression
Quantification of adverse effects	Sexual function score
No. of patients treated	88
Treatment period	No treatment
Age group	Young
Treatment consequences	Sexual dysfunction
Efficacy	36.2% prevalence in depressed men, 13.3% in controls
Randomization of patients	No
Study quality	**2–**
Reference	1565: Kockott G, Pfeiffer W. Sexual disorders in nonacute psychiatric outpatients. Compr Psychiatry 1996;37:56–61.
Language	English

Compound	Antidepressants (N06A)
Disease treated	Depression
Quantification of adverse effects	Sexual function score
No. of patients treated	49
Treatment period	No treatment
Age group	Young
Treatment consequences	Sexual dysfunction

2

Efficacy	48.2% prevalence in depressed men, 17.6 in controls
Randomization of patients	No
Study quality	**2–**
Reference	1564: Angst J: Sexual problems in healthy and depressed patients. Int Clin Psychopharmacol 1998;13: S1–S3.
Language	English

Compound	Antidepressants (N06A)
Disease treated	Depression
Quantification of adverse effects	Sexual function scores
No. of patients treated	Seven case-control studies quoted (40–264 patients)
Treatment period	No treatment
Age group	All ages
Treatment consequences	Sexual dysfunction
Efficacy	Prevalence up to 48.2% in depressed men
Randomization of patients	No
Study quality	**2++ (structured review)**
Reference	1031: Baldwin DS. Sexual dysfunction associated with antidepressant drugs. Expert Opin Drug Saf. 2004 Sep;3(5):457–70.
Language	English

Compound	Imipramine (N06AA02)
Disease treated	Depression
Quantification of adverse effects	Sexual function score
No. of patients treated	26; 41
Age group	Young
Treatment period	n.g.
Dose	200 mg
Treatment consequences	Sexual dysfunction as a side effect
Efficacy	30% in imipramin group, 6% in placebo group
Randomization of patients	Yes
Dose arms 1–3	Imipramine; placebo
Study quality	**1–**

Reference	1566: Harrison WM, Rabkin JG, Ehrhardt AA et al. Effects of antidepressant medication on sexual function : a controlled study. J Clin Phychopharmacol 1986;6: 144–149.
Language	English

Compound	Selective serotonin reuptake inhibitors (SSRI) (N06AB)
Disease treated	Depression
Quantification of adverse effects	Sexual dysfunction, self reported
No. of patients treated	596
Age group	Young
Treatment period	Various
Dose	Various
Treatment consequences	Sexual dysfunction
Efficacy	In 23.4% of patients clear association
Randomization of patients	No
Study quality	**3**
Reference	1449: Ashton AK, Hamer R, Rosen RC. Serotonin reuptake inhibitor-induced sexual dysfunction and its treatment: a large-scale retrospective study of 596 psychiatric outpatients. J Sex Marital Ther 1997;23: 165–173.
Language	English

Compound	Selective serotonin reuptake inhibitors (SSRI) in comparison with tricyclic antidepressants (N06AB)
Disease treated	Depression
Quantification of adverse effects	Sexual function score
No. of patients treated	34
Age group	Young
Treatment period	Various
Dose	Various
Treatment consequences	Sexual function, disturbance of various phases
Efficacy	Independent of type of antidepressant
Randomization of patients	No
Study quality	**3**

Reference	1429: Hsu JH, Shen WW. Male sexual side effects associated with antidepressants: a descriptive clinical study of 32 patients. Int J Psychiatry Med. 1995;25(2):191–201.
Language	English

Compound	**Selective serotonin reuptake inhibitors (SSRI) (N06AB)**
Disease treated	Depression
Quantification of adverse effects	Sexual function score
No. of patients treated	31
Age group	Young
Treatment period	Various
Dose	Various
Treatment consequences	Libido unaltered, erection/lubrication unaltered, orgasm quality impaired, sexual frequency unaltered
Efficacy	All patients
Randomization of patients	No
Study quality	**3**
Reference	1425: Labbate LA, Grimes JB, Arana GW. Serotonin reuptake antidepressant effects on sexual function in patients with anxiety disorders. Biol Psychiatry. 1998 Jun 15;43(12):904–7.
Language	English

Compound	**Selective serotonin reuptake inhibitors (SSRI) (N06AB)**
Disease treated	Depression
Quantification of adverse effects	Sexual function score
No. of patients treated	31
Age group	Young
Treatment period	3 months
Dose	Various
Treatment consequences	Orgasm quality, decreased
Efficacy	Most patients
Randomization of patients	No
Study quality	**3**
Reference	1416: Labbate LA, Grimes JB, Arana GW. Serotonin reuptake antidepressant effects on sexual function in patients with anxiety disorders. Biol Psychiatry. 1998 Jun 15;43(12):904–7.
Language	English

Compound	Selective serotonin reuptake inhibitors (SSRI) (N06AB)
Disease treated	Depression
Quantification of adverse effects	Erectile function
Age group	Old
Treatment consequences	Erectile function, impairment
Efficacy	Association by SSRI questionable, no controlled trials available
Study quality	**4 (review)**
Reference	1159: Fava M, Rankin M. Sexual functioning and SSRIs. J Clin Psychiatry. 2002;63 Suppl 5:13–6; discussion 23–5.
Language	English

Compound	Selective serotonin reuptake inhibitors (SSRI) (N06AB)
Disease treated	Depression
Quantification of adverse effects	Sexual functions
Age group	Young
Treatment consequences	Sexual dysfunction
Efficacy	Decreased libido in fluoxetine, abnormal ejaculation in venlafaxine
Study quality	**4 (review)**
Reference	1428: Margolese HC, Assalian P. Sexual side effects of antidepressants: a review. J Sex Marital Ther. 1996 Fall;22(3):209–17. McGill University, Canada.
Language	English

Compound	Fluoxetine (N06AB03)
Disease treated	Depression
Quantification of adverse effects	Sexual function score
No. of patients treated	190; 150
Age group	Young
Treatment period	Various
Dose	20 mg
Treatment consequences	Sexual dysfunction
Efficacy	No differences between drugs
Randomization of patients	Yes

Dose arms 1–3	Fluoxetine; mirtazapine
Study quality	**1+**
Reference	1568: Michelson D, Schmidt M, Lee J, Tepner R: Changes in sexual function during acute and six-month fluoxetine therapy: a prospective assessment. J Sex Marital Ther 2001;27: 289–302.
Language	English

Compound	Fluoxetine (N06AB03)
Disease treated	Depression
Quantification of adverse effects	Sexual function
No. of patients treated	160
Age group	All ages
Treatment period	Continuous
Dose	20–40 mg/day
Treatment consequences	Erectile function, impairment, libido, decrease
Efficacy	21 and 10% of patients
Randomization of patients	No
Study quality	**2+**
Reference	1474: Jacobsen FM. Fluoxetine-induced sexual dysfunction and an open trial of yohimbine. J Clin Psychiatry. 1992 Apr;53(4):119–22.
Language	English

Compound	Fluoxetine (N06AB03)
Disease treated	Erectile dysfunction, vascular
Quantification of adverse effects	Sexual function
No. of patients treated	3
Age group	Old
Treatment period	Continuous
Dose	n.g.
Treatment consequences	Erectile function, improvement
Efficacy	Moderate
Study quality	**3**

Reference	1473: Smith DM, Levitte SS. Association of fluoxetine and return of sexual potency in three elderly men. J Clin Psychiatry. 1993 Aug;54(8):317–9.
Language	English

Compound	Mianserin (N06AX03)
Disease treated	Depression and treatment with SSRI
Quantification of adverse effects	Sexual function score
No. of patients treated	15
Age group	Young
Treatment period	4 weeks
Dose	15 mg/day
Treatment consequences	Sexual function, improvement
Efficacy	Better orgasm and satisfaction
Randomization of patients	No
Study quality	**3**
Reference	1426: Aizenberg D, Gur S, Zemishlany Z, Granek M, Jeczmien P, Weizman A. Mianserin, a 5-HT2a/2c and alpha 2 antagonist, in the treatment of sexual dysfunction induced by serotonin reuptake inhibitors. Clin Neuropharmacol. 1997 Jun;20(3):210–4.
Language	English

Compound	Tradozone (N06AX05)
Disease treated	Erectile dysfunction
Quantification of adverse effects	Erectile function
No. of patients treated	396
Age group	Old
Treatment period	Single dose
Treatment consequences	Erectile function, improvement
Efficacy	Trazodone monotherapy appeared more likely than placebo to lead to a "positive treatment response", although this difference was not statistically significant.
Side effects	Specific adverse events with trazodone included dry mouth (19%), sedation (16%), dizziness (16%) and fatigue (15%).

Randomization of patients	Yes
Dose arms 1–3	200 mg/day; 50 mg/day; placebo
Study quality	**1+ (meta-analysis)**
Reference	1082: Fink HA, MacDonald R, Rutks IR, Wilt TJ. Trazodone for erectile dysfunction: a systematic review and meta-analysis. BJU Int. 2003 Sep;92(4):441–6.
Language	English

Compound	Tradozone (N06AX05)
Disease treated	Erectile dysfunction
Quantification of adverse effects	Sexual function score
No. of patients treated	79
Age group	Young
Treatment period	8 weeks
Dose	n.g.
Treatment consequences	Sexual function, improvement
Efficacy	60% of testosterone group, 69% of tradozone group, 39% of placebo Group
Side effects	Not mentioned
Randomization of patients	No
Dose arms 1–3	Tradozone; testosterone; placebo
Study quality	**2+**
Reference	1436: Aydin S, Odabas O, Ercan M, Kara H, Agargun MY. Efficacy of testosterone, trazodone and hypnotic suggestion in the treatment of non-organic male sexual dysfunction. Br J Urol. 1996 Feb;77(2):256–60.
Language	English

N07 Other Nervous System Drugs

Nicotine

Nicotine is not a drug for treating diseases, but it is a drug in the sense of the definition given by Goodman and Gilman (see above). In the following, it has to be considered that adverse effects of smoking may not be due to nicotine alone.

Sexual side effects have been well proven by multiple studies. In particular, the erectile function is compromised. Among the patients who complain of erectile dysfunction, there are more smokers and heavy smokers (40 vs 27.7%, and 39.2 vs 4%, respectively) than in the general population. The prevalence of erectile dysfunction in 1162 never smokers was 2.2%, in 1292 former smokers 2.0% and in 2008 current smokers 3.7% (Mannino et al. 1994).

The odds ratio (OR) for suffering from erectile dysfunction is significantly higher in smokers and in ex-smokers than in never smokers (OR 1.24–2.2, in all studies significantly enhanced). The association with pack-years suggested a dose–response pattern. Only one study published decribes no correlation of current cigarette smoking with erectile dysfunction, but the duration was positively correlated with erectile dysfunction ($p<0.01$; Bai et al. 2004). In men who are abstaining from smoking erectile function improved.

Current smokers showed impairment of subjective and objective erectile parameters; a higher number had abnormal nocturnal penile tumescences.

Cigarette smoking increased the incidence of erectile dysfunction in follow-up significantly (24 vs 14% in nonsmokers; Feldman et al. 2000). The relative risk of developing internal pudendal artery atherosclerosis for each 10 pack-years smoked is 1.31.

Overall level of evidence of adverse effects: B

Compound	Nicotine (N07BA01)
Disease treated	Erectile dysfunction
Quantification of adverse effects	IIEF
No. of patients treated	22,086
Age group	All ages
Treatment period	20 years
Dose	All doses

Treatment consequences	Erectile function, impairment
Efficacy	RR 1.5 (95% CI 1.3–1.7) in smokers as compared with non-smokers
Randomization of patients	No
Study quality	**2++**
Reference	1272: Bacon CG, Mittleman MA, Kawachi I, Giovannucci E, Glasser DB, Rimm EB. A prospective study of risk factors for erectile dysfunction. J Urol. 2006 Jul;176(1):217–21.
Language	English

Compound	Nicotine (N07BA01)
Disease treated	Erectile dysfunction in diabetes mellitus
Quantification of adverse effects	Erectile function
No. of patients treated	9670
Age group	20–70 years
Treatment period	Continuous
Dose	All doses
Treatment consequences	Erectile function, impairment
Efficacy	OR for smokers 1.4 (95% CI 1.3–1.6), OR for ex-smokers 1.5 (95% CI 1.3–1.6) as compared with non-smokers
Randomization of patients	No
Study quality	**2–**
Reference	1304: Bortolotti A, Fedele D, Chatenoud L, Colli E, Coscelli C, Landoni M, Lavezzari M, Santeusanio F, Parazzini F. Cigarette smoking: a risk factor for erectile dysfunction in diabetics. Eur Urol. 2001 Oct;40(4):392–6; discussion: 397.
Language	English

Compound	Nicotine (N07BA01)
Disease treated	Erectile dysfunction
Quantification of adverse effects	Erectile function, self-reported
No. of patients treated	8367
Age group	All ages
Treatment period	Continuous
Dose	All doses

Treatment consequences	Erectile function, impairment
Efficacy	OR 1.24 (CI 1.01–1.52, p=0.04) for smokers ≤20 cigarettes per day and 1.39 (CI 1.05–1.83) smokers >20 cigarettes per day as compared with non-smokers
Randomization of patients	No
Study quality	**2+**
Reference	1273: Millett C, Wen LM, Rissel C, Smith A, Richters J, Grulich A, de Visser R. Smoking and erectile dysfunction: findings from a representative sample of Australian men. Tob Control. 2006 Apr;15(2):136–9.
Language	English

Compound	Nicotine (N07BA01)
Disease treated	Erectile dysfunction
Quantification of adverse effects	Erectile function
No. of patients treated	4462
Age group	31–49 years
Treatment period	Continuous
Dose	All doses
Treatment consequences	Erectile function, impairment
Efficacy	Prevalence of erectile dysfunction in 1162 never smokers 2.2%, in 1292 former smokers 2.0%, in 2008 current smokers 3.7%
Randomization of patients	No
Study quality	**2++**
Reference	1309: Mannino DM, Klevens RM, Flanders WD. Cigarette smoking: an independent risk factor for impotence? Am J Epidemiol. 1994 Dec 1;140(11):1003–8.
Language	English

Compound	Nicotine (N07BA01)
Disease treated	Erectile dysfunction
Quantification of adverse effects	IIEF
No. of patients treated	4081
Age group	All ages
Treatment period	Continuous

2

Dose	All doses
Treatment consequences	Erectile function, impairment
Efficacy	Current smokers >10 cigarettes/day OR 1.4, former smokers OR 1.3 as compared with non-smokers
Randomization of patients	No
Study quality	**2–**
Reference	1284: Austoni E, Mirone V, Parazzini F, Fasolo CB, Turchi P, Pescatori ES, Ricci E, Gentile V; Andrology Prevention Week centres; Italian Society of Andrology. Smoking as a risk factor for erectile dysfunction: data from the Andrology Prevention Weeks 2001–2002 a study of the Italian Society of Andrology (s.l.a.). Eur Urol. 2005 Nov;48(5):810–7.
Language	English

Compound	Nicotine (N07BA01)
Disease treated	Erectile dysfunction
Quantification of adverse effects	Erectile function
No. of patients treated	3819
Age group	All ages
Treatment period	Continuous
Dose	All doses
Treatment consequences	Erectile function, impairment
Efficacy	40.1% of patients with erectile dysfunction are smokers, 27.7% of general population are smokers
Randomization of patients	No
Remarks	Study not controlled for other risk factors. Study population sought medical care for erectile dysfunction.
Study quality	**2–**
Reference	1189: Tengs TO, Osgood ND. The link between smoking and impotence: two decades of evidence. Prev Med. 2001 Jun;32(6):447–52.
Language	English

Compound	Nicotine (N07BA01)
Disease treated	Erectile dysfunction
Quantification of adverse effects	Erectile function
No. of patients treated	3143

Age group	50–70 years
Treatment period	Continuous
Dose	All doses
Treatment consequences	Erectile function, impairment
Efficacy	Current smoking OR=1.5 (95% CI: 0.9–2.2) as compared with non-smokers
Randomization of patients	No
Study quality	**2+**
Reference	1298: Shiri R, Koskimaki J, Hakama M, Hakkinen J, Huhtala H, Tammela TL, Auvinen A. Effect of life-style factors on incidence of erectile dysfunction. Int J Impot Res. 2004 Oct;16(5):389–94.
Language	English

Compound	Nicotine (N07BA01)
Disease treated	Erectile dysfunction
Quantification of adverse effects	Erectile function
No. of patients treated	2674
Age group	20–70 years
Treatment period	Continuous
Dose	All doses
Treatment consequences	Erectile function, impairment
Efficacy	Current smokers OR 2.41 (95% CI, 1.52–3.30), ex-smokers OR 2.15 (95% CI, 1.38–3.1) as compared with non-smokers
Randomization of patients	No
Study quality	**2+**
Reference	1301: Safarinejad MR. Prevalence and risk factors for erectile dysfunction in a population-based study in Iran. Int J Impot Res. 2003 Aug;15(4):246–52.
Language	English

Compound	Nicotine (N07BA01)
Disease treated	Erectile dysfunction
Quantification of adverse effects	Erectile function
No. of patients treated	2412
Age group	40–70 years

Treatment period	Continuous
Dose	All doses
Treatment consequences	Erectile function, impairment
Efficacy	OR=2.3 for >30 cigarettes/day for smokers as compared with non-smokers
Randomization of patients	No
Study quality	**2+**
Reference	1300: Nicolosi A, Glasser DB, Moreira ED, Villa M. Erectile Dysfunction Epidemiology Cross National Study Group. Prevalence of erectile dysfunction and associated factors among men without concomitant diseases: a population study. Int J Impot Res. 2003 Aug;15(4):253–7.
Language	English

Compound	Nicotine (N07BA01)
Disease treated	Erectile dysfunction
Quantification of adverse effects	IIEF
No. of patients treated	2226
Age group	20–86 years
Treatment period	Continuous
Dose	All doses
Treatment consequences	Erectile function, impairment
Efficacy	Current cigarette smoking not correlated with erectile dysfunction, while cigarette consumption and duration were positively correlated with erectile dysfunction ($p<0.01$).
Randomization of patients	No
Study quality	**2–**
Reference	1292: Bai Q, Xu QQ, Jiang H, Zhang WL, Wang XH, Zhu JC. Prevalence and risk factors of erectile dysfunction in three cities of China: a community-based study. Asian J Androl. 2004 Dec;6(4):343–8.
Language	English

Compound	Nicotine (N07BA01)
Disease treated	Erectile dysfunction
Quantification of adverse effects	Erectile function

No. of patients treated	2010
Age group	>18 years
Treatment period	Continuous
Dose	All doses
Treatment consequences	Erectile function, impairment
Efficacy	Current smokers OR of 1.7 (95% CI, 1.2–2.4), ex-smokers of 1.6 (95% CI, 1.1–2.3) as compared with non-smokers
Randomization of patients	No
Study quality	**2+**
Reference	1303: Mirone V, Imbimbo C, Bortolotti A, Cintio E di, Colli E, Landoni M, Lavezzari M, Parazzini F. Cigarette smoking as risk factor for erectile dysfunction: results from an Italian epidemiological study. Eur Urol. 2002 Mar;41(3):294–7.
Language	English

Compound	Nicotine (N07BA01)
Disease treated	Erectile dysfunction
Quantification of adverse effects	IIEF
No. of patients treated	1442
Age group	50–75 years
Treatment period	Continuous
Dose	All doses
Treatment consequences	Erectile function, impairment
Efficacy	Risk of erectile dysfunction non-significantly increased with smoking (OR=1.4)
Randomization of patients	No
Study quality	**2+**
Reference	1295: Shiri R, Hakama M, Hakkinen J, Tammela TL, Auvinen A, Koskimaki J. Relationship between smoking and erectile dysfunction. Int J Impot Res. 2005 Mar–Apr;17(2):164–9.
Language	English

Compound	Nicotine (N07BA01)
Disease treated	Erectile dysfunction
Quantification of adverse effects	Brief Male Sexual Function Inventory
No. of patients treated	1329

2

Age group	40–79 years
Treatment period	Continuous
Dose	All doses
Treatment consequences	Erectile function, impairment
Efficacy	Current smokers OR 2.74 (95% CI: 0.44, 16.89) as compared with non-smokers
Randomization of patients	No
Study quality	**2+**
Reference	1287: Gades NM, Nehra A, Jacobson DJ, McGree ME, Girman CJ, Rhodes T, Roberts RO, Lieber MM, Jacobsen SJ. Association between smoking and erectile dysfunction: a population-based study. Am J Epidemiol. 2005 Feb 15;161(4):346–51.
Language	English

Compound	Nicotine (N07BA01)
Disease treated	Erectile dysfunction
Quantification of adverse effects	Structured Interview (SIEDY)
No. of patients treated	1150
Age group	All ages
Treatment period	Continuous
Dose	All doses
Treatment consequences	Erectile function, impairment
Efficacy	Current smokers and past smokers showed impairment of subjective and objective (dynamic peak systolic velocity at penile duplex ultrasound) erectile parameters.
Randomization of patients	No
Study quality	**2–**
Reference	1285: Corona G, Mannucci E, Petrone L, Ricca V, Mansani R, Cilotti A, Balercia G, Chiarini V, Giommi R, Forti G, Maggi M. Psychobiological correlates of smoking in patients with erectile dysfunction. Int J Impot Res. 2005 Nov–Dec;17(6):527–34.
Language	English

Compound	Nicotine (N07BA01)
Disease treated	Erectile dysfunction
Quantification of adverse effects	IIEF
No. of patients treated	860
Age group	18–44 years
Treatment period	Continuous
Dose	All doses
Treatment consequences	Erectile function, impairment
Efficacy	337 patients >20 cigarettes/day (39.2%); in the general population only 4% are heavy smokers
Randomization of patients	No
Study quality	**2–**
Reference	1294: Natali A, Mondaini N, Lombardi G, Del Popolo G, Rizzo M. Heavy smoking is an important risk factor for erectile dysfunction in young men. Int J Impot Res. 2005 May–Jun;17(3):227–30.
Language	English

Compound	Nicotine (N07BA01)
Disease treated	Erectile dysfunction
Quantification of adverse effects	IIEF
No. of patients treated	819
Age group	31–60 years
Treatment period	Continuous
Dose	>20 cigarettes per day
Treatment consequences	Erectile function, impairment
Efficacy	OR 1.47 (CI 1.00–2.16) in smokers as compared with non-smokers
Randomization of patients	No
Study quality	**2+**
Reference	1280: Lam TH, Abdullah AS, Ho LM, Yip AW, Fan S. Smoking and sexual dysfunction in Chinese males: findings from men's health survey. Int J Impot Res. 2006 Jul–Aug;18(4):364–9.
Language	English

Compound	Nicotine (N07BA01)
Disease treated	Erectile dysfunction
Quantification of adverse effects	Erectile dysfunction
No. of patients treated	593
Age group	40–70 years
Treatment period	9 years observation period
Dose	Various risk factors
Treatment consequences	Development of erectile dysfunction
Efficacy	Changes in smoking and alcohol consumption were not associated with the incidence of erectile dysfunction.
Randomization of patients	No
Remarks	Midlife changes may be too late to reverse the effects of risk factors
Study quality	**2+**
Reference	1306: Derby CA, Mohr BA, Goldstein I, Feldman HA, Johannes CB, McKinlay JB. Modifiable risk factors and erectile dysfunction: Can lifestyle changes modify risk? Urology. 2000 Aug 1;56(2):302–6.
Language	English

Compound	Nicotine (N07BA01)
Disease treated	Erectile dysfunction
Quantification of adverse effects	Erectile function
No. of patients treated	513
Age group	40–70 years
Treatment period	Continuous
Dose	All doses
Treatment consequences	Erectile function, impairment
Efficacy	Cigarette smoking at baseline increased the likelihood of erectile dysfunction at follow-up (24 vs 14% in non-smokers).
Randomization of patients	No
Study quality	**2+**
Reference	1307: Feldman HA, Johannes CB, Derby CA, Kleinman KP, Mohr BA, Araujo AB, McKinlay JB. Erectile dysfunction and coronary risk factors: prospective results from the Massachusetts male aging study. Prev Med. 2000 Apr;30(4):328–38.

Language	English

Compound	Nicotine (N07BA01)
Disease treated	Erectile dysfunction
Quantification of adverse effects	IIEF
No. of patients treated	335
Age group	50–80 years
Treatment period	Continuous
Dose	All doses
Treatment consequences	Erectile function, impairment
Efficacy	OR 2.2 (CI 1.2–3.9) in smokers as compared with non-smokers; pack-years suggest a dose–response pattern.
Randomization of patients	No
Study quality	**2+**
Reference	1274: Polsky JY, Aronson KJ, Heaton JP, Adams MA. Smoking and other lifestyle factors in relation to erectile dysfunction. BJU Int. 2005 Dec;96(9):1355–9.
Language	English

Compound	Nicotine (N07BA01)
Disease treated	Erectile dysfunction
Quantification of adverse effects	IIEF
No. of patients treated	281
Age group	Middle-aged
Treatment period	Continuous
Dose	Cessation
Treatment consequences	Erectile function, improvement
Efficacy	After 1 year of cessation erectile function improved in >25% of ex-smokers but in none of the current smokers; 2.5% of ex-smokers and 6.8% of current smokers had deterioration in erectile dysfunction.
Randomization of patients	No
Study quality	**2–**
Reference	1291: Pourmand G, Alidaee MR, Rasuli S, Maleki A, Mehrsai A. Do cigarette smokers with erectile dysfunction benefit from stopping?: a prospective study. BJU Int. 2004 Dec;94(9):1310–3.

Language	English

Compound	Nicotine (N07BA01)
Disease treated	Erectile dysfunction in diabetes mellitus
Quantification of adverse effects	Erectile function
No. of patients treated	264
Age group	>21 years
Treatment period	Continuous
Dose	All doses
Treatment consequences	Erectile function, impairment
Efficacy	Incidence of erectile dysfunction within 10 years 25%; OR for smokers 2.41 (95% CI, 1.09–5.30) as compared with non-smokers
Randomization of patients	No
Study quality	**2+**
Reference	1290: Klein R, Klein BE, Moss SE. Ten-year incidence of self-reported erectile dysfunction in people with long-term type 1 diabetes. J Diabetes Complications. 2005 Jan–Feb;19(1):35–41.
Language	English

Compound	Nicotine (N07BA01)
Disease treated	Erectile dysfunction
Quantification of adverse effects	Nocturnal penile tumescence
No. of patients treated	207
Age group	Old
Treatment period	Continuous
Dose	All doses
Treatment consequences	Erectile function, impairment
Efficacy	122 (59%) patients had an abnormal NPT, 65 of 122 patients (53%) who smoked cigarettes
Randomization of patients	No
Study quality	**2–**

Reference	1308: McMahon CG, Touma K. Predictive value of patient history and correlation of nocturnal penile tumescence, colour duplex Doppler ultrasonography and dynamic cavernosometry and cavernosography in the evaluation of erectile dysfunction. Int J Impot Res. 1999 Feb;11(1):47–51.
Language	English

Compound	Nicotine (N07BA01)
Disease treated	Erectile dysfunction
Quantification of adverse effects	Selective pudendal angiography
No. of patients treated	200
Age group	Middle-aged
Treatment period	Continuous
Dose	All doses
Treatment consequences	Erectile function, impairment
Efficacy	RR 1.31 (CI 1.05; 1.64) of developing internal pudendal artery atherosclerosis for each 10 pack-years smoked
Randomization of patients	No
Study quality	**2+**
Reference	1312: Rosen MP, Greenfield AJ, Walker TG, Grant P, Dubrow J, Bettmann MA, Fried LE, Goldstein I. Cigarette smoking: an independent risk factor for atherosclerosis in the hypogastric–cavernous arterial bed of men with arteriogenic impotence. J Urol. 1991 Apr;145(4):759–63.
Language	English

Compound	Nicotine (N07BA01)
Disease treated	Erectile dysfunction
Quantification of adverse effects	Nocturnal penile tumescence and rigidity monitoring
No. of patients treated	109
Age group	44–51 years
Treatment period	Continuous
Dose	All doses
Treatment consequences	Erectile function, impairment

2

Efficacy	86% of smokers had abnormal NPTR testing compared with 55% of non-smokers (p=0.02). The average peak systolic velocity was 26.8 and 31.2 cm/s for smokers and non-smokers.
Randomization of patients	No
Study quality	**2–**
Reference	1296: Elhanbly S, Abdel-Gaber S, Fathy H, El-Bayoumi Y, Wald M, Niederberger CS. Erectile dysfunction in smokers: a penile dynamic and vascular study. J Androl. 2004 Nov–Dec;25(6):991–5.
Language	English

Compound	Nicotine (N07BA01)
Disease treated	Erectile dysfunction
Quantification of adverse effects	Sexual response to erotic film
No. of patients treated	42
Age group	18–44 years
Treatment period	Continuous
Dose	All doses
Treatment consequences	Rate of penile diameter change, decreased
Efficacy	Significantly with smoking high-nicotine cigarettes
Randomization of patients	No
Study quality	**1–**
Reference	1286: Gilbert DG, Hagen RL, D'Agostino JA. The effects of cigarette smoking on human sexual potency. Addict Behav. 1986;11(4):431–4.
Language	English

N07	Other Nervous System Drugs
	Opioids
	Buproprion showed a limited or no negative effect on erectile function. Methadone impaired sexual function, in particular the libido. **Overall level of evidence of adverse effects: D**

Compound	Buproprion (N07BA02)
Disease treated	Depression
Quantification of adverse effects	Sexual function score
No. of patients treated	120; 121
Age group	Young
Treatment period	n.g.
Dose	400 mg
Treatment consequences	Sexual dysfunction
Efficacy	15% in buproprion group, 10% in placebo group
Randomization of patients	Yes
Dose arms 1–3	Burproprion; placebo
Study quality	**1–**
Reference	1567: Croft H, Settle E, Houser T et al. A placebo-controlled comparison of the antidepresant efficacy and effect on sexual functioning of sustained-release buproprion and sertraline. Clin Ther 1999;21:643–58.
Language	English

Compound	Buproprion (N07BA02)
Disease treated	Depression and treatment with SSRI
Quantification of adverse effects	Sexual function score
No. of patients treated	42
Age group	All ages
Treatment period	4 weeks
Dose	150 mg/day
Treatment consequences	Libido increased, sexual activity improvement
Efficacy	Better in buproprione group

Randomization of patients	Yes
Dose arms 1–3	Buproprione; placebo
Study quality	**1+**
Reference	1431: Clayton AH, Warnock JK, Kornstein SG, Pinkerton R, Sheldon-Keller A, McGarvey EL. A placebo-controlled trial of bupropion SR as an antidote for selective serotonin reuptake inhibitor-induced sexual dysfunction. J Clin Psychiatry. 2004 Jan;65(1):62–7.
Language	English

Compound	Bupropion (N07BA02)
Disease treated	Depression and sexual dysfunction by SSRI
Quantification of adverse effects	Sexual function score
No. of patients treated	40
Age group	Young
Treatment period	3 weeks
Dose	n.g.
Treatment consequences	Sexual function rating scale, unaltered
Efficacy	No difference between groups
Randomization of patients	Yes
Dose arms 1–3	Buproprin; placebo
Study quality	**1+**
Reference	1421: Masand PS, Ashton AK, Gupta S, Frank B. Sustained-release bupropion for selective serotonin reuptake inhibitor-induced sexual dysfunction: a randomized, double-blind, placebo-controlled, parallel-group study. Am J Psychiatry. 2001 May;158(5):805–7.
Language	English

Compound	Buproprion (N07BA02)
Disease treated	Depression
Quantification of adverse effects	Sexual function questionnaire
No. of patients treated	14
Age group	Middle-aged
Treatment period	6 weeks
Dose	n.g.
Treatment consequences	Sexual activity, unaltered

Efficacy	No effects
Side effects	No effect on diabetes
Randomization of patients	No
Study quality	**3**
Reference	1623: Rowland DL, Myers L, Culver A, Davidson JM. Bupropion and sexual function: a placebo-controlled prospective study on diabetic men with erectile dysfunction. J Clin Psychopharmacol. 1997 Oct;17(5):350–7.
Language	English

Compound	Methadone (N07BC02)
Disease treated	Opiate addiction
Quantification of adverse effects	Sexual function score
No. of patients treated	92
Age group	Young
Treatment period	Continuous
Dose	Various
Treatment consequences	Sexual function, alteration
Efficacy	In 14% of patients sexual dysfunction was correlated to absolute dose.
Randomization of patients	No
Study quality	**3**
Reference	1397: Brown R, Balousek S, Mundt M, Fleming M. Methadone maintenance and male sexual dysfunction. J Addict Dis. 2005;24(2):91–106.
Language	English

Compound	Methadone (N07BC02)
Disease treated	Opiate addiction
Quantification of adverse effects	Sexual function
No. of patients treated	50
Age group	Young
Treatment period	Continuous
Dose	Various
Treatment consequences	Sexual function, alteration
Efficacy	In 33% of patients

2

Randomization of patients	No
Study quality	**3**
Reference	1270: Hanbury R, Cohen M, Stimmel B. Adequacy of sexual performance in men maintained on methadone. Am J Drug Alcohol Abuse. 1977;4(1):13–20.
Language	English

Compound	Methadone (N07BC02)
Disease treated	Opiate addiction
Quantification of adverse effects	Sexual function
No. of patients treated	31
Age group	Young
Treatment period	Continuous
Dose	Various
Treatment consequences	Sexual function, alteration
Efficacy	Daily methadone dose correlated significantly with frequency of ejaculation (-0.31).
Randomization of patients	No
Study quality	**3**
Reference	1269: Crowley TJ, Simpson R. Methadone dose and human sexual behavior. Int J Addict. 1978 Feb;13(2):285–95.
Language	English

N07 Other Nervous System Drugs

Others

There is an isolated case report of erectile dysfunction following cinnarizine.

Overall level of evidence of adverse effects: D

Compound	Cinnarizine (N07CA02)
Disease treated	Postural vertigo
Quantification of adverse effects	Erectile function
No. of patients treated	1

Age group	55 years
Treatment period	3 months
Dose	150 mg/day
Treatment consequences	Erectile function, impairment
Efficacy	"Complete impotence"
Remarks	No other reports in the literature
Study quality	**3**
Reference	1389: Sempere AP, Garcia FM, Duarte J, Mataix AL, Coria F, Claveria LE. Impotence associated with cinnarizine. Ann Pharmacother. 1993 Mar;27(3):370.
Language	English

R03 Drugs for Obstructive Airway Diseases

Terbutaline, a selective β-2 adrenergic agonist, and aminophylline, a bronchodilator, were used to resolve prolonged erection due to intracavernous injection.

Overall level of evidence of adverse effects: B

Compound	Terbutaline (R03AC03)
Disease treated	Erectile dysfunction
Quantification of adverse effects	Prolonged erection due to intracavernous injection
No. of patients treated	75
Age group	Middle-aged
Treatment period	Single dose
Treatment consequences	Detumescence
Efficacy	Detumescence in 36% (terbutaline) vs 12% (placebo)
Randomization of patients	Yes
Dose arms 1–3	Pseudoephedrine 60 mg; terbutaline sulfate 5 mg; sodium bicarbonate 648 mg as placebo
Remarks	Yes
Study quality	**1+**
Reference	1617: Lowe FC, Jarow JP. Placebo-controlled study of oral terbutaline and pseudoephedrine in management of prostaglandin E1-induced prolonged erections. Urology. 1993 Jul;42(1):51–3; discussion 53–4.
Language	English

Compound	Terbutaline (R03AC03)
Disease treated	Paraplegics
Quantification of adverse effects	Prolonged erection due to intracavernous injection
No. of patients treated	3
Age group	Middle-aged
Treatment period	Single dose
Dose	5 mg/day orally
Treatment consequences	Detumescence
Efficacy	Detumescence within 15 min
Randomization of patients	No
Study quality	**2–**
Reference	1616: Soni BM, Vaidyanathan S, Krishnan KR. Management of pharmacologically induced prolonged penile erection with oral terbutaline in traumatic paraplegics. Paraplegia. 1994 Oct;32(10):670–4.
Language	English

Compound	Terbutaline (R03AC03)
Disease treated	General anaesthesia
Quantification of adverse effects	Prolonged erection
No. of patients treated	n.g.
Age group	Middle-aged
Treatment period	Single dose
Dose	5 mg/day orally
Treatment consequences	Detumescence
Efficacy	Rapid detumescence
Study quality	**3**
Reference	1618: Shantha TR, Finnerty DP, Rodriquez AP. Treatment of persistent penile erection and priapism using terbutaline. J Urol. 1989 Jun;141(6):1427–9.
Language	English

Compound	Aminophyllin (R03DA05)
Disease treated	Cavernous tissue in vitro
Quantification of adverse effects	Muscle relaxation
No. of patients treated	16

Age group	42–68 years
Treatment period	In vitro
Dose	5×10^{-4}g
Treatment consequences	Cavernous tissue, relaxation
Efficacy	Good
Randomization of patients	No
Study quality	**3**
Reference	1438: Barbanti G, Beneforti P, Lapini A, Turini D. Relaxation of isolated corpus cavernosum induced by smooth-muscle relaxant drugs. A comparative study. Urol Res. 1988;16(4):299–302.
Language	English

Compound	Aminophyllin (R03DA05)
Disease treated	Erectile dysfunction
Quantification of adverse effects	Erectile function
No. of patients treated	14
Age group	Old
Treatment period	4 weeks
Dose	Cream containing aminophylline, isosorbide dinitrate and co-dergocrine mesylate
Treatment consequences	Erectile function, improvement
Efficacy	Moderate
Randomization of patients	No
Dose arms 1–3	Cream; placebo
Study quality	**3**
Reference	1437: Le Roux PJ, Naude JH. Topical vasoactive cream in the treatment of erectile failure: a prospective, randomized placebo-controlled trial. BJU Int. 1999 May;83(7):810–1.
Language	English

R06	Antihistamines for Systemic Use
	Two trials of antihistamines in treating erectile dysfunction are quoted. The effect is marginal.
	Overall level of evidence of adverse effects: C

Compound	Capsicain intraurethrally (not listed)
Disease treated	Erectile dysfunction
Quantification of adverse effects	Erectile function
No. of patients treated	20
Age group	Young
Treatment period	n.g.
Dose	10^{-5} mol, intraurethrally
Treatment consequences	Erectile function, improvement
Efficacy	Good success
Randomization of patients	No
Dose arms 1–3	Capsicaine; papaverine intracavernous; saline
Study quality	**2–**
Reference	1522: Lazzeri M, Barbanti G, Beneforti P, Turini D. Intraurethrally infused capsaicin induces penile erection in humans. Scand J Urol Nephrol. 1994 Dec;28(4):409–12.
Language	English

Compound	Loratadin (R06AX13)
Disease treated	Erectile dysfunction in severe depression
Quantification of adverse effects	IIEF
No. of patients treated	9
Age group	Young
Treatment period	2 weeks
Dose	10 mg/day
Treatment consequences	IIEF score, improvement
Efficacy	No effect
Randomization of patients	No
Study quality	**3**

Reference	1595: Aukst-Margetic B, Margetic B. An open-label series using loratadine for the treatment of sexual dysfunction associated with selective serotonin reuptake inhibitors. Prog Neuropsychopharmacol Biol Psychiatry. 2005 Jun;29(5):754–6.
Language	English

V03 All Other Therapeutic Products – Alcohol

Erectile dysfunction appears to be common in severe alcohol disease. The cessation of alcohol abuse improved erectile function in 25% of men studied, in particular in those with minor changes in the endocrine system. Also the impairment of nocturnal erections was found. The causative role of alcohol, however, appears to be minor compared with that of age: the percentage of alcoholics among patients with erectile dysfunction was not significantly higher than that of the general population. Sometimes it may be due to autonomic neuropathy.

The alcoholic hepatopathy appears to influence the steroid hormone levels and erectile function in a way different from that of other causes of hepatopathy. Breast swelling (gynaecomastia) has been observed in alcoholic cirrhosis but not in other forms of cirrhosis.

Overall level of evidence of adverse effects: B

Compound	Alcohol (V03AZ01)
Disease treated	Alcohol disease
Quantification of adverse effects	Erectile function by questionnaire
No. of patients treated	629
Age group	All ages
Treatment period	Continuous
Dose	Various
Treatment consequences	Erectile function, impairment
Efficacy	Using a multiple linear regression model, age and depression were found to be good predictors of erectile dysfunction but not alcohol abuse and panic disorder.
Randomization of patients	No
Study quality	**3**

Reference	1340: Okulate G, Olayinka O, Dogunro AS. Erectile dysfunction: prevalence and relationship to depression, alcohol abuse and panic disorder. Gen Hosp Psychiatry. 2003 May–Jun;25(3):209–13.
Language	English

Compound	Alcohol (V03AZ01)
Disease treated	Erectile dysfunction
Quantification of adverse effects	Erectile function
No. of patients treated	400
Age group	59 years (mean)
Treatment period	Continuous
Dose	Various
Treatment consequences	Erectile function, impairment
Efficacy	Prevalence of alcoholism was 7% in patients with erectile dysfunction
Randomization of patients	No
Study quality	**3**
Reference	1347: Slag MF, Morley JE, Elson MK, Trence DL, Nelson CJ, Nelson AE, Kinlaw WB, Beyer HS, Nuttall FQ, Shafer RB. Impotence in medical clinic outpatients. J Am Med Assoc. 1983 Apr 1;249(13):1736–40.
Language	English

Compound	Alcohol (V03AZ01)
Disease treated	Alcohol disease
Quantification of adverse effects	Erectile function
No. of patients treated	97
Age group	All ages
Treatment period	Continuous
Dose	Various
Treatment consequences	Erectile function, impairment
Efficacy	71% suffered from sexual dysfunction; among these, diminished sexual desire was 58%, erectile dysfunction 16%, premature ejaculation 4% and ejaculation deficiency 22%
Randomization of patients	No

Study quality	**3**
Reference	1349: Vijayasenan ME. Alcohol and sex. N Z Med J. 1981 Jan 14;93(675):18–20.
Language	English

Compound	Alcohol (V03AZ01)
Disease treated	Liver cirrhosis
Quantification of adverse effects	Hormones
No. of patients treated	78
Age group	All ages
Treatment period	Continuous
Dose	Various
Treatment consequences	Erectile function, impairment
Efficacy	Twelve of 21 patients with alcoholic cirrhosis, and 16 of 27 with postnecrotic cirrhosis, suffered from impotence. Both alcoholic groups had significantly lower levels of testosterone but higher levels of oestradiol and prolactin than the control group.
Randomization of patients	No
Dose arms 1–3	Alcohol cirrhosis; postnecrotic cirrhosis; no cirrhosis
Study quality	**2–**
Reference	1342: Wang YJ, Wu JC, Lee SD, Tsai YT, Lo KJ. Gonadal dysfunction and changes in sex hormones in postnecrotic cirrhotic men: a matched study with alcoholic cirrhotic men. Hepatogastroenterology. 1991 Dec;38(6):531–4.
Language	English

Compound	Alcohol (V03AZ01)
Disease treated	Alcohol disease
Quantification of adverse effects	Erectile function
No. of patients treated	60
Age group	All ages
Treatment period	Continuous
Dose	Cessation of alcohol
Treatment consequences	Erectile function, improvement after cessation

Efficacy	Twenty-five percent of the men studied experienced a spontaneous recovery. Indicators of recovery were absence of testicular atrophy and normal gonadotropin responses to GnRH.
Randomization of patients	No
Study quality	**3**
Reference	1348: Van Thiel DH, Gavaler JS, Sanghvi A. Recovery of sexual function in abstinent alcoholic men. Gastroenterology. 1983 Apr;84(4):677–82.
Language	English

Compound	Alcohol (V03AZ01)
Disease treated	Liver cirrhosis
Quantification of adverse effects	Hormones, erectile function
No. of patients treated	60
Age group	All ages
Treatment period	Continuous
Dose	Various
Treatment consequences	Erectile function, impairment
Efficacy	14 of 20 patients with alcohol cirrhosis, 10 of 40 non-alcoholic cirrhosis
Randomization of patients	No
Dose arms 1–3	Alcohol cirrhosis; other cirrhosis
Study quality	**2–**
Reference	1345: Cornely CM, Schade RR, Van Thiel DH, Gavaler JS. Chronic advanced liver disease and impotence: Cause and effect? Hepatology. 1984 Nov–Dec;4(6):1227–30.
Language	English

Compound	Alcohol (V03AZ01)
Disease treated	Alcohol disease
Quantification of adverse effects	Erectile function
No. of patients treated	35
Age group	Young
Treatment period	Continuous
Dose	Various

Treatment consequences	Erectile function, impairment
Efficacy	Erectile dysfunction not associated with hepatic disease, elevated SHBG or hyper-oestrogenism; free T 30% lower, total T 20% lower than in normal males
Randomization of patients	No
Study quality	**3**
Reference	1350: Farnsworth WE, Cavanaugh AH, Brown JR, Alvarez I, Lewandowski LM. Factors underlying infertility in the alcoholic. Arch Androl. 1978;1(2):193–5.
Language	English

Compound	Alcohol (V03AZ01)
Disease treated	Liver cirrhosis
Quantification of adverse effects	Hormones
No. of patients treated	26
Age group	All ages
Treatment period	Continuous
Dose	Various
Treatment consequences	Breast swelling, alteration
Efficacy	Gynaecomastia in alcoholic cirrhosis, not in other forms of cirrhosis; oestradiol level decreased
Randomization of patients	No
Dose arms 1–3	Alcohol cirrhosis; haemochromatosis; no cirrhosis
Study quality	**2–**
Reference	1343: Kley HK, Stremmel W, Niederau C, Hehrmann R, Shams O, Strohmeyer G, Kruskemper HL. Androgen and estrogen response to adrenal and gonadal stimulation in idiopathic hemochromatosis: evidence for decreased estrogen formation. Hepatology. 1985 Mar–Apr;5(2):251–6.
Language	English

Compound	Alcohol (V03AZ01)
Disease treated	Alcohol disease
Quantification of adverse effects	Erectile function
No. of patients treated	18
Age group	All ages

2

Treatment period	Continuous
Dose	Heavy drinkers
Treatment consequences	Erectile function, impairment
Efficacy	Sole clinical expression of autonomic neuropathy was impotence
Randomization of patients	No
Dose arms 1–3	Alcohol; no alcohol
Study quality	**2–**
Reference	1339: Ravaglia S, Marchioni E, Costa A, Maurelli M, Moglia A. Erectile dysfunction as a sentinel symptom of cardiovascular autonomic neuropathy in heavy drinkers. J Peripher Nerv Syst. 2004 Dec;9(4):209–14.
Language	English

Compound	Alcohol (V03AZ01)
Disease treated	Erectile dysfunction in alcohol disease
Quantification of adverse effects	Erectile function
No. of patients treated	13
Age group	All ages
Treatment period	Continuous
Dose	Various
Treatment consequences	Nocturnal erections
Efficacy	Seven had normal and 6 had impaired nocturnal erections.
Randomization of patients	No
Study quality	**3**
Reference	1346: Tan ET, Johnson RH, Lambie DG, Vijayasenan ME, Whiteside EA. Erectile impotence in chronic alcoholics. Alcohol Clin Exp Res. 1984;8(3):297–301.
Language	English

Renal Dialysis and Renal Transplantation (not listed in ATC/DDD)

Erectile dysfunction is highly prevalent for patients on haemodialysis; about 80% of patients suffer from impotence, with a clear increase of prevalence with age. Penile calcification has been observed in a number of patients. It is unclear as to whether the terminal renal insufficiency itself, or the treatment with dialysis, is the cause. Its prevalence also increases with additional diseases, e.g. diabetes mellitus or other vascular risk factors including hypertension.

Renal transplantation does not restore erectile function completely.

Overall level of evidence of adverse effects: C

Compound	Renal Dialysis
Disease treated	Terminal renal insufficiency
Quantification of adverse effects	Erectile function
No. of patients treated	302
Age group	Middle-aged
Treatment period	Continuing
Treatment consequences	Erectile function, impairment
Efficacy	In 82% for all HD subjects, in 45% severe erectile dysfunction; in subjects <50 years 63%, in subjects >50 years 90%
Randomization of patients	No
Study quality	**2–**
Reference	1258: Rosas SE, Joffe M, Franklin E, Strom BL, Kotzker W, Brensinger C, Grossman E, Glasser D, Feldman HI. Prevalence and determinants of erectile dysfunction in hemodialysis patients. Kidney Int. 2001 Jun;59(6):2259–66.
Language	English

Compound	Renal Dialysis
Disease treated	Terminal renal insufficiency
Quantification of adverse effects	Erectile function
No. of patients treated	187
Age group	Middle-aged

2

Treatment period	Continuing
Treatment consequences	Erectile function, impairment
Efficacy	The prevalence of erectile dysfunction for patients <50 years and ≥50 years was 74.5 and 86.6%, respectively.
Randomization of patients	No
Study quality	**3**
Reference	1255: Arslan D, Aslan G, Sifil A, Cavdar C, Celebi I, Gamsari T, Esen AA. Sexual dysfunction in male patients on hemodialysis: assessment with the International Index of Erectile Function (IIEF). Int J Impot Res. 2002 Dec;14(6):539–42.
Language	English

Compound	Renal Dialysis
Disease treated	Terminal renal insufficiency
Quantification of adverse effects	Erectile function
No. of patients treated	180
Age group	Middle-aged
Treatment period	Continuing
Dose	n.g.
Treatment consequences	Erectile function, impairment
Efficacy	Higher in patients with diabetes mellitus, higher in elevated haemoglobin A1c levels
Randomization of patients	No
Study quality	**2–**
Reference	1254: Miyata Y, Shindo K, Matsuya F, Noguchi M, Nishikido M, Koga S, Kanetake H. Erectile dysfunction in hemodialysis patients with diabetes mellitus: association with age and hemoglobin A1c levels. Int J Urol. 2004 Jul;11(7):530–4.
Language	English

Compound	Renal Dialysis
Disease treated	Terminal renal insufficiency
Quantification of adverse effects	Erectile function
No. of patients treated	174
Age group	Middle-aged

Treatment period	Continuing
Treatment consequences	Erectile function, impairment
Efficacy	Prevalence significantly higher than in controls
Randomization of patients	No
Study quality	**2–**
Reference	1257: Naya Y, Soh J, Ochiai A, Mizutani Y, Ushijima S, Kamoi K, Ukimura O, Kawauchi A, Fujito A, Ono T, Iwamoto N, Aoki T, Imada N, Marumo K, Murai M, Miki T. Significant decrease of the International Index of Erectile Function in male renal failure patients treated with hemodialysis. Int J Impot Res. 2002 Jun;14(3):172–7.
Language	English

Compound	Renal Dialysis
Disease treated	Terminal renal insufficiency
Quantification of adverse effects	Erectile function
No. of patients treated	118
Age group	Middle-aged
Treatment period	Continuing
Treatment consequences	Erectile function, impairment
Efficacy	In 86.4% of patients, more frequent in patients >50 years
Randomization of patients	No
Study quality	**3**
Reference	1256: Neto AF, Freitas Rodrigues MA de, Saraiva Fittipaldi JA, Moreira ED Jr. The epidemiology of erectile dysfunction and its correlates in men with chronic renal failure on hemodialysis in Londrina, southern Brazil. Int J Impot Res. 2002 Aug;14 Suppl 2:S19–26.
Language	English

Compound	Renal Dialysis
Disease treated	Terminal renal insufficiency
Quantification of adverse effects	Erectile function
No. of patients treated	75
Age group	Young
Treatment period	Continuing

Treatment consequences	Erectile function, impairment
Efficacy	Prevalence of erectile dysfunction <50 years 80%, in those >50 years 88%, while among controls it was 28 and 69.8%, respectively
Remarks	A complete health evaluation of male haemodialysis patients should include sexual functions.
Study quality	**3**
Reference	1253: Ali ME, Abdel-Hafez HZ, Mahran AM, Mohamed HZ, Mohamed ER, El-Shazly AM, Gadallah AM, Abbas MA. Erectile dysfunction in chronic renal failure patients undergoing hemodialysis in Egypt. Int J Impot Res. 2005 Mar–Apr;17(2):180–5.
Language	English

Compound	Renal Dialysis
Disease treated	Terminal renal insuffiency, age >60 years
Quantification of adverse effects	IIEF
No. of patients treated	58
Age group	>18 years
Treatment period	Various
Treatment consequences	Prevalence of erectile dysfunction as compared with healthy men
Efficacy	OR 6.23 (95% CI 2.06–18.8)
Randomization of patients	No
Study quality	**2–**
Reference	2202: Rosas SE, Joffe M, Franklin E, Strom BL, Kotzker W, Brensinger C, Grossman E, Glasser D, Feldman HI. Prevalence and determinants of erectile dysfunction in hemodialysis patients. Kidney Int. 2001 Jun;59(6):2259–66.
Language	English

Compound	Renal Dialysis
Disease treated	Terminal renal insufficiency
Quantification of adverse effects	Erectile function
No. of patients treated	32
Age group	Middle-aged
Treatment period	Continuing
Treatment consequences	Erectile function, impairment

Efficacy	Penile calcification in 6 of 32 patients
Randomization of patients	No
Study quality	**3**
Reference	1259: Dalal S, Gandhi VC, Yu AW, Bhate DV, Said RA, Rahman MA, Ing TS. Penile calcification in maintenance hemodialysis patients. Urology. 1992 Nov;40(5):422–4.
Language	English

Compound	Renal Dialysis
Disease treated	Terminal renal insufficiency
Quantification of adverse effects	Erectile function
No. of patients treated	n.g.
Age group	Young
Treatment period	Continuing
Treatment consequences	Erectile function, impairment
Efficacy	Complete impotence
Study quality	**3**
Reference	1344: Foulks CJ, Cushner HM. Sexual dysfunction in the male dialysis patient: pathogenesis, evaluation, and therapy. Am J Kidney Dis. 1986 Oct;8(4):211–22.
Language	English

Compound	Renal transplantation
Disease treated	Kidney recipients
Quantification of adverse effects	Erection, alprostadil response
No. of patients treated	54
Age group	n.g.
Treatment period	Continuous
Treatment consequences	Erectile function, impairment
Efficacy	More pronounced in patients with vascular risk factors
Randomization of patients	No
Study quality	**2–**
Reference	1455: Abdel-Hamid IA, Ereaky I, Fouda MA, Mansour OE. Role of penile vascular insufficiency in erectile dysfunction in renal transplant recipients. Int Impot Res 2002;14: 32–37.
Language	English

Compound	Renal transplantation
Disease treated	Terminal renal insufficiency
Quantification of adverse effects	Sexual function
No. of patients treated	50
Age group	45 years (mean)
Treatment period	16 months
Treatment consequences	Erectile function, maintenance
Efficacy	92% of patients
Randomization of patients	No
Study quality	**3**
Reference	1563: Burgos FJ, Pascual J, Gomez V, Orofino L, Liano F, Ortuno J. Effect of kidney transplantation and cyclosporine treatment on male sexual performance and hormonal profile: a prospective study. Transplant Proc. 1997 Feb–Mar;29(1–2):227–8.
Language	English

Compound	Renal transplantation
Disease treated	Terminal renal insufficiency
Quantification of adverse effects	Hormones
No. of patients treated	21; 15
Age group	Young
Treatment period	n.g.
Treatment consequences	Hormone levels, alteration
Efficacy	FSH, LH and prolactin levels higher in patients than in controls; T levels comparable
Randomization of patients	No
Study quality	**2–**
Reference	1380: Mendoza C, Carreras A, Ruiz E, Ortega E, Hervas J, Osorio C. Hypothalamo–hypophyseo–gonadal axis in individuals with chronic renal insufficiency subjected to hemodialysis. Rev Esp Fisiol. 1985 Dec;41(4):443–6.
Language	English

Compound	Renal transplantation
Disease treated	Terminal renal insufficiency
Quantification of adverse effects	Erectile function, IIEF and NPT
No. of patients treated	15
Age group	21–50 years
Treatment period	Transplantation after 4.3 years mean of dialysis
Treatment consequences	Hormone levels, alteration
Efficacy	Testosterone levels, decrease; IIEF increase in 11 cases, unchanged in 2 cases, worsened in 2 cases
Randomization of patients	No
Study quality	**3**
Reference	1275: Shamsa A, Motavalli SM, Aghdam B. Erectile function in end-stage renal disease before and after renal transplantation. Transplant Proc. 2005 Sep;37(7):3087–9.
Language	English

Compound	Renal transplantation
Disease treated	Terminal renal insufficiency
Quantification of adverse effects	Erectile function
No. of patients treated	n.g.
Age group	Young
Treatment consequences	Erectile function, impairment
Efficacy	Due to vascular mechanisms and cyclosporin(?)
Randomization of patients	No
Study quality	**3**
Reference	1032: Abdel-Hamid IA. Mechanisms of vasculogenic erectile dysfunction after kidney transplantation. BJU Int. 2004 Sep;94(4):497–500.
Language	English

2.5 Drugs Which Compromise Ejaculation

A10 Drugs Used in Diabetes

Diabetes mellitus and the treatments used do not appear to be a risk factor for premature ejaculation. There was no increase in the odds ratio in a large study.

Overall level of evidence of adverse effects: B.

Compound	Drugs used in diabetes (A10)
Disease treated	Diabetes mellitus
Quantification of adverse effects	Ejaculation history
No. of patients treated	569
Age group	All ages
Treatment consequences	Premature ejaculation
Efficacy	No association
Randomization of patients	No
Study quality	**2–**
Reference	1722: Basile Fasolo C, Mirone V, Gentile V, Parazzini F, Ricci E; Andrology Prevention Week centers; Italian Society of Andrology (SIA). Premature ejaculation: prevalence and associated conditions in a sample of 12,558 men attending the andrology prevention week 200: a study of the Italian Society of Andrology (SIA).J Sex Med. 2005 May;2(3):376–82.
Language	English

C01 Cardiac Therapy

There was no association of cardiac diseases and ejaculation disorders in cross-sectional prospective studies of large samples; however, a significant lower prevalence of premature ejaculation in men with sufficient physical activity could be shown (Stulhofer and Bajic 2006).

Overall level of evidence: B

Midodrine (C01CA17), an α-adrenergic agonist, was used in order to treat retrograde ejaculation. It was suggested to improve sperm transport in the vas deferens and contraction of the bladder neck. The effect is limited.

Overall level of evidence of adverse effects: B.

Compound	Cardiac therapy (C01)
Disease treated	Cardiac disease
Quantification of adverse effects	Ejaculation history
No. of patients treated	1155
Age group	50–80 years
Treatment consequences	Abnormal ejaculation
Efficacy	OR 1.98 (95% CI 1.28–3.06)
Randomization of patients	No
Study quality	**2+**
Reference	1724: Li MK, Garcia LA, Rosen R. Lower urinary tract symptoms and male sexual dysfunction in Asia: a survey of ageing men from five Asian countries. Br J Urol Int. 2005 Dec;96(9):1339–54.
Language	English

Substance (ATC code)	Midodrine (C01CA17)
Disease treated	Oligozoospermia
Quantification of dysfunction	Semen parameters
No. of patients treated	140
Age group	Young
Treatment period	Single dose
Dose	5–15 mg
Treatment consequences	Semen parameters, improvement
Efficacy	In 23 of 140 patients, sperm count improved by more than 10×10^6/ml sperm
Randomization of patients	No
Study quality	**3**
Reference	1994: Köhn FM, Schill WB. The alpha-sympathomimetic midodrin as a tool for diagnosis and treatment of sperm transport disturbances. Andrologia. 1994 Sep–Oct;26(5):283–7.

Language	English

Substance (ATC code)	Midodrine (C01CA17)
Disease treated	Retrograde ejaculation
Quantification of dysfunction	Ejaculation history
No. of patients treated	16
Age group	36 years (mean)
Treatment period	Single dose
Dose	2.5–20 mg
Treatment consequences	Antegrade ejaculation, induction
Efficacy	Ineffective in 8 patients
Randomization of patients	No
Study quality	**3**
Reference	1733: Blanchard-Dauphin A, Rigot JM, Thevenon A. Treatment of ejaculation disorders by midodrine (Gutron) per os. Retrospective study of about 16 subjects. Ann Readapt Med Phys. 2005 Feb;48(1):34–40.
Language	French

Substance (ATC code)	Midodrine (C01CA17)
Disease treated	Retrograde ejaculation in spinal injury
Quantification of dysfunction	Ejaculation history
No. of patients treated	14
Age group	25.8 years (mean)
Treatment period	
Dose	10–30 mg as infusion
Treatment consequences	antegrade ejaculation, induction
Efficacy	10 of 14 patients
Randomization of patients	No
Study quality	**3**
Reference	1782: Staerman F, Bryckaert PE, Youinou Y, Colin J, Brandt B, Lardennois B. Pharmacologic stimulation of ejaculation with midodrine hydrochloride (Gutron) for medically assisted reproduction in spinal injury. Prog Urol. 2001 Dec;11(6):1264–8.
Language	French

Substance (ATC code)	Midodrine (C01CA17)
Disease treated	Anejaculation after retroperitoneal lymphadenectomy
Quantification of dysfunction	Ejaculation history
No. of patients treated	12
Age group	Young
Treatment period	n.g.
Dose	10–30 mg/day
Treatment consequences	Antegrade ejaculation, induction
Efficacy	7 of 12 patients
Randomization of patients	No
Study quality	**3**
Reference	1995: Jonas D, Linzbach P, Weber W. The use of midodrin in the treatment of ejaculation disorders following retroperitoneal lymphadenectomy. Eur Urol. 1979;5(3):184–7.
Language	English

Substance (ATC code)	Midodrine (C01CA17)
Disease treated	Retrograde ejaculation
Quantification of dysfunction	Ejaculation history
No. of patients treated	6
Age group	Young
Treatment period	n.g.
Dose	n.g.
Treatment consequences	Ejaculation volume, increased
Efficacy	In most cases
Randomization of patients	Cross-over
Study quality	**2+**
Reference	1979: Riley AJ, Riley EJ. Partial ejaculatory incompetence: the therapeutic effect of midodrine, an orally active selective alpha-adrenoceptor agonist. Eur Urol. 1982;8(3):155–60.
Language	English

Substance (ATC code)	Amezinium (C01CA28)
Disease treated	Retrograde ejaculation
Quantification of dysfunction	Ejaculation history
No. of patients treated	3
Age group	Young
Treatment period	6 months
Dose	10 mg/day
Treatment consequences	Antegrade ejaculation, induction
Efficacy	In all cases up to 28.7 million/ml sperm
Randomization of patients	No
Study quality	**3**
Reference	1763: Ichiyanagi O, Sasagawa I, Suzuki Y, Matsuki S, Itoh K, Miura M, Tomita Y. Successful treatment of retrograde ejaculation with amezinium. Arch Androl. 2003 May–Jun;49(3):215–7.
Language	English

Compound	Cardiac therapy (C01)
Disease treated	Cardiac disease
Quantification of adverse effects	Ejaculation history
No. of patients treated	569
Age group	All ages
Treatment period	No treatment
Treatment consequences	Premature ejaculation
Efficacy	No association
Randomization of patients	No
Study quality	**2–**
Reference	1722: Basile Fasolo C, Mirone V, Gentile V, Parazzini F, Ricci E; Andrology Prevention Week centers; Italian Society of Andrology (SIA). Premature ejaculation: prevalence and associated conditions in a sample of 12,558 men attending the andrology prevention week 2001: a study of the Italian Society of Andrology (SIA).J Sex Med. 2005 May;2(3):376–82.
Language	English

Compound	Cardiac therapy (C01)
Disease treated	Low physical activity
Quantification of adverse effects	Sexual function questionnaire
No. of patients treated	30; 208
Age group	>36 years
Treatment period	No treatment
Treatment consequences	Premature ejaculation
Efficacy	OR 0.5 (95% CI 0.2–1.5)
Randomization of patients	No
Study quality	**2+**
Reference	1721: Stulhofer A, Bajic Z. Prevalence of erectile and ejaculatory difficulties among men in Croatia. Croat Med J. 2006 Feb;47(1):114–24.
Language	English

C02	**Antihypertensives**
C04	**Peripheral Vasodilators**
C07	**Beta-blocking Agents**
C10	**Lipid-modifying Agents**

Among antihypertensives, a report on amezinium for treatment of retrograde ejaculation is available. It worked in three of three cases. Some other reports of drugs with similar effects are of interest. The presence of hypertension or dyslipaemia itself was not associated with a greater risk of ejaculation disorders (Basile Fassolo et al. 2005; Li et al. 2005).

Overall level of evidence of adverse effects: C

Compound	Antihypertensives (C02)
Disease treated	Hypertension
Quantification of adverse effects	Ejaculation history
No. of patients treated	569
Age group	All ages

Treatment period	No treatment
Treatment consequences	Premature ejaculation
Efficacy	No association
Randomization of patients	No
Study quality	**2–**
Reference	1722: Basile Fasolo C, Mirone V, Gentile V, Parazzini F, Ricci E; Andrology Prevention Week centers; Italian Society of Andrology (SIA). Premature ejaculation: prevalence and associated conditions in a sample of 12,558 men attending the andrology prevention week 2001: a study of the Italian Society of Andrology (SIA).J Sex Med. 2005 May;2(3):376–82.
Language	English

Substance (ATC code)	Phenoxybenzamine (C04AX02)
Disease treated	Contraception
Quantification of dysfunction	Ejaculation history
No. of patients treated	n.g.
Age group	Young
Treatment period	n.g.
Dose	20 mg/day
Treatment consequences	Ejaculation after orgasm, blockade
Efficacy	After 2–3 days
Randomization of patients	No
Study quality	**3**
Reference	1949: Homonnai ZT, Shilon M, Paz GF. Phenoxybenzamine: an effective male contraceptive pill. Contraception. 1984 May;29(5):479–91.
Language	English

Substance (ATC code)	Labetalol (C07AG01)
Disease treated	Hypertension
Quantification of adverse effects	Ejaculation history
No. of patients treated	3
Age group	Old

Treatment period	Continuous
Dose	n.g.
Treatment consequences	Anejaculation, induction
Efficacy	Slow development
Randomization of patients	Case report
Study quality	**3**
Reference	1919: O'Meara J, White WB. Ejaculatory failure and urinary dysfunction secondary to labetalol. J Urol. 1988 Feb;139(2):371–2.
Language	English

Compound	Lipid-modifying agents (C10A)
Disease treated	Hypercholesterolaemia
Quantification of adverse effects	Ejaculation history
No. of patients treated	1155
Age group	50–80 years
Treatment consequences	Abnormal ejaculation
Efficacy	OR 0.84 (95% CI 0.59–1.19)
Randomization of patients	No
Study quality	**2+**
Reference	1724: Li MK, Garcia LA, Rosen R. Lower urinary tract symptoms and male sexual dysfunction in Asia: a survey of ageing men from five Asian countries. Br J Urol Int. 2005 Dec;96(9):1339–54.
Language	English

G04	Urologicals
	The use of specific α-adrenoreceptor agonists as well as 5-α-reductase inhibitors for lower urinary tract symptoms may impair ejaculation to a different extent. There are well-conducted studies on the whole group of drugs as well as on particular drugs.
	Overall level of evidence of adverse effects: B

Compound	Drugs used in benign prostatic hyperplasia (G04C)
Disease treated	Lower urinary tract symptoms (LUTS)
Quantification of adverse effects	Ejaculation history
No. of patients treated	1155
Age group	50–80 years
Treatment period	No treatment
Treatment consequences	Abnormal ejaculation
Efficacy	Increasing OR with LUTS severity
Randomization of patients	No
Study quality	**2+**
Reference	1724: Li MK, Garcia LA, Rosen R. Lower urinary tract symptoms and male sexual dysfunction in Asia: a survey of ageing men from five Asian countries. Br J Urol Int. 2005 Dec;96(9):1339–54.
Language	English

Compound	Drugs used in benign prostatic hyperplasia (G04C)
Disease treated	Lower urinary tract symptoms (LUTS)
Quantification of adverse effects	Sexual function inventory (SFI)
No. of patients treated	696
Age group	63 years (mean)
Treatment period	No treatment
Treatment consequences	Abnormal ejaculation
Efficacy	Correlation with age, correlation with IPSS
Randomization of patients	No
Study quality	**2–**

Reference	1726: Sak SC, Hussain Z, Johnston C, Eardley I. What is the relationship between male sexual function and lower urinary tract symptoms (LUTS)? Eur Urol. 2004 Oct;46(4):482–7.
Language	English

Substance (ATC code)	Alfuzosin (G04CA01)
Disease treated	Lower urinary tract symptoms
Quantification of adverse effects	International prostate symptom score (IPSS)
No. of patients treated	3076
Age group	65.9 years (mean)
Treatment period	Continuous
Dose	10 mg/day
Treatment consequences	IPSS, rigidity, ejaculation, improvement
Efficacy	Good
Randomization of patients	No
Study quality	**3**
Reference	1730: van Moorselaar RJ, Hartung R, Emberton M, Harving N, Matzkin H, Elhilali M, Alcaraz A, Vallancien G; ALF-ONE Study Group. Alfuzosin 10 mg once daily improves sexual function in men with lower urinary tract symptoms and concomitant sexual dysfunction. Br J Urol Int. 2005 Mar;95(4):603–8.
Language	English

Substance (ATC code)	Alfuzosin (G04CA01)
Disease treated	Healthy
Quantification of adverse effects	Ejaculation history
No. of patients treated	48
Age group	18–36 years
Treatment period	5 days
Dose	10 mg/days
Treatment consequences	Ejaculate volume, increased
Efficacy	By 0.3 ml
Randomization of patients	Yes, cross-over
Study quality	**1–**

Reference	1701: Giuliano F. Impact of medical treatments for benign prostatic hyperplasia on sexual function. Br J Urol Int. 2006 Apr;97 Suppl 2:34–8; discussion 44–5.
Language	English

Substance (ATC code)	Tamsulosin (G04CA02)
Disease treated	Healthy
Quantification of adverse effects	Ejaculation history
No. of patients treated	48
Age group	18–36 years
Treatment period	5 days
Dose	0.8 mg/day
Treatment consequences	Ejaculate volume, decreased
Efficacy	By 2.4 ml
Randomization of patients	Yes, cross-over
Study quality	**1–**
Reference	1701: Giuliano F. Impact of medical treatments for benign prostatic hyperplasia on sexual function. Br J Urol Int. 2006 Apr;97 Suppl 2:34–8; discussion 44–5.
Language	English

Substance (ATC code)	Tamsulosin (G04CA02)
Disease treated	Healthy
Quantification of adverse effects	Ejaculation history
No. of patients treated	48
Age group	Middle-aged
Treatment period	5 days
Dose	0.8 mg/days
Treatment consequences	Seminal volume, decreased by more than 20%
Efficacy	89% in tamsulosin, 20% in alfuzosin, 12% in placebo
Randomization of patients	Yes
Dose arms 1–3	Tamsulosin; alfuzosin; placebo
Study quality	**1+**
Reference	1986: Hellstrom WJ, Sikka SC. Effects of acute treatment with tamsulosin versus alfuzosin on ejaculatory function in normal volunteers. J Urol. 2006 Oct;176(4 Pt 1):1529–33.
Language	English

Substance (ATC code)	Tamsulosin (G04CA02)
Disease treated	Depression
Quantification of adverse effects	Ejaculation history
No. of patients treated	2
Age group	Young
Treatment period	n.g.
Dose	n.g.
Treatment consequences	Ejaculation quality, improvement
Efficacy	Prompt and complete resolution of pain
Randomization of patients	No
Study quality	**3**
Reference	1777: Demyttenaere K, Huygens R. Painful ejaculation and urinary hesitancy in association with antidepressant therapy: relief with tamsulosin. Eur Neuropsychopharmacol. 2002 Aug;12(4):337–41.
Language	English

Substance (ATC code)	Tamsulosin (G04CA02)
Disease treated	Lower urinary tract symptoms (LUTS)
Quantification of adverse effects	Ejaculation history
Age group	Old
Treatment consequences	Retrograde ejaculation, induction
Efficacy	4–11%
Randomization of patients	No
Study quality	**4 (review)**
Reference	1981: Schulman CC. Lower urinary tract symptoms/benign prostatic hyperplasia: minimizing morbidity caused by treatment. Urology. 2003 Sep;62(3 Suppl 1):24–33.
Language	English

Substance (ATC code)	Dutasteride (G04CB02)
Disease treated	Benign prostatic hyperplasia
Quantification of adverse effects	International prostate symptom score (IPSS)
No. of patients treated	2802
Age group	Old

Treatment period	2 years
Dose	n.g.
Treatment consequences	Sexual functions, impairment
Efficacy	In 6.1% of dutasterid group, in 3% of placebo group
Randomization of patients	Yes
Dose arms 1–3	Dutasteride; placebo
Study quality	**1+**
Reference	1747: Roehrborn CG, Marks LS, Fenter T, Freedman S, Tuttle J, Gittleman M, Morrill B, Wolford ET. Efficacy and safety of dutasteride in the four-year treatment of men with benign prostatic hyperplasia. Urology. 2004 Apr;63(4):709–15.
Language	English

Substance (ATC code)	α-adrenoreceptor agonists (G04CX)
Disease treated	Lower urinary tract symptoms
Quantification of adverse effects	Sexual function score
No. of patients treated	830
Age group	Old
Treatment period	12 weeks
Dose	Various
Treatment consequences	Abnormal ejaculation, induction
Efficacy	Similar rate in different α-blockers
Randomization of patients	Yes
Dose arms 1–3	Tamsulosin; alfuzosin; placebo
Study quality	**1+**
Reference	1812: Hofner K, Claes H, De Reijke TM, Folkestad B, Speakman MJ. Tamsulosin 0.4 mg once daily: effect on sexual function in patients with lower urinary tract symptoms suggestive of benign prostatic obstruction. Eur Urol. 1999 Oct;36(4):335–41.
Language	English

Substance (ATC code)	α-adrenoreceptor agonists (G04CX)
Disease treated	Lower urinary tract symptoms
Quantification of adverse effects	International prostate symptom score (IPSS)
Age group	Old

Treatment period	Continuous
Treatment consequences	Abnormal ejaculation
Efficacy	Similar rate in different α-blockers
Randomization of patients	No
Study quality	**4 (review)**
Reference	1725: Milani S, Djavan B. Lower urinary tract symptoms suggestive of benign prostatic hyperplasia: latest update on alpha-adrenoceptor antagonists. Br J Urol Int. 2005 Jun;95 Suppl 4:29–36.
Language	English

H01	**Pituitary and Hypothalamic Hormones and Analogues**
	Oxytocin was used in trials to improve emptying of the epididymis in the course of ejaculation in order to increase the sperm count in a semen sample. There was no effect.
	Overall level of evidence of adverse effects: B

Substance (ATC code)	Oxytocin (H01BB02)
Disease treated	Healthy
Quantification of dysfunction	Semen parameters
No. of patients treated	103
Age group	Young
Treatment period	Prior to ejaculation
Dose	16 IU intranasally
Treatment consequences	Seminal parameters, alteration
Efficacy	Ineffective
Randomization of patients	Yes
Dose arms 1–3	Oxytocin; placebo
Study quality	**1+**
Reference	1783: Walch K, Eder R, Schindler A, Feichtinger W. The effect of single-dose oxytocin application on time to ejaculation and seminal parameters in men. J Assist Reprod Genet. 2001 Dec;18(12):655–9.
Language	English

Substance (ATC code)	Oxytocin (H01BB02)
Disease treated	Infertility
Quantification of dysfunction	Semen parameters
No. of patients treated	49
Age group	Young
Treatment period	Prior to ejaculation
Dose	0.75 IU i.v.
Treatment consequences	Seminal parameters, alteration
Efficacy	Ineffective
Randomization of patients	Yes
Dose arms 1–3	Oxytocin; placebo
Study quality	**1+**
Reference	1985: Byrne MM, Rolf C, Depenbusch M, Cooper TG, Nieschlag E. Lack of effect of a single i.v. dose of oxytocin on sperm output in severely oligozoospermic men. Hum Reprod. 2003 Oct;18(10):2098–102.
Language	English

H03	Thyroid Therapy
	Thyroid hormone supplementation improved sexual functions in men with diseases of the thyroid gland. **Overall level of evidence of adverse effects: C**

Substance (ATC code)	Thyroid hormones (H03AA)
Disease treated	Thyroid diseases
Quantification of adverse effects	Sexual function score
No. of patients treated	48
Age group	Middle-aged
Treatment period	16 weeks
Dose	n.g.
Treatment consequences	Sexual functions, improvement
Efficacy	With thyroid hormone treatment
Randomization of patients	No

Study quality	**3**
Reference	1717: Carani C, Isidori AM, Granata A, Carosa E, Maggi M, Lenzi A, Jannini EA. Multicenter study on the prevalence of sexual symptoms in male hypo- and hyperthyroid patients. J Clin Endocrinol Metab. 2005 Dec;90(12):6472–9. Epub 2005 Oct 4.
Language	English

M03	**Muscle Relaxants**
	Baclofen intrathecally was able to inhibit ejaculation. **Overall level of evidence of adverse effects: C**

Substance (ATC code)	Baclofen intrathecal (M03BX01)
Disease treated	Spinal cord injury
Quantification of adverse effects	Ejaculation history
No. of patients treated	3
Age group	38.2 years (mean)
Treatment period	Continuous
Dose	290±68 µg/day
Treatment consequences	Anejaculation, induction
Efficacy	In 2 of 3 patients
Randomization of patients	No
Study quality	**3**
Reference	1830: Denys P, Mane M, Azouvi P, Chartier-Kastler E, Thiebaut JB, Bussel B. Side effects of chronic intrathecal baclofen on erection and ejaculation in patients with spinal cord lesions. Arch Phys Med Rehabil. 1998 May;79(5):494–6.
Language	English

N01	Anaesthetics
	Lidocain was topically applied to the glans penis prior to a coitus in order to improve ejaculation latency in premature ejaculation. A positive effect was shown in controlled studies, but the application was thought to be inconvenient. SS cream is another local anaesthetic ointment; its effect has not yet been proven in comparison studies.
	Overall level of evidence of adverse effects: B

Substance (ATC code)	Lidocaine locally (N01BB02)
Disease treated	Premature ejaculation
Quantification of dysfunction	Intravaginal ejaculation latency time (IELT)
No. of patients treated	42
Age group	18–50 years
Treatment period	60 days
Dose	Not mentioned
Treatment consequences	Ejaculation latency, improvement
Efficacy	From 1:49 to 8:45 min in verum, none in placebo
Randomization of patients	Yes
Dose arms 1–3	Lidocaine; placebo
Study quality	**1–**
Reference	1745: Busato W, Galindo CC. Topical anaesthetic use for treating premature ejaculation: a double-blind, randomized, placebo-controlled study. Br J Urol Int. 2004 May;93(7):1018–21.
Language	English

Substance (ATC code)	Lidocaine locally (N01BB02)
Disease treated	Premature ejaculation
Quantification of dysfunction	Intravaginal ejaculation latency time (IELT)
No. of patients treated	40
Age group	Young
Treatment period	Local
Dose	5% cream
Treatment consequences	Ejaculation latency, improvement

Side effects compromising effectiveness	Six patients loss of erection
Efficacy	To 6–8 min
Randomization of patients	Yes
Dose arms 1–3	20 min prior to coitus; 30 min prior to coitus; placebo
Study quality	**1–**
Reference	1771: Atikeler MK, Gecit I, Senol FA. Optimum usage of prilocaine–lidocaine cream in premature ejaculation. Andrologia. 2002 Dec;34(6):356–9.
Language	English

Substance (ATC code)	Lidocaine (N01BB02)
Disease treated	Premature ejaculation
Quantification of dysfunction	Ejaculation history
No. of patients treated	22
Age group	32.5 years (mean)
Treatment period	15 min before coitus
Dose	5% cream
Treatment consequences	Ejaculation latency, improvement
Efficacy	In 86% of patients
Randomization of patients	Yes
Dose arms 1–3	Sildenafil; sildenafil+EMLA; placebo
Study quality	**1–**
Reference	1703: Atan A, Basar MM, Tuncel A, Ferhat M, Agras K, Tekdogan U. Comparison of efficacy of sildenafil-only, sildenafil plus topical EMLA cream, and topical EMLA-cream-only in treatment of premature ejaculation. Urology. 2006 Feb;67(2):388–91.
Language	English

Substance (ATC code)	Lidocaine locally (N01BB02)
Disease treated	Premature ejaculation
Quantification of dysfunction	Intravaginal ejaculation latency time (IELT)
No. of patients treated	14
Age group	Young

Treatment period	On demand
Dose	7.5 mg aerosol
Treatment consequences	Ejaculation latency, improvement
Efficacy	From 1:24 to 11:21 min
Randomization of patients	No
Study quality	**2+**
Reference	1757: Henry R, Morales A. Topical lidocaine–prilocaine spray for the treatment of premature ejaculation: a proof of concept study. Int J Impot Res. 2003 Aug;15(4):277–81.
Language	English

N03	**Antiepileptics**
	A case report described anejaculation during treatment with gabapentin for seizure control.
	Overall level of evidence of adverse effects: C

Substance (ATC code)	Gabapentin (N03AX12)
Disease treated	Epilepsy
Quantification of adverse effects	Sexual function score
No. of patients treated	1
Age group	Young
Treatment period	1 month
Dose	900–1800 mg/day
Treatment consequences	Anejaculation, anorgasmia, induction
Efficacy	During treatment
Randomization of patients	No
Study quality	**3**
Reference	1813: Labbate LA, Rubey RN. Gabapentin-induced ejaculatory failure and anorgasmia. Am J Psychiatry. 1999 Jun;156(6):972.
Language	English

2

N05	Psycholeptics
	The treatmentof psychoses induced decrease in ejaculate volume or retrograde ejaculation.
	Overall level of evidence of adverse effects: B

Compound	Sertindole (N05AE03)
Disease treated	Schizophrenia
Quantification of adverse effects	Ejaculation history
No. of patients treated	282
Age group	Young
Treatment period	Continuous
Dose	24 mg/day
Treatment consequences	Ejaculation volume, decreased
Efficacy	In 33 of 282 patients, with haloperidol in 6 of 252
Randomization of patients	Yes
Dose arms 1–3	Sertindole; haloperidole
Study quality	**1+**
Reference	1990: Lewis R, Bagnall A-M, Leitner M. Sertindole for schizophrenia. The Cochrane Database of Systematic Reviews 2006 Issue 4
Language	English

Substance (ATC code)	Risperidone (N05AX08)
Disease treated	Schizophrenia
Quantification of adverse effects	Ejaculation history
No. of patients treated	2
Age group	Young
Treatment period	Continuous
Dose	Continuous
Treatment consequences	Retrograde ejaculation, induction
Efficacy	During treatment
Randomization of patients	No
Study quality	**3**
Remarks	Risperidone has also a adrenergic blocking effects

Reference	1761: Holtmann M, Gerstner S, Schmidt MH. Risperidone-associated ejaculatory and urinary dysfunction in male adolescents. J Child Adolesc Psychopharmacol. 2003 Spring;13(1):107–9.
Language	English

Substance (ATC code)	Risperidone (N05AX08)
Disease treated	Schizophrenia
Quantification of adverse effects	Retrograde ejaculation
No. of patients treated	1
Age group	51 years
Treatment period	Continuous
Dose	8 mg/day
Treatment consequences	Retrograde ejaculation induction
Efficacy	During treatment
Randomization of patients	No
Study quality	**3**
Reference	1746: Loh C, Leckband SG, Meyer JM, Turner E. Risperidone-induced retrograde ejaculation: case report and review of the literature. Int Clin Psychopharmacol. 2004 Mar;19(2):111–2.
Language	English

Substance (ATC code)	Risperidone (N05AX08)
Disease treated	Schizophrenia
Quantification of adverse effects	Ejaculation history
No. of patients treated	1
Age group	Young
Treatment period	Continuous
Dose	5 mg
Treatment consequences	Anejaculation, development
Efficacy	Slow development
Randomization of patients	No
Study quality	**3**
Reference	1810: Raja M. Risperidone-induced absence of ejaculation. Int Clin Psychopharmacol. 1999 Sep;14(5):317–9.
Language	English

2

N06	Psychoanaleptics
	Numerous reports indicate ejaculation disorders induced by psychoanaleptics used for the treatment of depression. The retardation of ejaculation is regularly observed. Following this observation, specific serotonin reuptake inhibitors (SSRI) were used to control ejaculation in premature ejaculation. A prominent author is M.D. Waldinger (The Hague, The Netherlands). The efficacy of this treatment has been demonstrated in a number of controlled studies. As adverse effects a "sertoninergic syndrome" has been described, characterized by headache, nausea, sweating, dizziness and, in rare severe cases, by hyperthermia, rigidity, delirium and coma (Montague et al. 2004). **Overall level of evidence of adverse effects: A**

Substance (ATC code)	Clomipramine (N06AA04)
Disease treated	Premature ejaculation
Quantification of dysfunction	Ejaculation history
No. of patients treated	50
Age group	Young
Treatment period	6 weeks
Dose	20 mg/day
Treatment consequences	Ejaculation latency, improvement
Efficacy	Significantly
Randomization of patients	Yes
Dose arms 1–3	Clomipramine; placebo
Study quality	**1+**
Reference	1972: Girgis SM, El-Haggar S, El-Hermouzy S. A double-blind trial of clomipramine in premature ejaculation. Andrologia. 1982 Jul–Aug;14(4):364–8.
Language	English

Substance (ATC code)	Clomipramine (N06AA04)
Disease treated	Premature ejaculation
Quantification of dysfunction	Sexual function score
No. of patients treated	34
Age group	Young

Treatment period	2 weeks
Dose	25 mg
Treatment consequences	Ejaculation latency, improvement; control over orgasm, improvement
Efficacy	Good; poor in placebo
Randomization of patients	Yes
Dose arms 1–3	Clomipramine; placebo
Study quality	**1+**
Reference	1980: Strassberg DS, Gouveia Brazao CA de, Rowland DL, Tan P, Slob AK. Clomipramine in the treatment of rapid (premature) ejaculation. J Sex Marital Ther. 1999 Apr–Jun;25(2):89–101.
Language	English

Substance (ATC code)	Clomipramine (N06AA04)
Disease treated	Obsessive–compulsive disorder
Quantification of dysfunction	Sexual function score
No. of patients treated	33
Age group	Young
Treatment period	Continuous
Dose	25 mg
Treatment consequences	Orgasm, delayed
Efficacy	24 of 24 total or partial anorgasmia in verum group
Randomization of patients	Yes
Dose arms 1–3	Clomipramine; placebo
Study quality	**1–**
Reference	1996: Monteiro WO, Noshirvani HF, Marks IM, Lelliott PT. Anorgasmia from clomipramine in obsessive–compulsive disorder. A controlled trial. Br J Psychiatry. 1987 Jul;151:107–12.
Language	English

Substance (ATC code)	Amoxapine (N06AA17)
Disease treated	Depression
Quantification of adverse effects	Ejaculation history
No. of patients treated	1

2

Age group	33
Treatment period	7 days
Dose	150 mg/days
Treatment consequences	Ejaculation after orgasm, blockade
Efficacy	Significantly
Randomization of patients	No
Study quality	**3**
Reference	1977: Schwarcz G. Case report of inhibition of ejaculation and retrograde ejaculation as side effects of amoxapine. Am J Psychiatry. 1982 Feb;139(2):233–4.
Language	English

Substance (ATC code)	Selective serotonin reuptake inhibitor (SSRI) (N06AB)
Disease treated	Depression
Quantification of adverse effects	Sexual function score
No. of patients treated	139
Age group	41 years (mean)
Treatment period	Continuous
Dose	Various
Treatment consequences	Ejaculation latency, improvement
Efficacy	In 22.6%
Randomization of patients	No
Study quality	**3**
Reference	1842: Montejo Al, Llorca G, Izquierdo JA, Ledesma A, Bousono M, Calcedo A, Carrasco JL. Sexual dysfunction secondary to SSRIs. A comparative analysis in 308 patients. Actas Luso Esp Neurol Psiquiatr Cienc Afines. 1996 Nov–Dec;24(6):311–21.
Language	Spanish

Substance (ATC code)	Selective serotonin reuptake inhibitor (SSRI) (N06AB)
Disease treated	Premature ejaculation
Quantification of dysfunction	Intravaginal ejaculation latency time (IELT)
No. of patients treated	60
Age group	Young
Treatment period	6 weeks

Dose	Various
Treatment consequences	Ejaculation latency, improvement
Efficacy	Best in paroxetine
Randomization of patients	Yes
Dose arms 1–3	Paroxetine; fluoxetin; placebo
Study quality	**1+**
Reference	1824: Waldinger MD, Hengeveld MW, Zwinderman AH, Olivier B. Effect of SSRI antidepressants on ejaculation: a double-blind, randomized, placebo-controlled study with fluoxetine, fluvoxamine, paroxetine, and sertraline. J Clin Psychopharmacol. 1998 Aug;18(4):274–81.
Language	English

Substance (ATC code)	Selective serotonin reuptake inhibitor (SSRI) (N06AB)
Disease treated	Premature ejaculation
Quantification of dysfunction	Intravaginal ejaculation latency time (IELT)
No. of patients treated	36
Age group	44 years (mean)
Treatment period	4 weeks
Dose	Various
Treatment consequences	Ejaculation latency, improvement
Efficacy	From 0:36 to 5:45 min in chlorpromazine
Randomization of patients	Yes
Dose arms 1–3	Fluoxetine; chlomipramine; placebo
Study quality	**1+**
Reference	1825: Kim SC, Seo KK. Efficacy and safety of fluoxetine, sertraline and clomipramine in patients with premature ejaculation: a double-blind, placebo controlled study. J Urol. 1998 Feb;159(2):425–7.
Language	English

Substance (ATC code)	Selective serotonin reuptake inhibitor (SSRI) (N06AB)
Disease treated	Premature ejaculation
Quantification of dysfunction	Intravaginal ejaculation latency time (IELT)
No. of patients treated	30
Age group	Young

Treatment period	4 weeks
Treatment consequences	Ejaculation latency, improvement
Efficacy	4.05-fold by clomipramine, 1.41-fold by placebo
Randomization of patients	Yes
Dose arms 1–3	Clomipramide 25 mg; paroxetine 20 mg
Study quality	**1+**
Reference	1737: Waldinger MD, Zwinderman AH, Olivier B. On-demand treatment of premature ejaculation with clomipramine and paroxetine: a randomized, double-blind fixed-dose study with stopwatch assessment. Eur Urol. 2004 Oct;46(4):510–5; discussion 516.
Language	English

Substance (ATC code)	Selective serotonin reuptake inhibitor (SSRI) (N06AB)
Disease treated	Premature ejaculation
Quantification of dysfunction	Intravaginal ejaculation latency time (IELT)
No. of patients treated	24
Age group	Young
Treatment period	6 weeks
Treatment consequences	Ejaculation latency, improvement
Efficacy	From 15 to 119 s in paroxetine, from 23 to 28 s in mirtazapine
Randomization of patients	Yes
Dose arms 1–3	Paroxetine 20 mg/day; mirtazapine 30 mg/day
Study quality	**1+**
Reference	1752: Waldinger MD, Zwinderman AH, Olivier B. Antidepressants and ejaculation: a double-blind, randomized, fixed-dose study with mirtazapine and paroxetine. J Clin Psychopharmacol. 2003 Oct;23(5):467–70.
Language	English

Substance (ATC code)	Selective serotonin reuptake inhibitor (SSRI) (N06AB)
Disease treated	Premature ejaculation
Quantification of dysfunction	Intravaginal ejaculation latency time (IELT)
No. of patients treated	24
Age group	Young

Treatment period	Continuous
Dose	Various
Treatment consequences	Ejaculation latency, improvement
Efficacy	Significant
Side effects compromising effectiveness	Headache, nausea, sweating, dizziness
Randomization of patients	Yes
Study quality	**1+ (guideline)**
Reference	1992: Montague DK, Jarow J, Broderick GA, Dmochowski RR, Heaton JP, Lue TF, Nehra A, Sharlip ID; AUA Erectile Dysfunction Guideline Update Panel. AUA guideline on the pharmacologic management of premature ejaculation. J Urol. 2004 Jul;172(1):290–4.
Language	English

Substance (ATC code)	Selective serotonin reuptake inhibitor (SSRI) (N06AB)
Disease treated	Premature ejaculation
Quantification of dysfunction	Ejaculation history
Age group	Young
Treatment period	On demand
Treatment consequences	Ejaculation latency, improvement
Efficacy	On-demand SSRI treatment has less ejaculation-delaying effects than daily SSRI treatment
Randomization of patients	No
Study quality	**4 (review)**
Reference	1707: Waldinger MD, Schweitzer DH, Olivier B. On-demand SSRI treatment of premature ejaculation: pharmacodynamic limitations for relevant ejaculation delay and consequent solutions. J Sex Med. 2005 Jan;2(1):121–31.
Language	English

Substance (ATC code)	Fluoxetine (N06AB03)
Disease treated	Premature ejaculation
Quantification of dysfunction	Intravaginal ejaculation latency time (IELT)
No. of patients treated	80

Age group	36 years (mean)
Treatment period	3 months
Dose	n.g.
Treatment consequences	Ejaculation latency, improvement
Efficacy	From 0.5 to 3.57 min in both groups
Randomization of patients	Yes
Dose arms 1–3	Fluoxetine 20 mg/day; fluoxetine 90 mg/week
Study quality	**1+**
Reference	1762: Manasia P, Pomerol J, Ribe N, Gutierrez del Pozo R, Alcover Garcia J. Comparison of the efficacy and safety of 90 mg versus 20 mg fluoxetine in the treatment of premature ejaculation. J Urol. 2003 Jul;170(1):164–5.
Language	English

Substance (ATC code)	Fluoxetine (N06AB03)
Disease treated	Premature ejaculation
Quantification of dysfunction	Intravaginal ejaculation latency time (IELT)
No. of patients treated	78
Age group	Young
Treatment period	3 months
Dose	Various
Treatment consequences	Ejaculation latency, improvement
Efficacy	Better when lidocain gel added
Randomization of patients	No
Study quality	**2+**
Reference	1714: Metin A, Kayigil O, Ahmed SI. Does lidocaine ointment addition increase fluoxetine efficacy in the same group of patients with premature ejaculation? Urol Int. 2005;75(3):231–4.
Language	English

Substance (ATC code)	Fluoxetine (N06AB03)
Disease treated	Premature ejaculation
Quantification of dysfunction	Ejaculation history
No. of patients treated	57

Age group	27 years (mean)
Treatment period	8 weeks
Dose	40 mg/day
Treatment consequences	Ejaculation latency, improvement
Efficacy	In 72%
Randomization of patients	Yes
Dose arms 1–3	Fluoxetine; placebo
Study quality	**1+**
Reference	1805: Murat Basar M, Atan A, Yildiz M, Baykam M, Aydoganli L. Comparison of sertraline to fluoxetine with regard to their efficacy and side effects in the treatment of premature ejaculation. Arch Esp Urol. 1999 Nov;52(9):1008–11.
Language	English

Compound	Fluoxetine (N06AB03)
Disease treated	Premature ejaculation
Quantification of dysfunction	Sexual function
No. of patients treated	40
Age group	Young
Treatment period	2 weeks
Dose	10 mg/day
Treatment consequences	Ejaculation latency, increase
Efficacy	Good
Side effects compromising effectiveness	No major side effects
Randomization of patients	Yes
Dose arms 1–3	Fluoxetine; placebo
Study quality (SIGN 50)	**1–**
Reference and year	1471: Haensel SM, Klem TM, Hop WC, Slob AK. Fluoxetine and premature ejaculation: a double-blind, crossover, placebo-controlled study. J Clin Psychopharmacol. 1998 Feb;18(1):72–7.
Language	English

2

Substance (ATC code)	Fluoxetine (N06AB03)
Disease treated	Premature ejaculation
Quantification of dysfunction	Ejaculation history
No. of patients treated	26
Age group	19–48 years
Treatment period	8 weeks
Dose	20 mg/days
Treatment consequences	Ejaculation latency, improvement
Efficacy	In 31% with fluoxetine, in 53% with fluoxetine+local anaesthetic
Randomization of patients	Yes
Dose arms 1–3	Fluoxetine; fluoxetine+local anaesthetic
Study quality	**1+**
Reference	1797: Atan A, Basar MM, Aydoganli L. Comparison of the efficacy of fluoxetine alone vs fluoxetine plus local lidocaine ointment in the treatment of premature ejaculation. Arch Esp Urol. 2000 Nov;53(9):856–8.
Language	English

Substance (ATC code)	Citalopram (N06AB04)
Disease treated	Premature ejaculation
Quantification of dysfunction	Ejaculation history, IELT, IIEF
No. of patients treated	58
Age group	Young
Treatment period	12 weeks
Dose	20 mg/day
Treatment consequences	IELT, increase
Efficacy	In verum 32–268 s, in placebo from 28 to 38 s
Randomization of patients	Yes
Dose arms 1–3	Citalopram; placebo
Study quality	**1+**
Reference	1984: Safarinejad MR, Hosseini SY. Safety and efficacy of citalopram in the treatment of premature ejaculation: a double-blind placebo-controlled, fixed dose, randomized study. Int J Impot Res. 2006 Mar–Apr;18(2):164–9.
Language	English

Substance (ATC code)	Citalopram (N06AB04)
Disease treated	Premature ejaculation
Quantification of dysfunction	Intravaginal ejaculation latency time (IELT)
No. of patients treated	26
Age group	Young
Treatment period	4 weeks
Dose	20 mg
Treatment consequences	Ejaculation latency, improvement
Efficacy	In 70% in citalopram, in 7.7% in placebo
Randomization of patients	Yes
Dose arms 1–3	Citalopram; placebo
Study quality	**1+**
Reference	1769: Atmaca M, Kuloglu M, Tezcan E, Semercioz A. The efficacy of citalopram in the treatment of premature ejaculation: a placebo-controlled study. Int J Impot Res. 2002 Dec;14(6):502–5.
Language	English

Substance (ATC code)	Citalopram (N06AB04)
Disease treated	Depression
Quantification of adverse effects	Ejaculation history
No. of patients treated	1
Age group	43
Treatment period	Discontinuation
Dose	20 mg
Treatment consequences	Premature ejaculation
Efficacy	As a consequence of discontinuation
Randomization of patients	No
Study quality	**3**
Reference	1750: Adson DE, Kotlyar M. Premature ejaculation associated with citalopram withdrawal. Ann Pharmacother. 2003 Dec;37(12):1804–6.
Language	English

Substance (ATC code)	Paroxetine (N06AB05)
Disease treated	Premature ejaculation
Quantification of adverse effects	Intravaginal ejaculation latency time (IELT)
No. of patients treated	80
Age group	34 years (mean)
Treatment period	6 months
Dose	10–20mg/day
Treatment consequences	Ejaculation latency, improvement
Efficacy	Better in group with addition of sildenafil
Randomization of patients	No
Dose arms 1–3	Paroxetine; paroxetine+sildenafil; placebo
Study quality	**2+**
Reference	1772: Salonia A, Maga T, Colombo R, Scattoni V, Briganti A, Cestari A, Guazzoni G, Rigatti P, Montorsi F. A prospective study comparing paroxetine alone versus paroxetine plus sildenafil in patients with premature ejaculation. J Urol. 2002 Dec;168(6):2486–9.
Language	English

Substance (ATC code)	Paroxetine (N06AB05)
Disease treated	Premature ejaculation
Quantification of adverse effects	Intravaginal ejaculation latency time (IELT)
No. of patients treated	42
Age group	40.5 years (mean)
Treatment period	3 weeks
Dose	10 mg/day+20 mg on demand
Treatment consequences	Ejaculation latency, improvement
Efficacy	Increase from 0.3 to 3.5 min; in placebo 0.3 to 0.6 min
Randomization of patients	Yes
Dose arms 1–3	Paroxetine; placebo
Study quality	**1+**
Reference	1814: McMahon CG, Touma K. Treatment of premature ejaculation with paroxetine hydrochloride as needed: two single-blind placebo controlled crossover studies. J Urol. 1999 Jun;161(6):1826–30.
Language	English

Substance (ATC code)	Paroxetine (N06AB05)
Disease treated	Premature ejaculation
Quantification of dysfunction	Ejaculation history
No. of patients treated	31
Age group	Young
Treatment period	3–5 h prior to coitus
Dose	Various
Treatment consequences	Ejaculation latency, improvement
Efficacy	Best in paroxetine
Randomization of patients	Yes
Dose arms 1–3	Paroxetine; sildenafil; pause-squeeze technique
Study quality	1+
Reference	1790: Abdel-Hamid IA, El Naggar EA, El Gilany AH. Assessment of as needed use of pharmacotherapy and the pause-squeeze technique in premature ejaculation. Int J Impot Res. 2001 Feb;13(1):41–5.
Language	English

Substance (ATC code)	Paroxetine (N06AB05), citalopram
Disease treated	Premature ejaculation
Quantification of adverse effects	Intravaginal ejaculation latency time (IELT)
No. of patients treated	30
Age group	Young
Treatment period	5 weeks
Dose	20 mg/days
Treatment consequences	Ejaculation latency, improvement
Efficacy	8.9-fold with prilocaine, 1.8-fold in citalopram
Randomization of patients	Yes
Dose arms 1–3	Paroxetine; citalopram
Study quality	1+
Reference	1785: Waldinger MD, Zwinderman AH, Olivier B. SSRIs and ejaculation: a double-blind, randomized, fixed-dose study with paroxetine and citalopram. J Clin Psychopharmacol. 2001 Dec;21(6):556–60.
Language	English

2

Substance (ATC code)	Paroxetine (N06AB05)
Disease treated	Premature ejaculation
Quantification of adverse effects	Intravaginal ejaculation latency time (IELT)
No. of patients treated	26
Age group	39.5 years (mean)
Treatment period	On demand
Dose	20 mg
Treatment consequences	Ejaculation latency, improvement
Efficacy	Increase from 0.3 to 3.2 min; in placebo 0.3 to 0.45 min
Randomization of patients	Yes
Dose arms 1–3	Paroxetine on demand
Study quality	**1+**
Reference	1814: McMahon CG, Touma K. Treatment of premature ejaculation with paroxetine hydrochloride as needed: two single-blind placebo controlled crossover studies. J Urol. 1999 Jun;161(6):1826–30.
Language	English

Substance (ATC code)	Paroxetine (N06AB05)
Disease treated	Premature ejaculation
Quantification of adverse effects	Intravaginal ejaculation latency time (IELT)
No. of patients treated	14
Age group	Young
Treatment period	3 weeks
Dose	20 mg
Treatment consequences	Ejaculation latency, improvement
Efficacy	From 0.4 to 5.8 min in paroxetine on demand
Randomization of patients	No
Dose arms 1–3	Paroxetine daily 20 mg; paroxetine on demand; placebo
Study quality	**2+**
Reference	1719: Rivera P, Gonzalez R, Gonzalez F, Storme O. Use of paroxetine on-demand in premature ejaculation. Actas Urol Esp. 2005 Apr;29(4):387–91.
Language	Spanish

Substance (ATC code)	Sertraline (N06AB06)
Disease treated	Premature ejaculation
Quantification of adverse effects	Ejaculation history
No. of patients treated	37
Age group	Young
Treatment period	4 weeks
Dose	50 mg
Treatment consequences	Ejaculation latency, improvement
Efficacy	Significant
Randomization of patients	Yes
Dose arms 1–3	Sertraline; placebo
Study quality	**1–**
Reference	1819: Biri H, Isen K, Sinik Z, Onaran M, Kupeli B, Bozkirli I. Sertraline in the treatment of premature ejaculation: a double-blind placebo controlled study. Int Urol Nephrol. 1998;30(5):611–5.
Language	English

Substance (ATC code)	Antidepressants, tricyclic (N06AX)
Disease treated	Depression
Quantification of adverse effects	Ejaculation history
No. of patients treated	4
Age group	Young
Treatment period	3 weeks
Dose	Various
Treatment consequences	Ejaculation quality, painful
Efficacy	Resolve of pain after withdrawal of medication
Randomization of patients	No
Study quality	**3**
Reference	1895: Aizenberg D, Zemishlany Z, Hermesh H, Karp L, Weizman A. Painful ejaculation associated with antidepressants in four patients. J Clin Psychiatry. 1991 Nov;52(11):461–3.
Language	English

Substance (ATC code)	Dapoxetine (not listed)
Disease treated	Premature ejaculation
Quantification of dysfunction	Ejaculation history
No. of patients treated	In various stages of development
Age group	Young
Treatment period	On demand
Dose	Various
Treatment consequences	Ejaculation latency, improvement
Efficacy	Rapid onset, rapid clearance after orgasm
Randomization of patients	No
Study quality	**3**
Reference	1705: Andersson KE, Mulhall JP, Wyllie MG. Pharmacokinetic and pharmacodynamic features of dapoxetine, a novel drug for "on–demand" treatment of premature ejaculation. Br J Urol Int. 2006 Feb;97(2):311–5.
Language	English

Substance (ATC code)	Dapoxetine (not listed)
Disease treated	Premature ejaculation
Quantification of dysfunction	Ejaculation history
No. of patients treated	n.g.
Age group	Young
Treatment period	4 weeks
Dose	30 mg/day
Treatment consequences	Ejaculation latency, improvement
Efficacy	Rapid onset, rapid clearance after orgasm
Randomization of patients	Yes
Dose arms 1–3	Dapoxetine 30 mg; dapoxetine 60 mg
Study quality	**1+**
Reference	1982: Modi NB, Dresser MJ, Simon M, Lin D, Desai D, Gupta S. Single- and multiple-dose pharmacokinetics of dapoxetine hydrochloride, a novel agent for the treatment of premature ejaculation. J Clin Pharmacol. 2006 Mar;46(3):301–9.
Language	English

Substance (ATC code)	Dapoxetine (not listed)
Disease treated	Premature ejaculation
Quantification of dysfunction	Ejaculation history
No. of patients treated	24
Age group	Young
Treatment period	4 weeks
Dose	60 mg/day
Treatment consequences	Pharmacokinetic in the combination with sildenafil and tadalafil
Efficacy	sildenafil increased area under curve of dapoxetine serum levels by 22%
Randomization of patients	Cross-over
Dose arms 1–3	Dapoxetine+tadalafil; dapoxetine+sildenafil; dapoxetine
Study quality	**1+**
Reference	1983: Dresser MJ, Desai D, Gidwani S, Seftel AD, Modi NB. Dapoxetine, a novel treatment for premature ejaculation, does not have pharmacokinetic interactions with phosphodiesterase-5 inhibitors. Int J Impot Res. 2006 Jan–Feb;18(1):104–10.
Language	English

Substance (ATC code)	Tradozone (not listed)
Disease treated	Depression
Quantification of adverse effects	Ejaculation history
No. of patients treated	1
Age group	Middle-aged
Treatment period	n.g.
Dose	n.g.
Treatment consequences	Dry orgasm
Efficacy	During treatment
Randomization of patients	No
Study quality	**3**
Reference	1946: Jones SD. Ejaculatory inhibition with trazodone. J Clin Psychopharmacol. 1984 Oct;4(5):279–81.
Language	English

N07	**Other Nervous System Drugs**
V03	**All Other Therapeutic Products**
	Treatment with bethanechol was able to act against ejaculation retardation induced by clomipramine. Nicotine abuse as well as alcohol drinking was not associated with an increased incidence of premature ejaculation.
	Overall level of evidence of adverse effects: B

Substance (ATC code)	Bethanechol (N07AB02)
Disease treated	Panic disorder, clomipramine-treated
Quantification of adverse effects	Ejaculation history
No. of patients treated	12
Age group	Young
Treatment period	14 days
Dose	20 mg
Treatment consequences	Ejaculation delay induced by clomipramine
Efficacy	Improvement
Randomization of patients	Yes
Dose arms 1–3	Bethanecol; placebo
Study quality	**1–**
Reference	1735: Bernik M, Vieira AH, Nunes PV. Bethanecol chloride for treatment of clomipramine-induced orgasmic dysfunction in males. Rev Hosp Clin Fac Med Sao Paulo. 2004 Dec;59(6):357–60. Epub 2005 Jan 11.
Language	English

Substance (ATC code)	Bethanechol (N07AB02)
Disease treated	Bulimia, treated with antidepressants
Quantification of adverse effects	Ejaculation history
No. of patients treated	1
Age group	43
Treatment period	On demand
Dose	20 mg
Treatment consequences	Ejaculation delay induced by antidepressants
Efficacy	Improvement

Randomization of patients	No
Study quality	**3**
Reference	1736: Yager J. Bethanechol chloride can reverse erectile and ejaculatory dysfunction induced by tricyclic antidepressants and mazindol: case report. J Clin Psychiatry. 1986 Apr;47(4):210–1.
Language	English

Compound	Nicotine (N07BA01)
Disease treated	Healthy
Quantification of adverse effects	Sexual function questionnaire
No. of patients treated	17; 240
Age group	>36 years
Treatment period	Various
Dose	Various
Treatment consequences	Premature ejaculation
Efficacy	OR 0.9 (95% CI 0.5–2.3)
Randomization of patients	No
Study quality	**2+**
Reference	1721: Stulhofer A, Bajic Z. Prevalence of erectile and ejaculatory difficulties among men in Croatia. Croat Med J. 2006 Feb;47(1):114–24.
Language	English

Compound	Alcohol (V03AZ01)
Disease treated	Healthy
Quantification of adverse effects	Sexual function questionnaire
No. of patients treated	7; 178
Age group	>36 years
Treatment period	Various
Dose	Various
Treatment consequences	Premature ejaculation
Efficacy	OR 0.2 (95% CI 0.1–0.6)
Randomization of patients	No
Study quality	**2+**

2

Reference	1721: Stulhofer A, Bajic Z. Prevalence of erectile and ejaculatory difficulties among men in Croatia. Croat Med J. 2006 Feb;47(1):114–24.
Language	English

Medicinal Plants (not listed in ATC/DDD)

Two Korean publications describe the effect of SS-cream, which contains extracts of venenum bufonis, radix alba ginseng radix alba, radix angelicae gigantea, cortex cinnamoni, flos caryophylli, radix asiasari, herba cistanchis, semen torilidis and fructus zanthoxylli.

Overall level of evidence of positive effects: C

Substance (ATC code)	SS cream (not listed)
Disease treated	Premature ejaculation
Quantification of dysfunction	Intravaginal ejaculation latency time (IELT)
No. of patients treated	186
Age group	Young
Treatment period	1 h before coitus
Dose	0.1 g
Treatment consequences	Ejaculation latency, improvement
Efficacy	Significantly prolonged to more than 10 min
Side effects compromising effectiveness	In 5.9% of patients local irritation. Cortex cinnamoni and flos caryophylli are potent allergens.
Randomization of patients	No
Study quality	**3**
Reference	1837: Xin ZC, Choi YD, Lee SH, Choi HK. Efficacy of a topical agent SS-cream in the treatment of premature ejaculation: preliminary clinical studies. Yonsei Med J. 1997 Apr;38(2):91–5.
Language	English

Substance (ATC code)	SS cream (not listed)
Disease treated	Premature ejaculation
Quantification of dysfunction	Vibratory threshold

No. of patients treated	53
Age group	37.3 years (mean)
Treatment period	1 h prior to vibration
Dose	Various concentrations
Treatment consequences	Ejaculation latency, improvement
Efficacy	Dose dependent
Randomization of patients	Yes
Dose arms 1–3	SS cream; placebo
Study quality	**1–**
Reference	1803: Xin ZC, Choi YD, Lee WH, Choi YJ, Yang WJ, Choi HK, Kim DK. Penile vibratory threshold changes with various doses of SS-cream in patients with primary premature ejaculation. Yonsei Med J. 2000 Feb;41(1):29–33.
Language	English

Retroperitoneal Lymph Node Surgery

Lymph node surgery in the retroperitoneum for metastatic testicular tumors implies the risk of ejaculation impairment. The consequence is a failure of emission of the semen into the posterior urethra, not a retrograde ejaculation. Nerve-sparing surgical techniques have been shown to minimize the risk.

Overall level of evidence of adverse effects: C

Substance (ATC code)	Retroperitoneal lymph node dissection
Disease treated	Testicular cancer
Quantification of adverse effects	Ejaculation history
No. of patients treated	61
Age group	Young
Treatment consequences	Dry orgasm
Efficacy	In 54 of 61 patients
Randomization of patients	No
Study quality	**3**

Reference	1941: Brenner J, Vugrin D, Whitmore WF Jr. Effect of treatment on fertility and sexual function in males with metastatic nonseminomatous germ cell tumors of testis. Am J Clin Oncol. 1985 Apr;8(2):178–82.
Language	English

Substance (ATC code)	Retroperitoneal lymph node dissection
Disease treated	Testicular cancer
Quantification of adverse effects	Ejaculation history
No. of patients treated	39
Age group	Young
Treatment consequences	Ejaculation disorder
Efficacy	In none of 14 patients after nerve sparing
Randomization of patients	No
Study quality	**2+**
Reference	1988: Castelli E, Terrone C, Luca S de, Rossetti SR. Retroperitoneal lymphadenectomy for testicular cancer and genito-sexual conditions: retrospective study. Prog Urol. 2000 Sep;10(4):578–82.
Language	French

Substance (ATC code)	Retroperitoneal lymph node dissection
Disease treated	Testicular cancer
Quantification of adverse effects	Ejaculation history
No. of patients treated	38
Age group	Young
Treatment consequences	Dry orgasm
Efficacy	In 50% of patients
Randomization of patients	No
Study quality	**3**
Reference	1943: Porst H, Altwein JE, Mayer R, Bach D. Erection and ejaculation disorders following retroperitoneal lymphadenectomy in non-seminomatous testicular tumors. Urologe A. 1984 Nov;23(6):324–8.
Language	German

Substance (ATC code)	Retroperitoneal lymph node dissection
Disease treated	Testicular cancer
Quantification of adverse effects	Ejaculation history
No. of patients treated	15
Age group	Young
Treatment consequences	Dry orgasm
Efficacy	In 51of 61 patients
Randomization of patients	No
Study quality	**3**
Reference	1940: Fossa SD, Ous S, Abyholm T, Loeb M. Post-treatment fertility in patients with testicular cancer. I. Influence of retroperitoneal lymph node dissection on ejaculatory potency. Br J Urol. 1985 Apr;57(2):204–9.
Language	English

Substance (ATC code)	Retroperitoneal lymph node dissection
Disease treated	Testicular cancer
Quantification of adverse effects	Ejaculation history
No. of patients treated	6
Age group	Young
Treatment consequences	Ejaculation disorder
Efficacy	One of six after nerve-sparing surgery
Randomization of patients	No
Study quality	**2–**
Reference	1987: Arai Y, Ishitoya S, Okubo K, Aoki Y, Okada T, Maeda H, Suzuki Y. Nerve-sparing retroperitoneal lymph node dissection for metastatic testicular cancer. Int J Urol. 1997 Sep;4(5):487–92.
Language	English

2.6 Database of Drugs

The classification of drugs included in the database of this book was performed according to the ATC/DDD system (Table 2.6.1). This system was developed by modifying and extending the European Pharmaceutical Market Research Association (EPhMRA) classification system by Norwegian researchers and was called the Anatomical Therapeutic Chemical (ATC) classification. In 1982, the WHO Collaborating Centre for Drug Statistics Methodology was established in Oslo and is funded by the Norwegian government. In 1996, WHO started to develop use of the ATC/DDD system as an international standard for drug utilization studies. Access to stan-

Table 2.6.1 Classification system of ATC/DDD

Level	Main group	Level	Main group
A	Alimentary tract and metabolism	L	Antineoplastic and immunomodulating agents
B	Blood and blood-forming organs	M	Musculoskeletal system
C	Cardiovascular system	N	Nervous system
D	Dermatologicals	P	Antiparasitic products
G	Genito-urinary system and sex hormones	R	Respiratory system
H	Systemic hormonal preparations	S	Sensory organs
J	Antiinfectives for systemic use	V	Various

First level: At the broadest level, drugs are divided into one of the following 14 anatomical groups. The first level of the code is based on a letter, e.g. "B" for blood and blood-forming organs.
Second level: either a pharmacological or therapeutic subgroup (e.g. "B03" for anti-anemic preparations).
Third level: a chemical or therapeutic or pharmacological subgroup (e.g. "B03A" for iron preparations).
Fourth level: a chemical, therapeutic or pharmacological subgroup. This is the level used to count "number of different drugs", as it is the level which aggregates drugs just above their descriptive chemical substance (e.g. "B03AA" for iron, bivalent, oral preparations). A count of an individual's drugs at the fourth level of ATC gives the researcher a categorical option with which to stratify and then describe pharmaceutical users. It approximates a measure of comorbidity.
Fifth level: the subgroup for the chemical substance (e.g. "B03AA07" ferrous sulphate).

dardized and validated information on drug use was found to be essential to allow identification of problems connected with drug utilization and monitoring of the outcomes of the interventions.

The purpose of the ATC/DDD system is to serve as a tool for drug utilization research. The classification of a substance in the ATC/DDD system is not a recommendation for use, nor does it imply any judgements about efficacy or relative efficacy of drugs and groups of drugs.

A search for the code of each drug is possible at the Web address http://www.whocc.no/atcddd.
The German version of the ATC/DD classification is available at: http://www.dimdi.de/static/de/klassi/atcddd.

Table 2.6.2 Drugs Used for Searches

Drug (chemical substance)	ATC code	ATC classification, second level	Code
(N(G)-nitro-L-arginine methyl ester	Not listed	Urologicals	G04
1,3 butadiene	Not listed	Environmental toxicants	
19-nortestosterone	G03FA05	Sex hormones and modulators of the genito-urinary system	G03
2, 2-bis(p-hydroxyphenyl)-1,1,1-trichloroethane (HPTE)	Not listed	Environmental toxins	
2-Methoxyethanol	Not listed	Antineoplastic agents (in vitro)	L01
4-tert-octyphenol	Not listed	Environmental toxicants	
5-amino salicylic acid	J04AA01	Antimycobacterials	J04
7-α-methyl-nortestosterone (MENT)	Not listed	Sex hormones and modulators of the genito-urinary system	G03
Acetaminophen	Not listed	Analgesics	N02
Acetylcysteine	R05CB01	Cough and cold preparations	R05
Aciclovir	J05AB01	Antivirals for systemic use	J05
Acridinyl anisidide	Not listed	Antineoplastic drugs	L01
Adriamycin	Not listed	Antineoplastic drugs	L01
Albuterol	Not listed	Beta-blocking agent	C07
Alcohol (Ethanol)	V03AZ01	All other therapeutic products	V03
Alfuzosin	G04CA01	Urologicals	G04
Allopurinol	M04AA01	Antigout preparations	M04
Alprostadil	G04BE01	Urologicals	G04
Ambroxol	R02AD05	Throat preparations	R02
Amezinum	Not listed	Psychoanaleptics	N06

Drug (chemical substance)	ATC code	ATC classification, second level	Code
Aminophyllin	R03DA05	Drugs for obstructive airway diseases	R03
Amiodarone	C01BD01	Cardiac therapy	C01
Amitriptyline	N06AA09	Psychoanalptics	N06
amoxapine	N06AA17	Psychoanaleptics	N06
Amoxicillin	J01CA04	Antibacterials for systemic use	J01
Amphetamine	Not listed	Other nervous system drugs	N07
Ampicillin	J01CA01	Antibacterials for systemic use	J01
Anandamide	Not listed	Other nervous system drugs	N07
Angiotensin II	Not listed	Agents acting on the renin–angiotensin system	C09
Antipyrine	Not listed	Sex hormones and modulators of the genito-urinary system	G03
Apomorphin	G04BE07	Urologicals	G04
Asparaginase	L01XX02	Antineoplastic agents	L01
Aspirin	N02BA01	Analgesics	N02
Atenolol	C07AB03	Beta-blocking agents	C07
Atorvastin	Not listed	Lipid-modifying agents	C10
Azathioprine	L04AX01	Immunosuppressive agents	L04
Baclofen	M03BX01	Muscle relaxants	M03
Benzodiazepine	N05BA	Psycholeptics	N05
Bethanecol	Not listed	Other nervous system drugs	N07
Bezafibrate	C10AB02	Lipid-modifying agents	C10
Boron	Not listed	Environmental toxins	
Bromhexine	R05CB02	Cough and cold preparations	R05
Bromine vapor	Not listed	Environmental toxins	
Bromocriptin	N04BC01	Anti-Parkinson drugs	N04
Bufexamac	M01AB17	Antiinflammatory and antirheumatic products	M01
Buprenorphine	N02AE01	Analgesics	N02
Buproprion	N07BA02	Other nervous system drugs	N07
Buserelin	L02AE01	Endocrine therapy	L02
Calcitonin-gene related peptide	Not listed	Peripheral vasodilator	C04
Capsicain	Not listed	Antihistamines for systemic use	R06
Captopril	C09AA01	Agents acting on the renin–angiotensin system	C09
Carbamazepine	N03AF01	Antiepileptics	N03
Carbidopa	N04BA10	Anti-Parkinson drugs	N04

Drug (chemical substance)	ATC code	ATC classification, second level	Code
Carbon disulfide	Not listed	Environmental toxins	
Casodex	Not listed	Urologicals	G04
Cefaclor	J01DC04	Antibacterials for systemic use	J01
Cetirizine	R06AE07	Antihistamines for systemic use	R06
Cetrorelix	H01CC02	Pituitary and hypothalamic hormones and analogues	H01
Chlorambucil	L01AA02	Antineoplastic agents	L01
Chlorcarbacine	Not listed	Antineoplastic agents	L01
Chlormadinone	G03DB06	Sex hormones and modulators of the genito-urinary system	G03
Chloroform	N01AB02	Anaesthetics	N01
Chlorohydrine	Not listed	Sex hormones and modulators of the genito-urinary system	G03
Chlorpheniramine	R06AB02	Antihistamines for systemic use	R06
Cimetidine	A02BA01	Drugs for acid-related disorders	A02
Ciprofloxacin	J01AM02	Antibacterials for systemic use	J01
Cisplatin	L01XA01	Antineoplastic drugs	L01
Citalopram	N06AB04	Psychoanaleptics	N06
Clobutinol	R05DB03	Cough and cold preparations	R05
Clomiphen	Not listed	Sex hormones and modulators of the genito-urinary system	G03
Clomipramin	N06AA04	Psychoanaleptics	N06
Clonazepam	N03AE01	Antiepileptics	N03
Clonidine	C02AC01	Antihypertensives	C02
Clotrimazole	D01AC01	Antifungals for dermatological use	D01
Colchicine	M04AC01	Antigout preparations	M04
Copper	Not listed	Environmental toxicants	
Cortisone	H02AB10	Corticosteroids for systemic use	H02
Co-trimoxazole	Not listed	Antibacterials for systemic use	J01
Cyclophosphamide	L01AA01	Antineoplastic drugs	L01
Cyproterone acetate	G03HA01	Sex hormones and modulators of the genito-urinary system	G03
Dapoxetine	Not listed	Psychoanaleptics	N06
Deoxyadenosin	Not listed	Peripheral vasodilators	C04
Desogestrel	G03AC09	Sex hormones and modulators of the genito-urinary system	G03

Drug (chemical substance)	ATC code	ATC classification, second level	Code
Diazepam	N05BA01	Psycholeptics	N05
Dibromochloropropane	Not listed	Environmental toxins	
Dichlorobenzylindazol	Not listed	Sex hormones and modulators of the genito-urinary system	G03
Diclofenac	M01AB05	Antiinflammatory and antirheumatic products	M01
Diethylstibestrol	L02AA01	Endocrine therapy	L02
Digitoxin	C01AA04	Cardiac therapy	C01
Digoxin	C01AA05	Cardiac therapy	C01
Dihydroergotamine	N02CA01	Analgesics	N02
Dithiothreitol	Not listed	Sex hormones and modulators of the genito-urinary system	G03
Doxacosin	Not listed	Urologicals	G04
Doxyrubicine	Not listed	Antineoplastic drugs	L01
Dutasteride	G04CB02	Urologicals	G04
Efalizumab	L04AA21	Immunosuppressive agents	L04
Endothelin-1	Not listed	Peripheral vasodilators	C04
Enoxacin	J01MA04	Antibacterials for systemic use	J01
Ergotamine	N02CA02	Analgesics	N02
Erythromycin	J01FA01	Antibacterials for systemic use	J01
Erythropoietin	B03XA01	Antianemic preparations	B03
Escin	C05CA07	Vasoprotectives	C05
Estradiol	G03CA03	Sex hormones and modulators of the genito-urinary system	G03
Etenorgestrel	Not listed	Sex hormones and modulators of the genito-urinary system	G03
Ethosuximide	N03AD01	Antiepileptics	N03
Etilefrine	C01CA01	Cardiac therapy	C01
Etofibrate	C10AB09	Lipid-modifying agents	C10
Etretinate	D05BB01	Antipsoriatics	D05
Famotidine	A02BA03	Drugs for acid-related disorders	A02
Fenofibrat	C10AB05	Lipid-modifying agents	C10
Fentanyl	N01AH01	Analgesics	N02
Finasteride	G04CB01	Urologicals	G04
Finrozole	Not listed	Sex hormones and modulators of the genito-urinary system	G03
Fluconazol	J02AC01	Antimycotics for systemic use	J02
Fluoxetine	N06AB03	Psychoanaleptics	N06

2

Drug (chemical substance)	ATC code	ATC classification, second level	Code
Fluoxymesterone	G03BA01	Sex hormones and modulators of the genito-urinary system	G03
Fluvastatin	C10AA04	Lipid-modifying agents	C10
Follicle-stimulating hormone (FSH)	G03GA04	Sex hormones and modulators of the genito-urinary system	G03
Forskolin	Not listed	Peripheral vasodilator	C04
Foscarnet	J05AD01	Antivirals for systemic use	J05
Fulvestrant	L02BA03	Endocrine therapy	L02
Furosemide	C03CA01	Diuretics	C03
Gabapentin	N03AX12	Antiepileptics	N03
Gancyclovir	J05AB06	Antivirals for systemis use	J05
Gemcitabine	L01BC05	Antineoplastic drugs	L01
Gestrinone	G03XA02	Sex hormones and modulators of the genito-urinary system	G03
Ginsenoide	Not listed	Sex hormones and modulators of the genito-urinary system	G03
Glibencamide	A10BB01	Drugs used in diabetes	A10
GnRH	L02AE	Endocrine therapy	L02
Goserelin	L02AE03	Endocrine therapy	L02
Gossypol	Not listed	Sex hormones and modulators of the genito-urinary system	G03
Griseofulvin	D01AA08	Antifungals for dermatological use	D01
Guanthedine	C02CC02	Antihypertensives	C02
Haloperidol	N05AD01	Psycholeptics	N05
Halothane	N01AB01	Anaesthetics	N01
Heparin	B01AB01	Antithrombotic agents	B01
Heroin	Not listed	Analgesics	N02
Hetastarch	B05AA07	Blood substitutes and perfusion substitutes	B05
Hexadione	Not listed	Environmental toxins	
Human chorionic gonadotropin (hCG)	G03GA01	Sex hormones and modulators of the genito-urinary system	G03
Hyaluronic acid	M09AX01	Other drugs for disorders of the musculoskeletal system	M09
Hydralazine	C02DB02	Antihypertensives	C02
Ibuprofen	M01AE01	Antiinflammatory and antirheumatic products	M01
Imatinib	L01XX28	Antineoplastic agents	L01
Imipramine	N06AA02	Psychoanaleptics	N06

Drug (chemical substance)	ATC code	ATC classification, second level	Code
Imiquimod	D06BB10	Antibiotics and chemotherapeutics for dermatological use	C06
Indometacin	M01AB01	Antiinflammatory and antirheumatic products	M01
Infliximab	L04AA12	Immunosuppressive agents	L04
Isoniazid	J04AC01	Antimycobacterials	J04
Isosorbide	C01DA08	Cardiac therapy	C01
Isotretinoin	D10AD04	Antiacne preparations	D10
Itraconazole	J02AC02	Antimycotics for systemic use	J02
Kallikrein	Not listed	Sex hormones and modulators of the genito-urinary system	G03
Kan Yang	Not listed	Sex hormones and modulators of the genito-urinary system	G03
Ketoconazole	J02AB02	Antimycotics for systemic use	J02
Ketotifen	R06AX17	Antihistamines for systemic use	R06
Labetalol	C07AG01	Beta-blocking agents	C07
Lacidipine	C08CA09	Calcium channel blockers	C08
Lamotrigine	N03AX09	Antiepileptics	N03
Lansoprazole	A02BC03	Drugs for acid-related disorders	A02
Lead	Not listed	Environmental toxins	
Leflunomide	L04AA13	Immunosuppressive agents	L04
Letrozole	L02BG04	Endocrine therapy	L02
leuprolide	Not listed	Pituitary and hypothalamic hormones and analogues	H01
Levodopa	N04BA02	Antiparkinson drugs	N04
Levonorgestrel	G03AC03	Sex hormones and modulators of the genito-urinary system	G03
Lidocaine	N01BB02	Anaesthetics	N01
Lindane	P03AB02	Ectoparasiticides	P03
Linsidomine	C01DX18	Cardiac therapy	C01
Lisinopril	C09AA03	Agents acting on the renin–angiotensin system	C09
Lithium	N05AN01	Psycholeptics	N05
Loperamide	A07DA03	Antidiarrhoeals, intestinal antiinflammatory/antiinfective agents	A07
Loratadine	R06AX13	Antihistamines for systemic use	R06

2

Drug (chemical substance)	ATC code	ATC classification, second level	Code
Losartan	C09CA01	Agents acting on the renin–angiotensin system	C09
Lovastatin	C10AA02	Lipid-modifying agents	C10
Mebeverine	A03AA04	Drugs for functional gastrointestinal disorders	A03
Mechloretamine	Not listed	Antineoplastic agent	L01
Medroxprogesterone acetate	Not listed	Sex hormones and modulators of the genito-urinary system	G03
Meloxicam	M01AC06	Antiinflammatory and antirheumatic products	M01
Mesalazine	A07EC02	Antidiarrhoeals, intestinal antiinflammatory/antiinfective agents	A07
Mesterolone	G03BB01	Sex hormones and modulators of the genito-urinary system	G03
Metamizol	N02BB02	Analgesics	N02
Metandienone	Not listed	Anabolic agents for systemic use	A14
Metformin	A10BA02	Drugs used in diabetes	A10
Methadone	N07BC02	Other nervous system drugs	N07
Methotrexate	L01BA01	Antineoplastic agents	L01
Methyl bromide	D04AA33	Antipruritics	D04
Methyl mercury	D08AK05	Antiseptics and disinfectants	D08
Methyldopa	C02AB02	Antihypertensives	C02
Metoclopramide	A03FA01	Drugs for functional gastrointestinal disorders	A03
Metoprolol	C07AB02	Beta-blocking agents	C07
Metronidazole	G01AF01	Urologicals	G04
Mianserin	N06AX03	Psychoanaleptics	N06
Midazolam	N05CD08	Psycholeptics	N05
Midodrine	C01CA17	Cardiac therapy	C01
Minoxidil	C02DC01	Antihypertensives	C02
Mitoxanthone	L01DB07	Antineoplastic agents	L01
Molsidomine	C01DX12	Cardiac therapy	C01
Morphine	N02AA01	Analgesics	N02
Moxonidine	C02AC05	Antihypertensives	C02
Mustard gas	Not listed	Antineoplastic agents	L01
Naproxen	M01AE02	Antiinflammatory and antirheumatic products	M01
Neostigmine	N07AA01	Other nervous system drugs	N07

Drug (chemical substance)	ATC code	ATC classification, second level	Code
Nicotine	N07BA01	Other nervous system drugs	N07
Nifedipine	C08CA05	Calcium channel blockers	C08
Niridazol	P02BX02	Antihelminthics	P02
Nitrendipine	C08CA08	Calcium channel blockers	C08
Nitrofurantoin	J01XE01	Antibacterials for systemic use	J01
Nitroglycerine	C01DA02	Cardiac therapy	C01
Nogalamycin	Not listed	Antineoplastic agents	L01
Nonoxinol	Not listed	Sex hormones and modulators of the genito-urinary system	G03
Norephedrine	Not listed	Other nervous system drugs	N07
Norepinephrine	C01CA03	Cardiac therapy	C01
Norethisterone enanthate	G03AC01	Sex hormones and modulators of the genito-urinary system	G03
Norfloxacin	J01MA06	Antibacterials for systemic use	J01
Nystatin	D01AA01	Antifungals for dermatological use	D91
Ofloxacin	J01MA01	Antibacterials for systemic use	J01
Olanzapine	N05AH03	Psycholeptics	N05
Omeprazole	A02BC01	Drugs for acid-related disorders	A02
Opioids	N02A	Analgesics	N02
Oxybutynin	G04BD04	Urologicals	G04
Oxcarbazepine	Not listed	Psychoanaleptics	N06
Oxytocin	H01BB02	Pituitary and hypothalamic hormones and analogues	H01
Pantoprazole	A02BC02	Drugs for acid-related disorders	A02
Papaverine	G04BE02	Urologicals	G04
Paroxetine	N06AB05	Psychoanaleptics	N06
Penicillamine	M01CC01	Antiinflammatory and antirheumatic products	M01
Penicillin	J01C	Antibacterials for systemic use	J01
Pentoxifylline	C04AD03	Peripheral vasodilators	C04
Phenobarbital	N03AA02	Antiepileptics	N03
Phenoxybenzamin	C04AX02	Peripheral vasodilators	C04
Phentolamine	G04BE05	Urologicals	G04
Phenylephrine	C01CA06	Cardiac therapy	C01
Phenytoin	N03AB02	Antiepileptics	N03
Pimecrolimus	D11AX15	Other dermatological preparations	D11

Drug (chemical substance)	ATC code	ATC classification, second level	Code
Piracetam	N06BX03	Psychoanaleptics	N06
Pirenzepine	A02BX03	Drugs for acid-related disorders	A02
Piroxicam	M01AC01	Antiinflammatory and antirheumatic products	M01
Polybromobisphenyl	Not listed	Environmental toxins	
Pravastatin	C10AA03	Lipid-modifying agents	C10
Prazosin	C02CA01	Antihypertensives	C02
Prednisone	H02AB07	Corticosteroids for systemic use	H02
Procarbazine	L01XB01	Antineoplastic agents	L01
Progesterone	G03DA04	Sex hormones and modulators of the genito-urinary system	G03
Propafenone	C01BC03	Cardiac therapy	C01
Propranolol	C07AA05	Beta-blocking agents	C07
Quinagolide	G02CB04	Gynaecologicals	G02
Raloxifen	G03XC01	Sex hormones and modulators of the genito-urinary system	G03
Ranitidine	A02BA02	Drugs for acid-related disorders	A02
Remoxipiride	N05AL04	Psycholeptics	N05
Rifampicin	J04AB02	Antimycobacterials	J04
Risperidone	N05AX08	Psycholeptics	N05
Roxithromycin	J01FA06	Antibacterials for systemic use	J01
Selective serotonin reuptake inhibitors	N06AB	Psychoanaleptics	N06
Sertraline	N06AB06	Psychoanaleptics	N06
Sildenafil	G04BE03	Urologicals	G04
Simvastatin	C10AA01	Lipid-modifying agents	C10
Sirolimus	L04AA10	Immunosuppressive agents	L04
S-nitroso-N-acetylpenicillamine	Not listed	Urologicals	G04
Somatotropin	H01AC01	Pituitary and hypothalamic hormones and analogues	H01
SS cream	Not listed	Plant extract	
Styrene maleic anhydride	Not listed	Urologicals	G04
Sulfasalazine	A07EC01	Antidiarrhoeals, intestinal antiinflammatory/antiinfective agents	A07
Sulpiride	N05AL01	Psycholeptics	N05
Tadalafil	G04BE08	Urologicals	G04

Drug (chemical substance)	ATC code	ATC classification, second level	Code
Tamoxifen	L02BA01	Endocrine therapy	L02
Tamsulosin	G04CA02	Urologicals	G04
Terbutaline	R03AC03	Drugs for obstructive airway diseases	R03
Testosterone	G03BA03	Sex hormones and modulators of the genito-urinary system	G03
Tetracycline	A01AB13	Antibacterials for systemic use	J01
Tetrahydrocannabinol	Not listed	Other nervous system drugs	N07
Theophylline	R03DA04	Drugs for obstructive airway diseases	R03
Thiazide	C03AA	Diuretics	C03
Thioridazine	N05AC02	Psycholeptics	N05
Thyroid hormone	H03AA	Thyroid therapy	H03
Tilidine	N02AX01	Analgesics	N02
Tolazoline	C04AB02	Peripheral vasodilators	C04
Tolbutamide	A10BB03	Drugs used in diabetes	A10
Torasemide	C03CA04	Diuretics	C03
Tradozone	N06AX05	Psychoanaleptics	N06
Tramadol	N02AX02	Analgesics	N02
Tranilast	Not listed	Antihistamines for systemic use	R06
Trastuzumab	L01XC03	Antineoplastic agents	L01
Trichlormethiazide	C03AA06	Diuretics	C03
Trimethoprim	J01EA0	Antibacterials for systemic use	J01
Triterpenoid	Not listed	Environmental toxins	
Valproate	N03AG01	Antiepileptics	N03
Venlafaxine	N06AX16	Psychoanaleptics	N06
Verapamil	C08DA01	Calcium channel blockers	C08
Vinblastine	L01CA01	Antineoplastic drugs	L01
Vinclozolin	Not listed	Environmental toxins	
Vincristine	L01CA02	Antineoplastic drugs	L01
Xylometazoline	R01AA07	Nasal preparations	R01
Yohimbine	Not listed	Antihypertensives	C02
Zolpidem	N05CF02	Psycholeptics	N05

The list of drugs as given in Table 2.6.2 was compiled from Goodman and Gilman's *The Pharmacological Basis of Therapeutics* (11th edition), from Meyler's *Side Effects of Drugs* (13th edition), from the textbook by Müller-Oerlinghausen et al. (1999), from Mach et al. (2006) and the "Rote Liste" 2006.

The drugs of Table 2.6.2 were used for Medline and Scopus searches. The Medline and Scopus searches were performed using a drug as MESH terms and combining it with the MESH terms "sperm", "testosterone", "impotence" and "ejaculation". By these searches, more than 2000 articles were identified in which the effects of drugs on male sexual health are mentioned. Not all drugs listed in Table 2.6.2 produced hits in the literature databases. In addition, secondary literature was used.

The articles were evaluated using a standardized protocol (see Table 2.6.3) and the results were collected in a Microsoft Excel file, from which the tables as given in the

Table 2.6.3 Parameters extracted from references. (From Follmann et al. 2005)

Study number
No. of patients
Age group
Disease treated
Treatment period
Side effects
Quantification of dysfunction
Randomization of patients
Treatment
Dosage
Dose arm 1
Dose arm 2
Dose arm 3
Efficacy
Kind of study
Study quality
Remarks
Financing
Language
Reference

Table 2.6.4 SIGN grading system for clinical studies (Scottish Intercollegiate Guidelines Network, http://www.sign.ac.uk/)

Levels of evidence							
1++	1+	1–	2++	2+	2–	3	4
High-quality meta-analyses, systematic reviews of RCTs, or RCTs with a very low risk of bias	Well-conducted meta-analyses, systematic reviews of RCTs, or RCTs with a low risk of bias	Meta-analyses, systematic reviews of RCTs, or RCTs with a high risk of bias	High-quality systematic reviews of case-control or cohort studies High quality case-control or cohort studies with a very low risk of confounding, bias, or chance and a high probability that the relationship is causal	Well-conducted case-control or cohort studies with a low risk of confounding, bias or chance, and a moderate probability that the relationship is causal	Case-control or cohort studies with a high risk of confounding, bias or chance, and a significant risk that the relationship is not causal	Non-analytic studies, e.g. case reports, case series	Expert opinion

Table 2.6.5 SIGN levels of recommendation as designed for guidelines

Grade of recommendation	
A	At least one meta-analysis, systematic review or RCT rated as 1++, and directly applicable to the target population
	A systematic review of RCTs or a body of evidence consisting principally of studies rated as 1+, directly applicable to the target population and demonstrating overall consistency of results
B	A body of evidence including studies rated as 2++, directly applicable to the target population, and demonstrating overall consistency of results
	Extrapolated evidence from studies rated as 1++ or 1+
C	A body of evidence including studies rated as 2+, directly applicable to the target population and demonstrating overall consistency of results
	Extrapolated evidence from studies rated as 2++
D	Evidence level 3 or 4
	Extrapolated evidence from studies rated as 2+

Chaps. 2.3–2.5 were extracted. Dose and patient number are not always given in reviews, meta-analyses and animal experimental studies. The evaluation considered only descriptions of clinical effects; no considerations of pharmacodynamics and pharmacokinetics were made. The very important information on financing of studies could not be included in the database, because only a negligible number of studies considered this topic. In the case of drugs used for improving male sexual functions, e.g. phosphodiesterase 5-inhibitors in order to treat insufficient erectile function, the adverse effects on other organ systems were collected as "side effects" as a burden of male sexual health.

The rating of studies was performed in analogy to the SIGN 50 grading system (Table 2.6.4).

From the studies evaluated, an overall level of evidence of adverse effects and positive effects was deduced analogue to the SIGN levels of recommendation (Table 2.6.5), which were originally designed for the compilation of treatment guidelines.

In this book ADEs and other effects of drugs on sexual functions are listed. The drugs are arranged in chapters according to the second ATC level (see above). Within the chapters, they are arranged according to the ACT code, beginning with studies concerning the total group of drugs. Within the chapters for single drugs, the studies are arranged according to the disease treated and, secondarily, to the number of patients included in a descending sequence. Reviews are usually posted at the end of the list of studies dealing with a drug, but if they are useful for basic understanding of adverse drug effects, they may also be found at the beginning of the chapter. If disorders of sexual functions do not only occur as adverse effects to drugs in a particular disease, but also as the consequence of the disease itself (e.g. erectile dysfunction in treated and untreated depression), studies which quote the prevalence of the disorder are referenced at the end of a chapter.

References

1. Dukes MNG et al. (Eds) Meyler's side effects of drugs, 13th Ed. Elsevier, Amsterdam, etc1996
2. Goodman LS, Gilman A. The pharmacological basis of therapeutics, 11th Ed. Laurence L. Brunton, New York u.a.: McGraw-Hill, 2006
3. Follmann M, Sterry W, Rzany B, Psoriasis-Leitlinienkerngruppe; Deutsche Dermatologische Gesellschaft (DDG). Development of the evidence-based guidelines for psoriasis: a project of the German Dermatological Society (DDG), JDDG 2005;3: 678–89
4. Mach MA von, Kaes J, Solak E, Lauterbach M, Weilemann LS. Unerwünschte Arzneimittelwirkungen. Dtsch Ärztebl 2006;103(11):A694–700
5. Müller-Oerlinghausen B, Lasek R, Düppenbecker H, Munter KH, Hrsg. Handbuch der unerwünschten Arzneimittelwirkungen. Urban and Fischer, München, 1999
6. Rote Liste, Rote Liste Service GmbH, Frankfurt/Main 2006

Subject Index

MIX
Papier aus verantwortungsvollen Quellen
Paper from responsible sources
FSC® C105338

If you have any concerns about our products,
you can contact us on
ProductSafety@springernature.com

In case Publisher is established outside the EU,
the EU authorized representative is:
Springer Nature Customer Service Center GmbH
Europaplatz 3, 69115 Heidelberg, Germany

Printed by Libri Plureos GmbH
in Hamburg, Germany